AF425558

SURGICAL EXAM CASES

Q&A

SURGICAL EXAM CASES

Q&A

Charles Tan

Adjunct Assistant Professor, Department of Surgery,
Yong Loo Lin School of Medicine, National University of Singapore

World Scientific

NEW JERSEY · LONDON · SINGAPORE · GENEVA · BEIJING · SHANGHAI · TAIPEI · CHENNAI

Published by

World Scientific Publishing Co. Pte. Ltd.

5 Toh Tuck Link, Singapore 596224

USA office: 27 Warren Street, Suite 401-402, Hackensack, NJ 07601

UK office: 57 Shelton Street, Covent Garden, London WC2H 9HE

British Library Cataloguing-in-Publication Data
A catalogue record for this book is available from the British Library.

SURGICAL EXAM CASES
Q&A

Copyright © 2025 by World Scientific Publishing Co. Pte. Ltd.

All rights reserved. This book, or parts thereof, may not be reproduced in any form or by any means, electronic or mechanical, including photocopying, recording or any information storage and retrieval system now known or to be invented, without written permission from the publisher.

For photocopying of material in this volume, please pay a copying fee through the Copyright Clearance Center, Inc., 222 Rosewood Drive, Danvers, MA 01923, USA. In this case permission to photocopy is not required from the publisher.

ISBN 978-981-98-0706-2 (hardcover)
ISBN 978-981-98-0756-7 (paperback)
ISBN 978-981-98-0707-9 (ebook for institutions)
ISBN 978-981-98-0708-6 (ebook for individuals)

For any available supplementary material, please visit
https://www.worldscientific.com/worldscibooks/10.1142/14155#t=suppl

Typeset by Stallion Press
Email: enquiries@stallionpress.com

To
my parents

To
Audra, Craig and Claire

Thank you for the support, encouragement and love.

Contents

Acknowledgements

I am indebted to the patients whom we have managed, and from whom we can humbly learn from to make us all better doctors.

I am grateful for the contributions of my colleagues who have shared their cases to help make this book possible.

Addy Tan Yong Hui
Mathew Yeo Sze Wei
Foo Chek Siang
Benjamin Chua Soo Yeng
Thomas Ho Wai Thong
Liau Kui Hin
Andrew Loy Heng Chian
Ong Lin Yin
Terence Goh Lin Hon
Timothy Shim Weng Hoh
Png Keng Siang
Lee Cheng Kiang
Lim Khong Hee
Nor Azhari Bin Mohd Zam
Tricia Kuo Li Chuen
Steven Kum Wei Cheong
Leonard Ho Ming Li

Teo Kejia
Kim Guo Wei
Lee Kuo Ann
Koong Heng Nung
James Mok Wan Loong
Yim Heng Boon
Toh Bin Chet
Stephen Tsao Kin Kwok
Eric Wee Wei Loong
Chin Chong Min
Ng Chee Kwan
Joe Lee King Chien
Melanie Seah Dee Wern
Chang Guohao
Ho Siew Hong
Tan Ker Kan

And to many others who have contributed in one form or another, a heartfelt thank you.

Proof reading — Audra Fong
Book cover and chapter illustrations — Craig and Claire Tan

Preface

This book is written for both undergraduate and post-graduate students as a learning resource to use alongside other standard textbooks to crystallize one's surgical knowledge. There are multiple surgical cases of different specialties organised in a question-and-answer format.

Learning though cases encourage students to apply factual knowledge to what they encounter in clinical practice. The case scenarios run through a logical sequence of interpreting history and clinical findings, generating differential diagnoses, formulating investigation options and administering management plans.

When I was a young surgical trainee, Low Cheng Hock used to share this quote by Sir William Osler: "He who studies medicine without books sails an uncharted sea, but he who studies medicine without patients does not go to sea at all." Besides actual bedside encounters with patients, this book aims to provide an avenue for students to recognize pathology and to learn from each unique scenario.

Within this collection are pictures of the many patients I have been given the privilege of caring for over 30 years of surgical practice. It is my heartfelt desire that the lessons gleaned can now be shared with a larger readership.

The inspiration for the inception of this simple book are my two children, Craig and Claire, who are medical students now, as well as the multitude of students that I have tutored over the decades.

May this book be useful to help make us all better doctors.

Charles Tan.

General

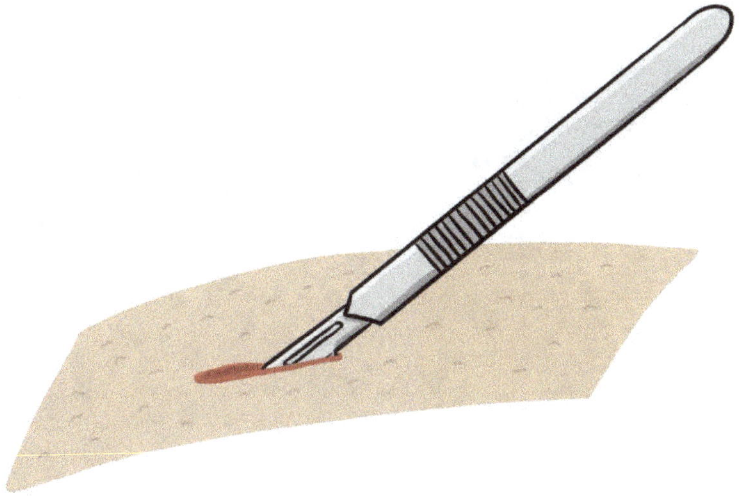

Q1.1

This is a 50-year-old male who presented with fever and a painful lump over his upper back.

1. Describe what is seen in the picture.
2. What is likely to be detected on physical examination?
3. What is the diagnosis?
4. What is the management?
5. What is seen one month later?

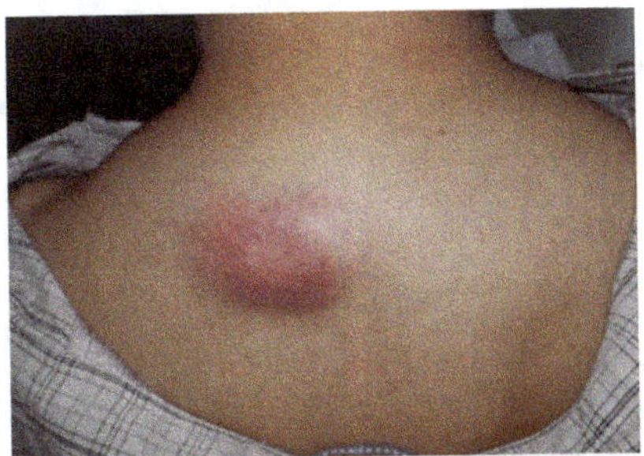

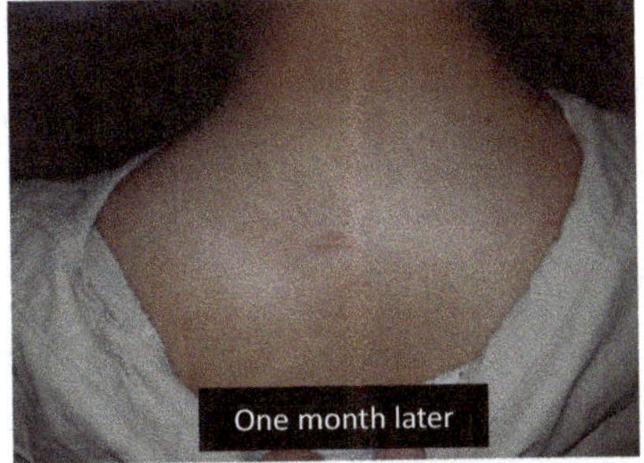

Q1.2

This is a 70-year-old male who presented with a lump over the back of the neck.

1. What is seen at his neck?
2. What radiological investigation was performed and what does it show?
3. What is the diagnosis?
4. What is the natural history of the lesion?

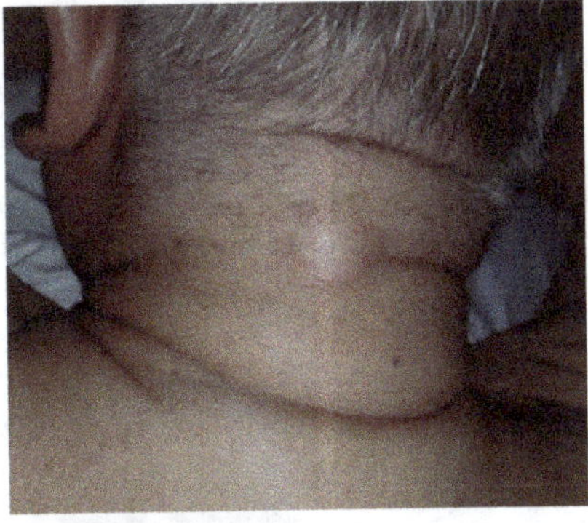

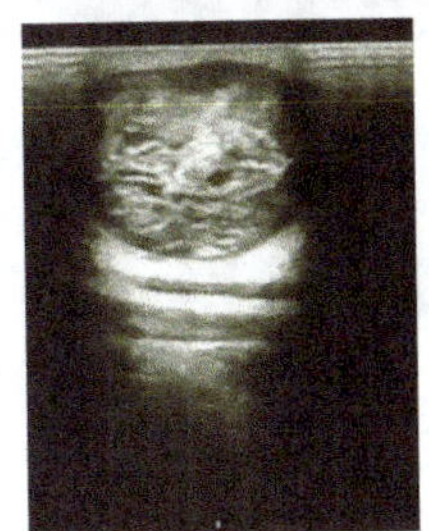

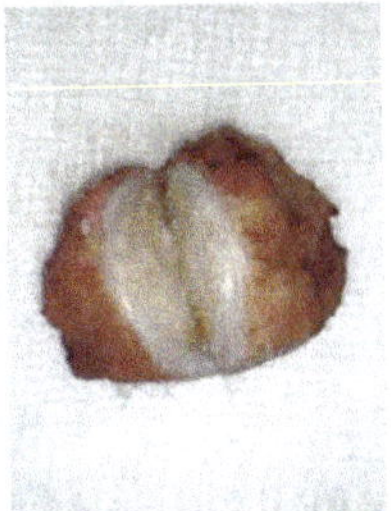

A1.1

1. There is an oval shaped mass over the left upper back. The overlying skin is red.

2. The lump will be painful and tender. The patient may be febrile.

3. Skin abscess. Infected epidermal cyst.

4. Surgical drainage of the pus and allowing the wound to heal by secondary intention.

5. The wound has healed by secondary intention.

A1.2

1. There is a well-circumscribed circular lesion at the back of the neck. It is not erythematous and there are no surrounding skin changes.

2. An ultrasound scan was performed. It shows a well-circumscribed, circular shaped, cystic mass with a thick hyperechoic focus, and a hypoechoic rim.

3. Skin/epidermal cyst.

4. The lesion can increase, remain the same or decrease in size. If the cyst persists, it can get infected and develop into an abscess.

Q1.3

These are pictures of 2 different patients with the same pathology.

1. What is the diagnosis?
2. What is the pathophysiology?
3. What is their clinical presentation?
4. What is the management?

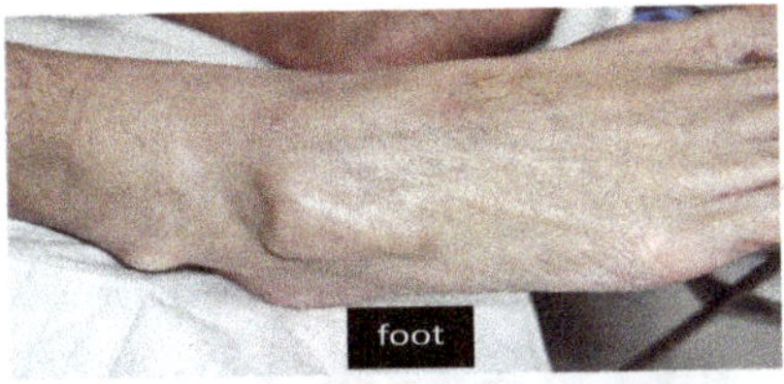

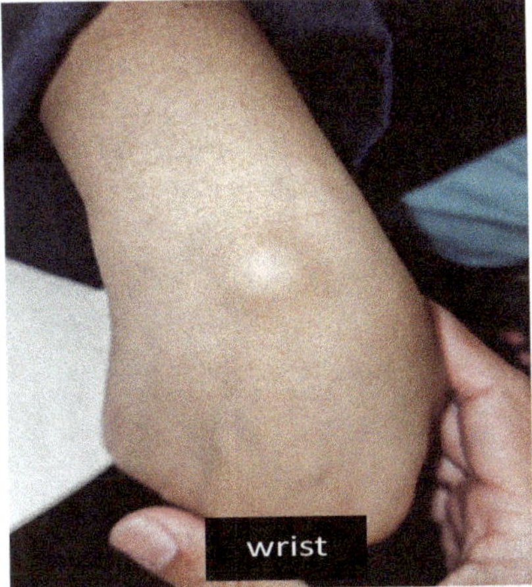

Q1.4

This is a 48-year-old male. There was a history of blunt trauma to the left elbow.

1. Describe the abnormality in picture A.
2. What is the diagnosis?
3. What is the clinical presentation?
4. What procedure was performed on him picture B?

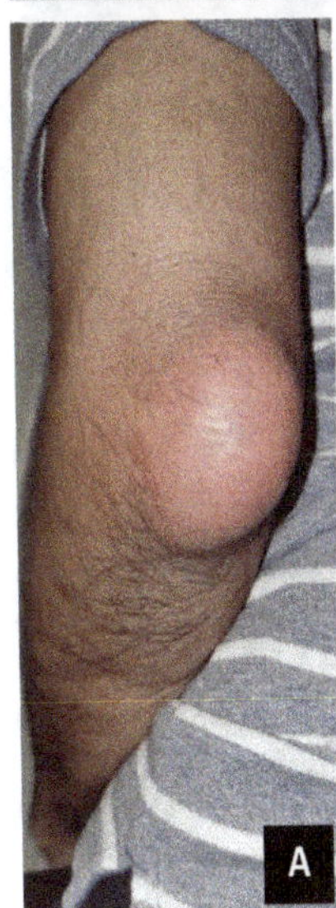

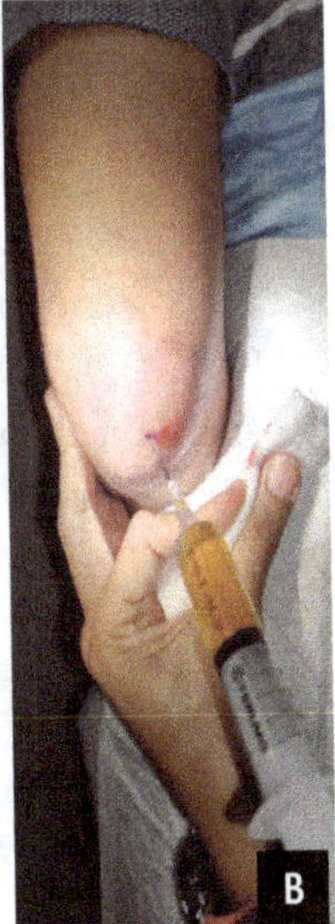

A1.3

1.   Ganglion cysts.

2.   They are mucin filled cysts arising from synovial joints.

3.   Most ganglion cysts are asymptomatic. Patients may present with pain, tenderness, or weakness that is exacerbated by joint motion. The cysts are firm and well-circumscribed.

4.   Asymptomatic patients can be managed conservatively. Some ganglion cysts may spontaneously regress. Aspiration is an option but is associated with a higher recurrence rate. Surgical excision down to the pedicle of the cyst has a lower recurrence rate.

A1.4

1.   There is a large erythematous swelling the size of a golf ball over the left elbow.

2.   Olecranon bursitis.

3.   The swelling often restricts elbow movement. If there is an underlying infection, it may be tender and the patient may be febrile.

4.   Aspiration of the bursa.

Q1.5

This is a 40-year-old female who presents with a lump over her left upper back. She has had previous surgery over the same area 5 years ago.

1. Describe what you see over her left upper back.

2. What scan was done to investigate the mass?

3. What is the diagnosis?

4. How was this pathology managed as seen in the specimen picture?

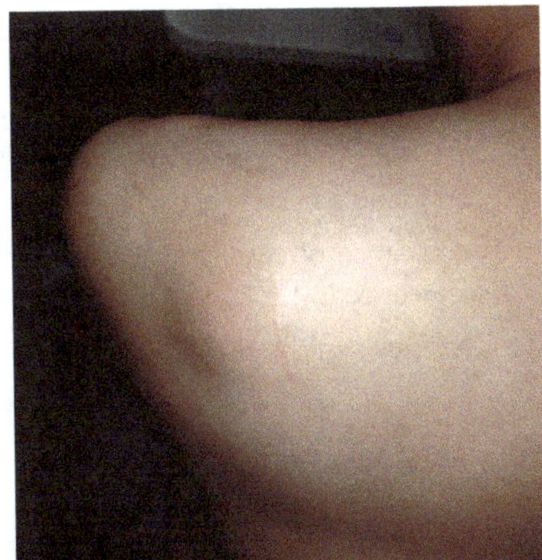

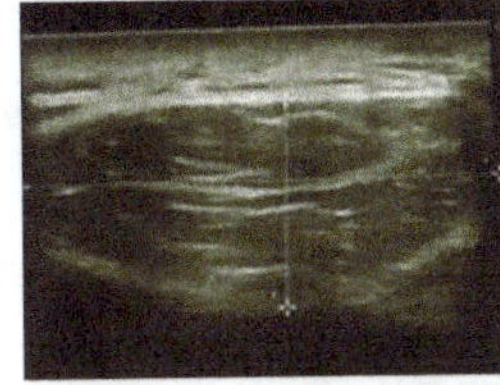

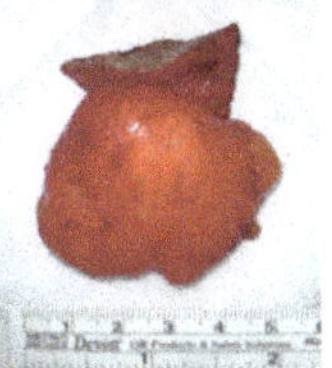

Q1.6

This is a 60-year-old male.

1. What is seen in the CT scan?

2. What is seen in the surgical picture?

3. What is the most likely diagnosis?

4. What is the adjuvant treatment after surgery?

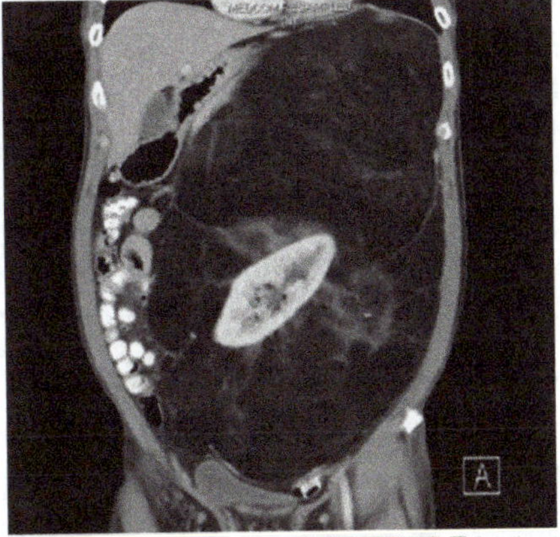

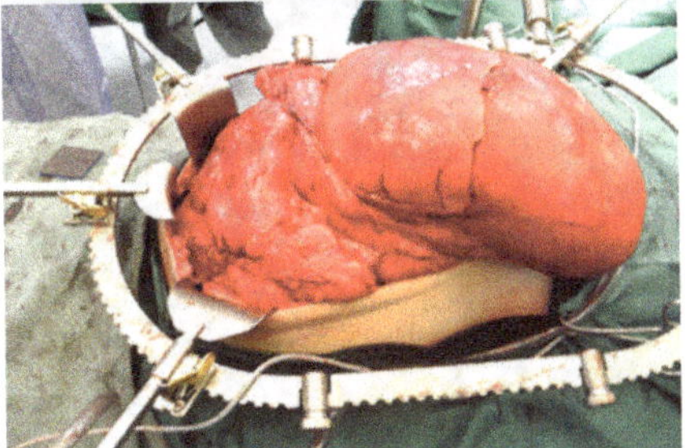

A1.5

1. There is a circular lesion over the left upper back. There are no surrounding skin changes. There is a surgical scar over the lesion.

2. An ultrasound scan. It shows an elliptical mass parallel to the skin surface and contains linear echogenic lines.

3. Recurrence of the lipoma that was previously entirely resected. Chance of recurrence is 1%.

4. The recurrent lipoma was resected.

A1.6

1. The coronal section of the CT scan shows a large hypodense mass in the abdominal cavity. In the middle of the lesion is a viable kidney. The mass displaces the intraperitoneal intestines to the right side.

2. The large mass is delivered through a large midline laparotomy incision.

3. A large liposarcoma arising from the retroperitoneal space.

4. Surgical excision is the mainstay of treatment. Radiation therapy may be a valuable adjunct to surgery. Liposarcoma response to chemotherapy is poor. Long-term follow-up is recommended due to the high rate of recurrence.

Q1.7

This is a 45-year-old female who presents with left axillary lymphadenopathy as seen in the CT scan.

1. What clinical examination should we perform?

2. What are common reasons for lymphadenopathy?

3. Describe the lymph nodes removed as seen in the surgical specimen.

4. What is the management of this patient?

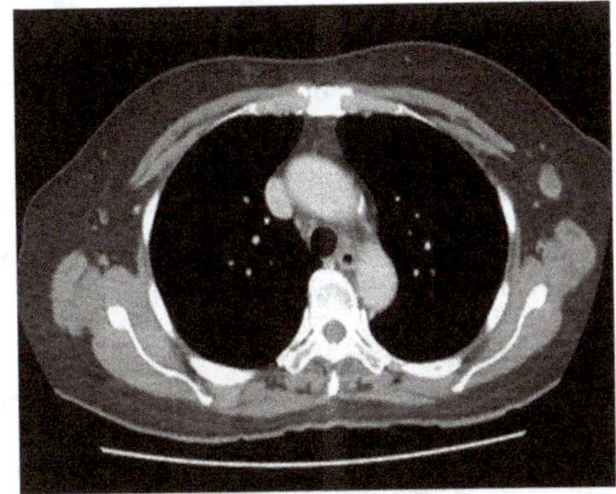

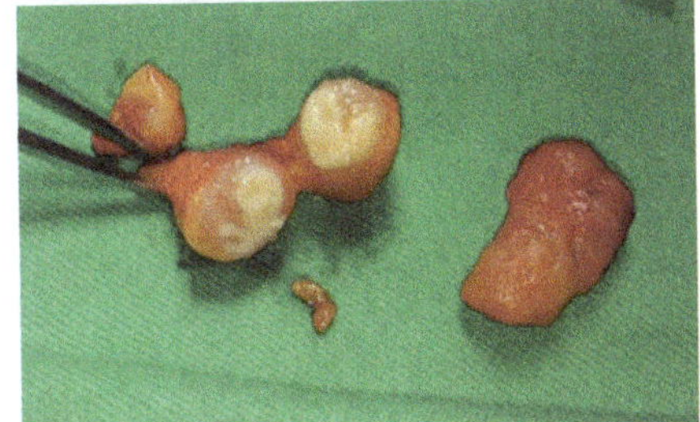

Q1.8

This is a 60-year-old male.

1. Describe the pathology.

2. What are his likely symptoms?

3. What is the diagnosis?

4. What are differential diagnoses that we need to exclude?

5. How can we manage the problem?

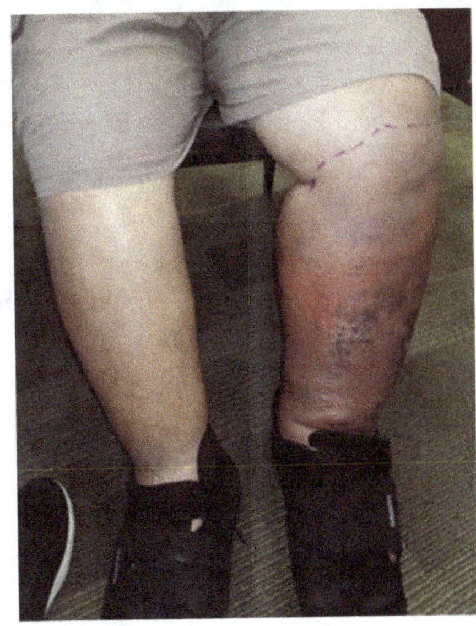

A1.7

1. Areas to be examined:
   Field of drainage of the axillary lymph node — breast and upper limb.
   Lymphadenopathy elsewhere — cervical, inguinal and contralateral axilla.

2. Infections and malignancies are the 2 most common causes. Others include storage diseases and drug reactions.

3. The lymph nodes are well circumscribed. The cut surface reveals collections of yellowish areas of caseating necrosis suggestive of Mycobacterium tuberculosis infection.

4. Tuberculosis is treated with multidrug therapy for a period of six to 12 months. The most common regime is isoniazid in combination with three other drugs — Rifampin, Pyrazinamide and Ethambutol.

A1.8

1. The left lower limb below the knee is circumferentially swollen and red.

2. A painful and warm left lower limb. He may be febrile.

3. Cellulitis — inflammation of the skin and subcutaneous tissue.

4. Deep vein thrombosis and necrotizing fasciitis.

5. The cellulitis can be initially treated with antibiotics and elevation of the lower limb. If there is any suggestion of progression to necrotizing fasciitis, aggressive surgical debridement of the infected tissue is imperative.

Q1.9

This is a 50-year-old female who had an excision of a skin lump over her back.

1. How was the surgical wound closed?

2. What are the phases of wound healing?

3. What is seen 2 weeks later when the stitches were removed?

4. What are factors that contribute to poor wound healing?

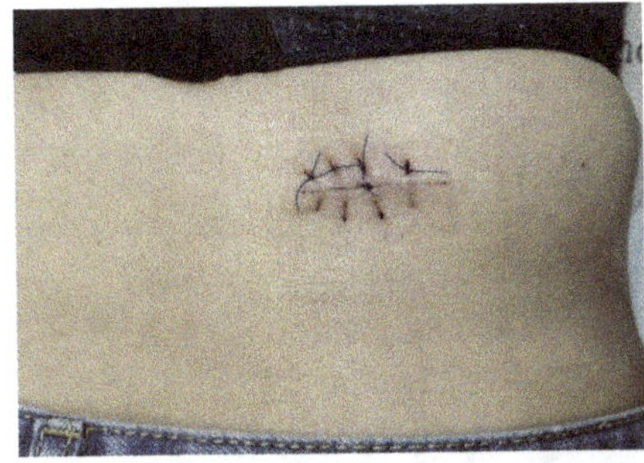

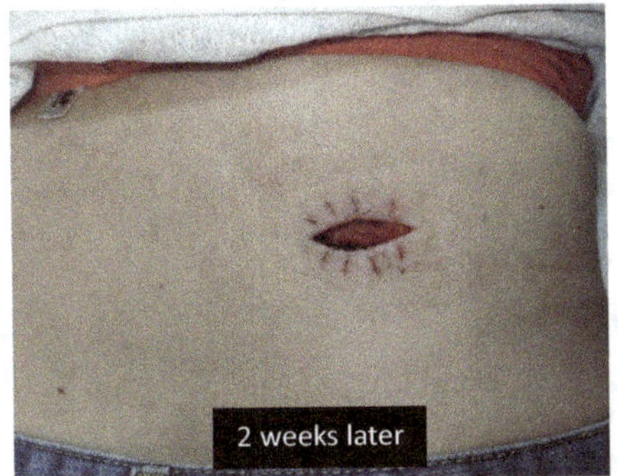

Q1.10

This is a 70-year-old male who had bilateral groin hernia surgery.

1. What complication has developed at post-op day 10?

2. What is his clinical presentation?

3. What is the pathogenesis?

4. How is this problem managed?

5. What would be of particular concern if the complication does not resolve?

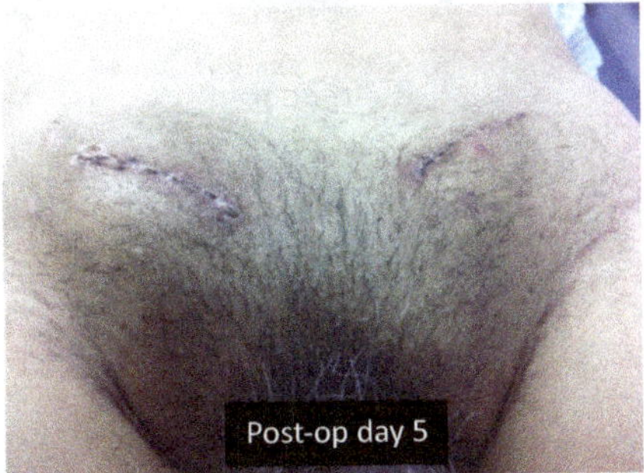

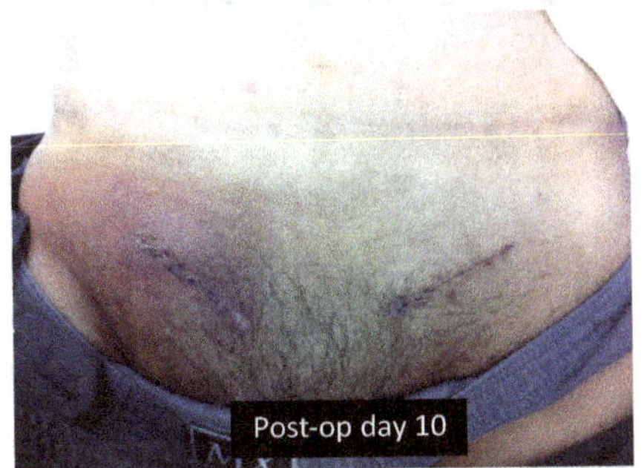

A1.9

1. It was closed with interrupted sutures.
2. The three phases are inflammation, proliferation, and maturation.
3. The wound has dehisced after removal of the stitches.
4. Surgeon factors: poor technique.
    Patient factors: poor vascular supply to the wound, infection, diabetes, malnutrition.

A1.10

1. Surgical site infection (SSI).
2. The right groin wound is swollen, painful, inflamed, and tender. He may have a fever.
3. The development of an SSI depends on contamination of the wound site during a surgical procedure (pathogenicity and inoculum of the microorganisms present) balanced against the host's immune response.
4. If the infection is superficial, it can be treated with intravenous antibiotics. If there are deeper collections of pus, removal of stitches and surgical drainage is necessary.
5. The patient had the hernia surgically repaired with a mesh. When there is infection in the presence of a foreign body, the mesh may need to be explanted.

Q1.11

This is a 40-year-old male.

1. Describe the abnormality.
2. What is the diagnosis?
3. What would you examine for?
4. What is the natural history of the problem?
5. What is the management?

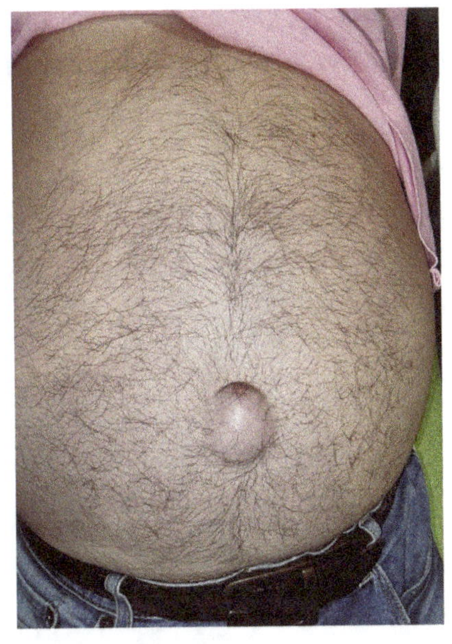

Q1.12

This is a 70-year-old male.

1. Describe the abnormality.
2. What is the diagnosis?
3. What are his symptoms?
4. What can be detected on clinical examination?
5. What is a concern during surgical repair?

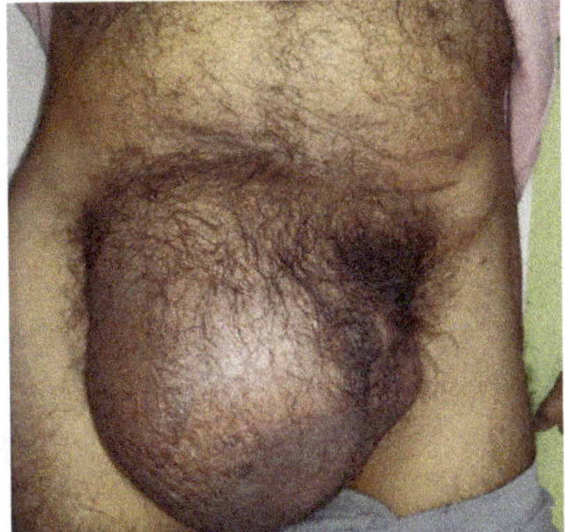

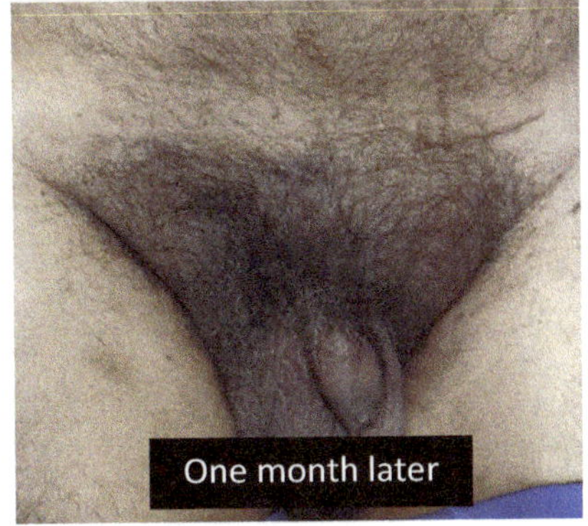

A1.11

1. There is a spherical lump over the umbilicus. There are no overlying skin changes.

2. Umbilical hernia.

3. Reducibility of the hernia and tenderness if it is not reducible.

4. All abdominal wall hernias will enlarge and become more symptomatic with time. This is due to the daily activities that increase intra-abdominal pressure, pushing out the visceral contents in the abdominal cavity through the hernia neck.

5. Surgical repair with a mesh to prevent incarceration.

A1.12

1. A large right inguinal scrotal mass. There is a surgical scar over the left groin.

2. A right inguinal scrotal hernia. Previous left inguinal hernia repair.

3. There will be pain and discomfort in the right groin/scrotum due to the large mass. If there is bowel in the hernia sac, intestinal obstruction can occur.

4. The hernia is unlikely to be reducible. Peristalsis may be felt on palpation and bowel sounds present on auscultation.

5. Reduction of the contents of the right inguinal hernia into the abdominal cavity may cause increase in intra-abdominal pressure and lead to abdominal compartment syndrome. Occasionally the bowel in the hernia sac may need to be sacrificed.

Q1.13

This is a 60-year-old male with a surgical complication.

1. What surgery was likely performed on him?
2. What is the abnormality in the abdominal wall?
3. What are factors that predispose to developing this?
4. What is the management?

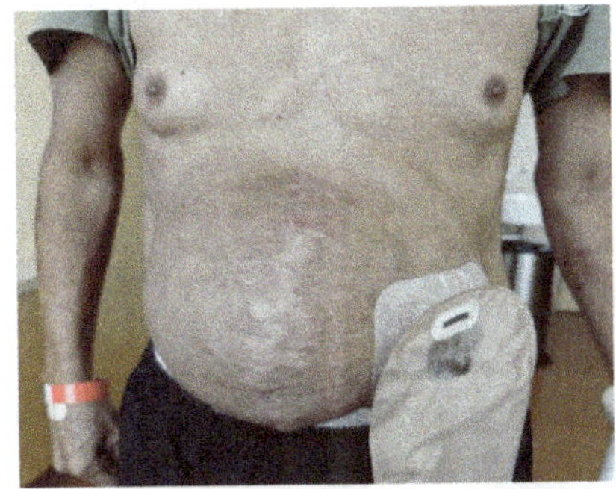

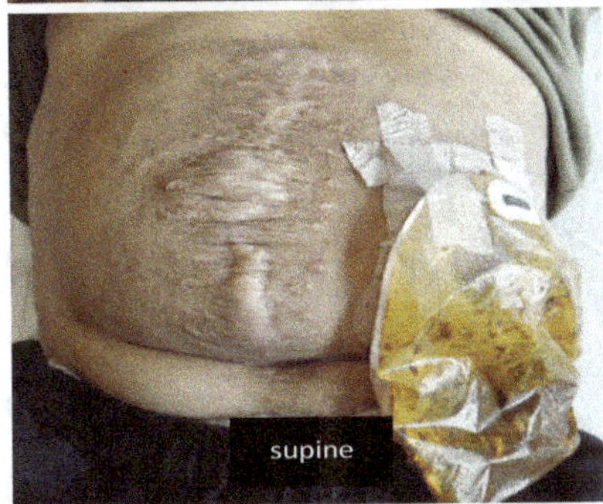

Q1.14

This is a 32-year-old female in supine position.

1. What is seen in her groin?
2. What is the most likely diagnosis?
3. Is it more common in males or females?
4. What is seen during laparoscopic surgery?
5. Why does this pathology have a higher chance of irreducibility?

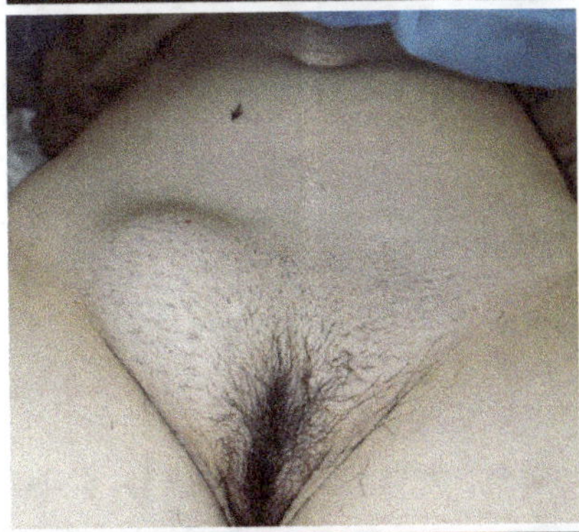

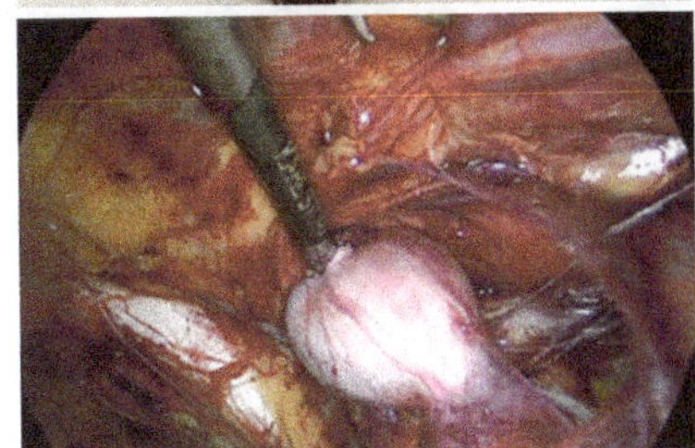

A1.13

1. A colostomy was performed, with or without resection of the colon, via a midline laparotomy.

2. There is a large incisional hernia and a colostomy bag.

3. **Patient-related factors** that impair proper wound healing and affect the strength of the new tissue to support the abdominal wall, e.g. obesity, malnutrition.
   Disease-related factors including incision site, timing and urgency of procedure, surgical complications, and the underlying disease. The most common is wound infection.
   Technical factors related to the surgical technique or suture materials used for closure.

4. Surgical repair of the hernia.

A1.14

1. There is a right groin lump that is irreducible in the supine position.

2. Right femoral hernia.

3. It is 10 times more common in women.

4. The hernia sac, which is made up of the peritoneal lining, is reduced from the neck of the hernia.

5. The femoral canal, which is bordered by the inguinal ligament anterosuperiorly, Cooper's ligament inferiorly, the femoral vein laterally and lacunar ligament medially is tight and does not allow expansion (unlike an inguinal hernia).

Q1.15

This is a 40-year-old female.

1. What is seen in the AXR?

2. What is the diagnosis?

3. What are some common causes?

4. What is the clinical presentation?

5. What are the findings during surgery for this patient?

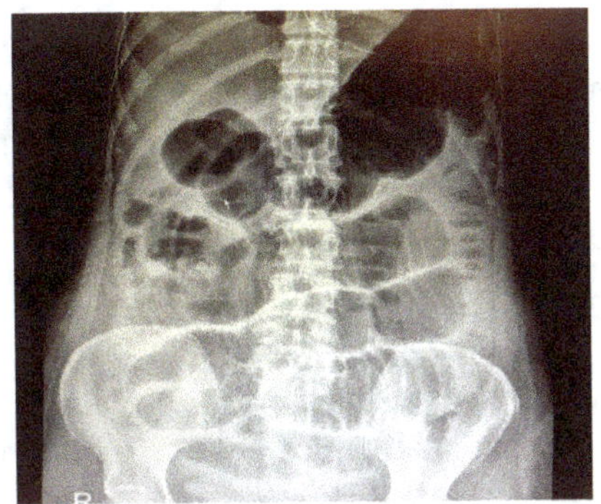

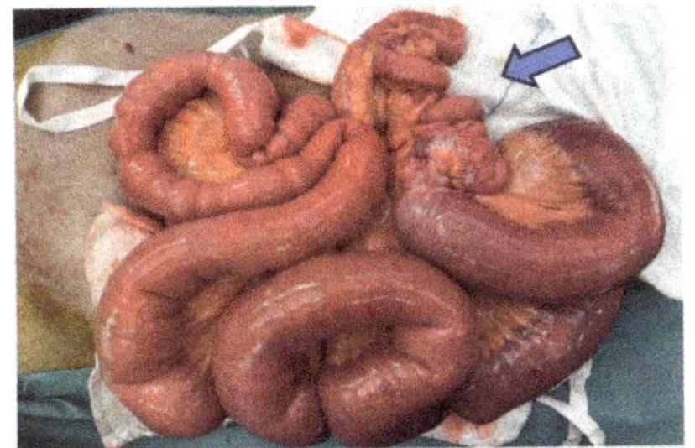

Q1.16

This 50-year-old male had emergency surgery. He has a history of a previous laparotomy for resection of retroperitoneal fibrosis.

1. What is seen in the surgical picture?

2. What is the most likely cause for the pathology to occur?

3. What is the likely clinical presentation?

4. What was likely performed during surgery?

5. What are the nutritional concerns if the patient survives?

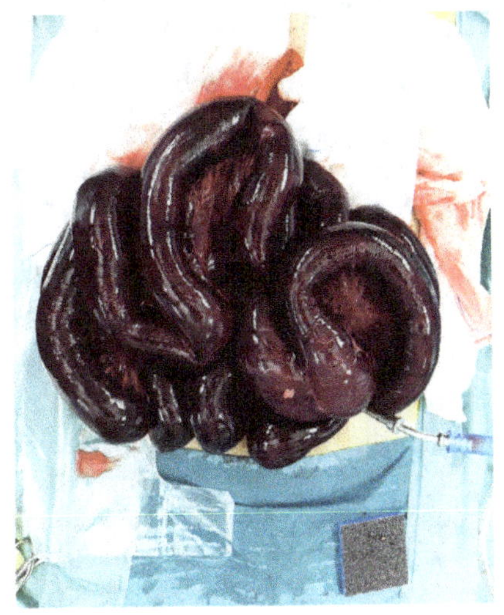

A1.15

1. The small bowel is dilated in the AXR. Small bowel is identified by its central position in the abdominal cavity and valvulae conniventes (plica circulares) seen.

2. Small bowel obstruction.

3. The most common cause is post-surgical adhesions in patients with previous abdominal surgery. Incarcerated hernias are the most common cause for patients with no history of surgery. Other aetiologies include malignancy, inflammatory bowel disease (Crohn's disease) and foreign bodies.

4. Central abdominal pain, which may start as intermittent due to peristalsis against an obstruction. Subsequently there will be abdominal distention with vomiting. The bowel sounds may be reduced and high pitched.

5. There is a transition point (arrow) between the dilated and decompressed small bowel. This is due to a malignant tumour. This patient had a carcinoid tumour of the small bowel causing obstruction.

A1.16

1. Long segment of ischaemic small bowel.

2. The mesentery of the small bowel may have been distorted from the previous surgery, causing the small bowel to twist and strangulate, leading to infarction.

3. Sepsis with severe abdominal pain and peritonitis.

4. Resection of the ischaemic segment of bowel.

5. Patients with bowel gangrene have higher mortality rates. This patient survived.

   With the resection of extensive small bowel, patients are at risk of developing short bowel syndrome. This will lead to intestinal malabsorption due to the loss of intestinal absorptive surface area and more rapid intestinal transit. Patients will need nutritional and fluid supplements.

Q1.17

These are 2 different patients with the same pathology.

1. What is seen in picture A?
2. What are the rules of 2 associated with this?
3. What are the clinical presentations?
4. What is the management?
5. What is seen in picture B?

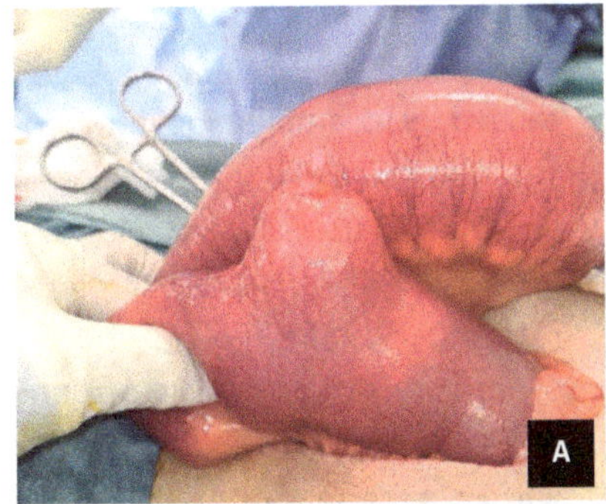

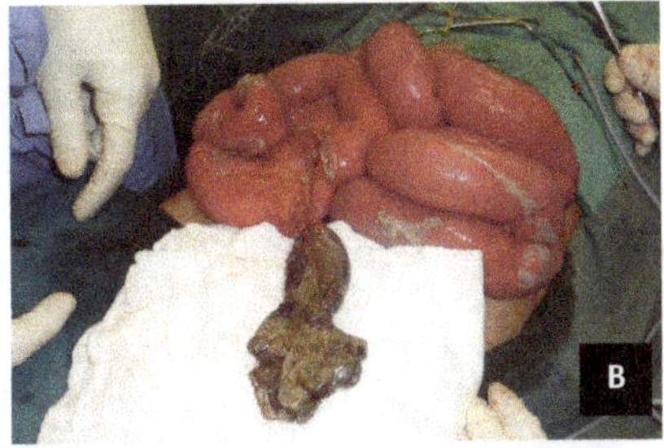

Q1.18

This 70-year-old male presented with back pain.

1. What are the names of this clinical sign?
2. What does this sign indicate?
3. What pathologies can give rise to this sign?

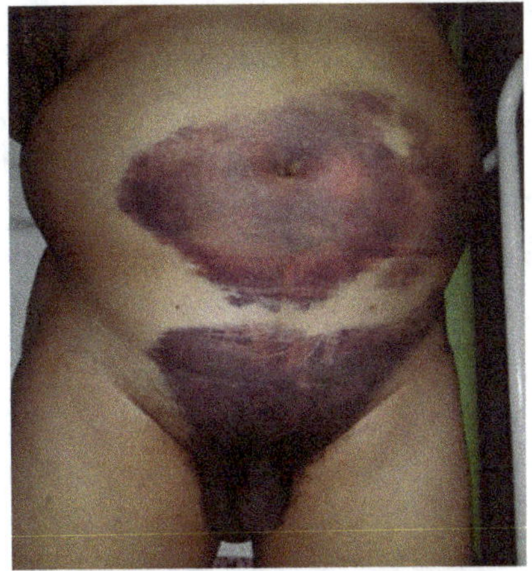

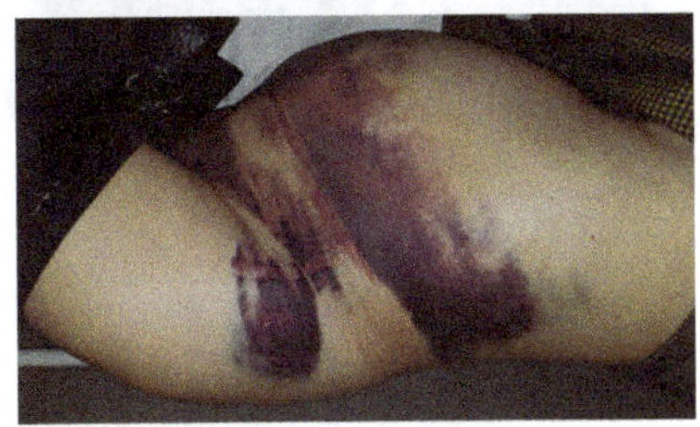

A1.17

1. A Meckel's diverticulum. It is a congenital abnormality of the small intestine caused by incomplete obliteration of the vitelline (omphalomesenteric) duct.

2. They occur in 2% of the population, 2% are symptomatic, children are usually less than 2 years old, male:female ratio 2:1, usually located 2 feet proximal to the ileocecal valve and are 2 inches long.

3. Majority are asymptomatic.
    Symptomatic patients can present with bleeding, intestinal obstruction and diverticulitis.

4. Surgical resection of the diverticulum to prevent potential complications.

5. The Meckel's diverticulum has twisted on itself (strangulated) and become necrotic.

A1.18

1. Grey Turner and Cullen's sign.

2. Haemorrhage into the retroperitoneal space manifest as subcutaneous ecchymosis or discoloration of the flank (Grey Turner) and/or periumbilical (Cullen's) region.

3. Rupture of any retroperitoneal blood vessel (e.g. aortic aneurysm or splenic or renal artery), haemorrhagic pancreatitis or rupture of a renal tumour.

Q1.19

This is a 40-year-old male.

1. What is the pathology seen in picture A?
2. What is the likely clinical presentation?
3. What is the likely diagnosis?
4. What was performed for the patient as seen in picture B?

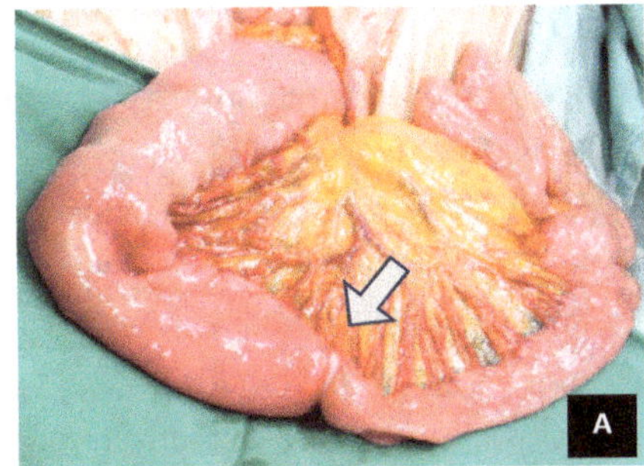

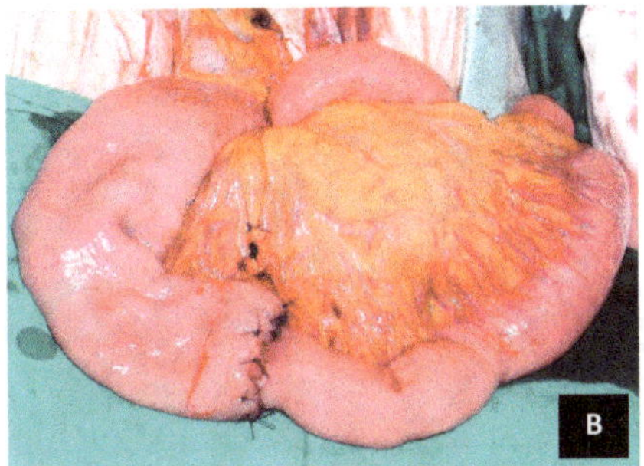

Q1.20

This is a 60-year-old male who presented with generalized abdominal pain.

1. What is the abnormality seen in the CT scan?
2. What is the clinical presentation?
3. What is the management?
4. Based on the surgical specimen, what is the likely cause?

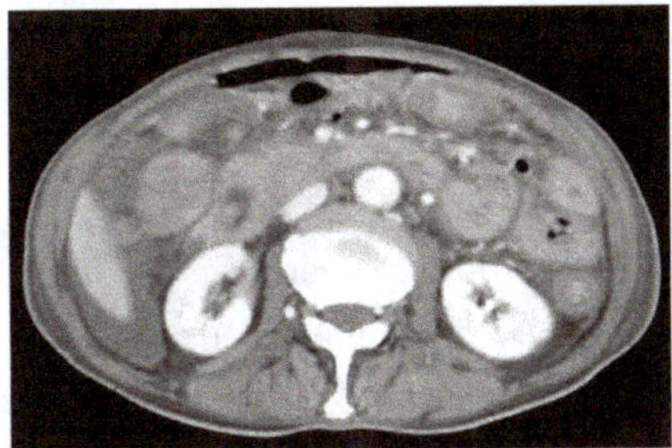

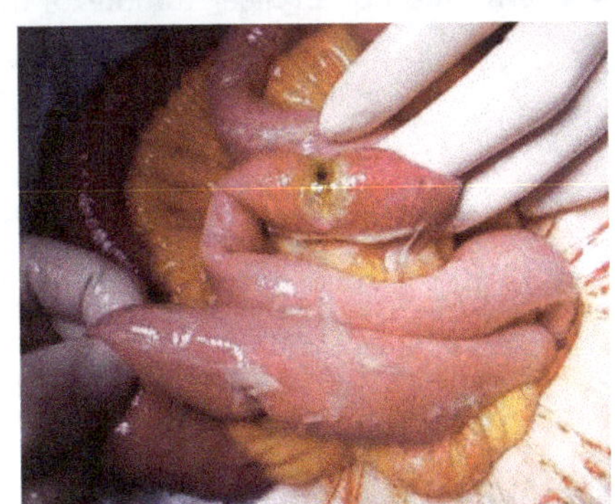

A1.19

1. There is a constriction in the small bowel causing proximal dilatation and distal decompression.

2. Signs and symptoms of intestinal obstruction. He will have colicky abdominal pain and a distended abdomen.

3. Small bowel carcinoma.

4. Resection of the tumour with adequate proximal and distal margins, followed by end-to-end anastomosis performed with interrupted sutures.

A1.20

1. There is "free gas" in the peritoneal cavity. "Free gas" is gas not in the bowel.

2. He will have generalized peritonitis. The patient will have abdominal pain associated with a distended tender guarded abdomen. He may be in septic shock due to severe bacteriemia.

3. Stabilization of the circulatory system of the patient, followed by emergency laparotomy to identify the source of visceral perforation.

4. Perforation of an ulcer/tumour of the small bowel.

Q1.21

This is a 35-year-old male.

1. What abnormality is seen in the CT scan?

2. What is the diagnosis?

3. What surgery was performed?

4. What are the common aetiologies that could lead to this condition in adults?

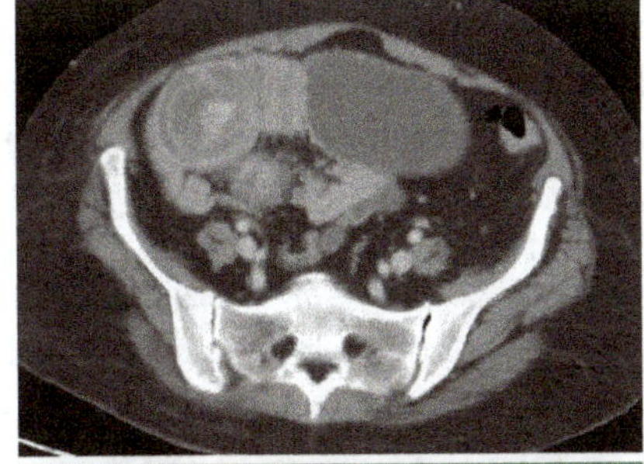

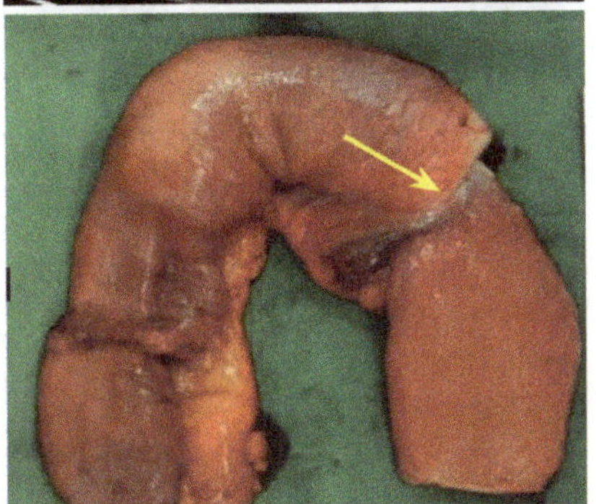

Q1.22

This is a 60-year-old male.

1. What was detected on rectal examination?

2. What is the initial management of the patient?

3. What was detected during endoscopy in the duodenum?

4. What is the management?

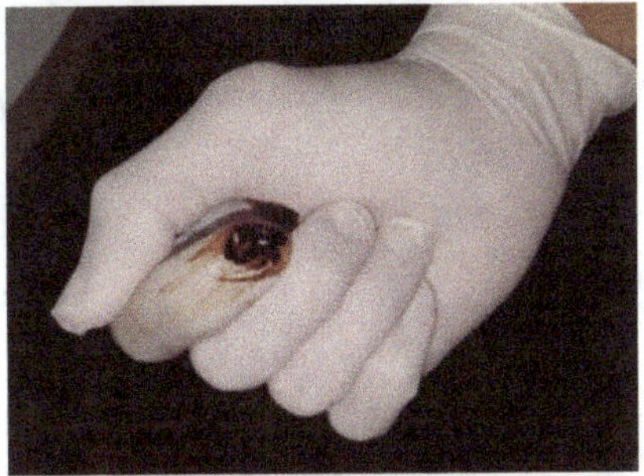

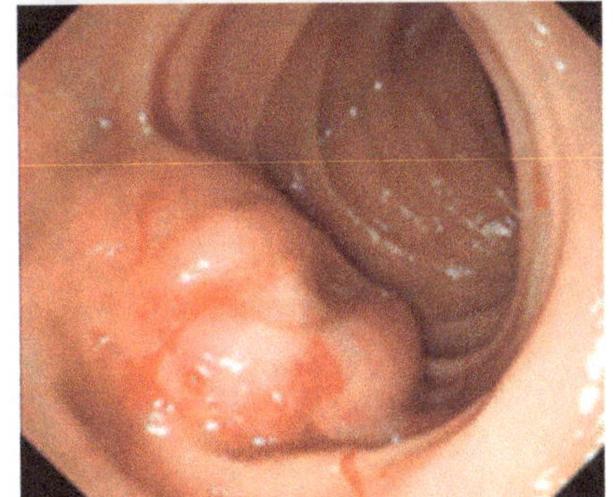

A1.21

1. There is a "doughnut shape" created by the hyperdense central core of bowel and mesentery surrounded by the hypodense outer oedematous bowel. There is associated proximal bowel dilatation.

2. Intussusception of the small bowel. It occurs when one segment of bowel telescopes into an adjacent bowel segment, causing intestinal obstruction and potentially, intestinal ischemia.

3. Initial surgical approach is to attempt reduction of the intussusception. If reduction fails, resection of the involved bowel segment is performed.

4. In adults, a lead point is sometimes present. These include a polyp, hamartoma, Meckel's diverticulum, enlarged lymph node or malignancy.

A1.22

1. Melena. It has a characteristic tarry colour and offensive smell, and is often difficult to flush away.

2. Ensure that the patient is haemodynamically stable.
   Check the haemoglobin levels. Transfusion may be necessary if there is significant blood loss.
   Investigate the cause of bleeding.

3. There is a tumour that is actively bleeding.

4. Surgical resection of the tumour.

Q1.23

This is a 60-year-old female who presented with right sided abdominal discomfort.

1. What is seen on clinical inspection of her abdomen?

2. What are the potential organs the pathology could arise from?

3. What is seen in the intra-op photos?

4. What is the diagnosis?

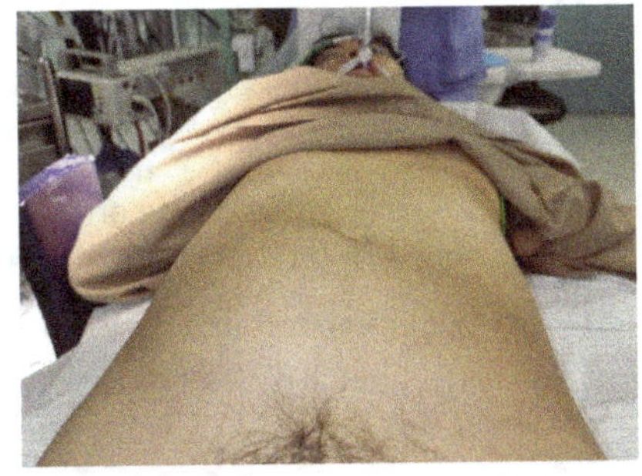

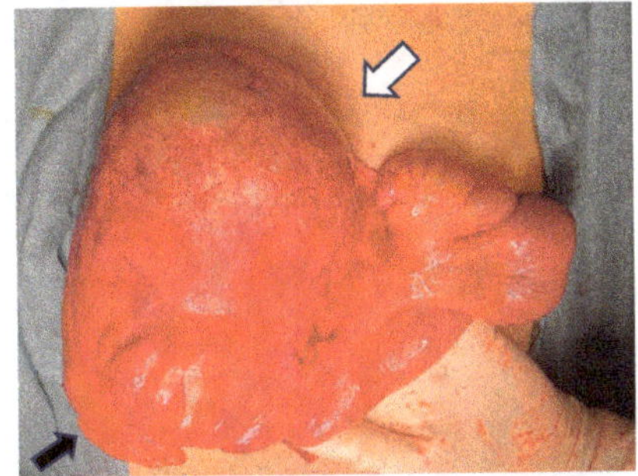

Q1.24

This is a 50-year-old male who had abdominal surgery.

1. What is seen in picture A?

2. What is seen in picture B?

3. What is the diagnosis?

4. What is the management?

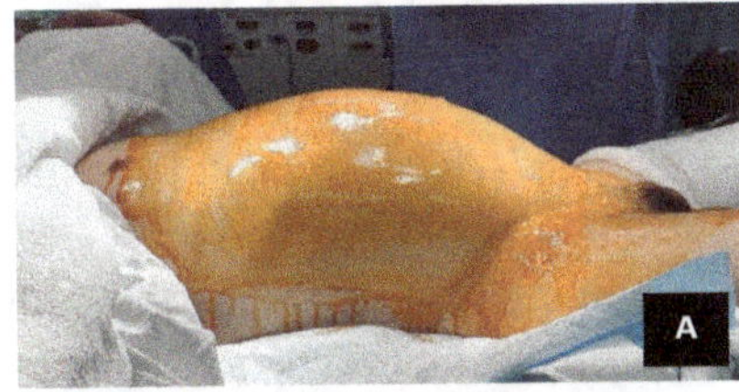

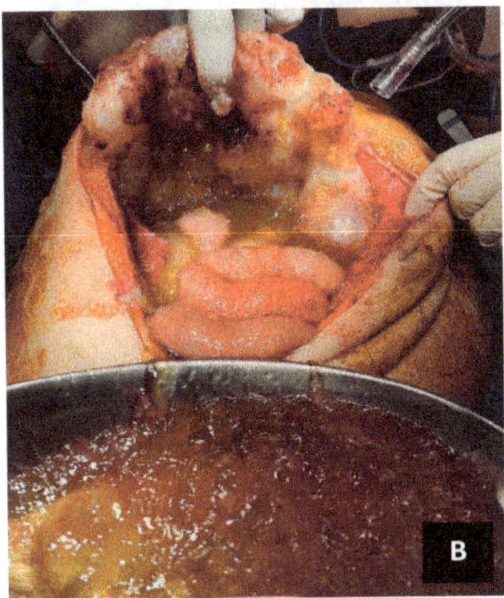

A1.23

1. There is a large mass in the right lower quadrant of the abdomen.
2. Colon, ileum and ovary.
3. There is a large mass (white arrow) bordered by ascending colon (right side), the appendix (black arrow) and terminal ileum.
4. Large mucinous cyst arising from the appendix.

A1.24

1. The abdomen is very distended.
2. There is "caking" of the omentum. The abdominal cavity is filled with gelatinous material, so called "jelly belly."
3. Pseudomyxoma peritonei (PMP). It is a rare clinical entity characterized by diffuse intra-abdominal gelatinous ascites with mucinous deposits on peritoneal surfaces.
4. Current recommended standard treatment for PMP consists of complete cytoreduction surgery (CRS) and hyperthermic intraperitoneal chemotherapy (HIPEC).

Q1.25

This is a 60-year-old female who had an open right hemicolectomy 2 months ago. There is persistent discharge from the wounds.

1. What is the diagnosis?

2. What is the pathogenesis?

3. How can we classify the discharge?

4. What are some factors preventing healing of the wounds?

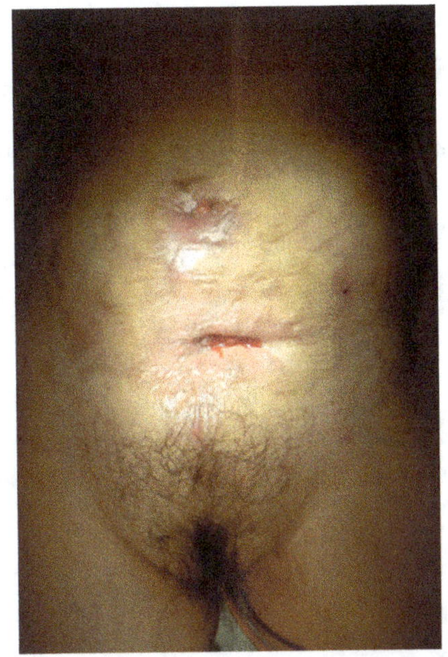

Q1.26

This is an underweight 55-year-old female.

1. What is seen in the coronal section of the CT scan?

2. What is the likely clinical presentation?

3. What is abnormal on the axial section of CT scan?

4. What is the diagnosis?

5. What is the management?

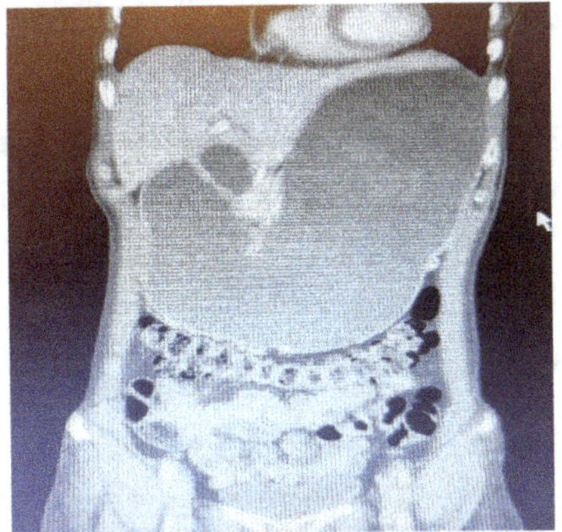

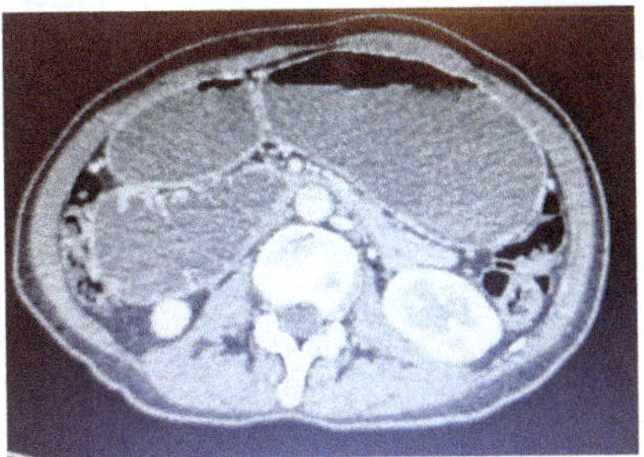

A1.25

1. Enterocutaneous fistula. It is an abnormal communication between the small or large bowel and the skin.

2. It is often due to an infection/pathology causing inflammation and poor abdominal wall wound healing. Common causes include bowel anastomosis leak, an inadvertent enterotomy or accidental bowel sutured to the abdominal wall on closure.

3. Depending on the volume of discharge output — high vs low.

4. Foreign body
   Radiation
   Inflammation/infection /IBD
   Epithelialization of the fistula tract
   Neoplasm
   Distal obstruction
   High output discharge

A1.26

1. There is a severely dilated stomach. The small bowel is of normal calibre.

2. Distended upper abdomen with vomiting.

3. The axial cut is at the level T12. The duodenum D3 is dilated and tapers towards D4.

4. Superior mesenteric artery syndrome. It is due to the compression of the third portion of the duodenum between the abdominal aorta and the superior mesenteric artery.

5. Initial treatment is usually conservative. The patient can lie in the lateral position to open the aortomesenteric angle to allow food to transit. A nasogastric tube can be inserted for gastric decompression.
   The patient is encouraged to eat small meals and engage in postural therapy.
   In patients who fail conservative therapy, surgical intervention (gastrojejunostomy) is necessary.

Q1.27

This is a 40-year-old female with metastatic cancer who had abdominal surgery.

1. What is seen in picture A?

2. What is seen in picture B?

3. What extensive surgical procedure has been carried out?

4. What are the indications for these extensive procedures?

5. What are the complications of this surgery?

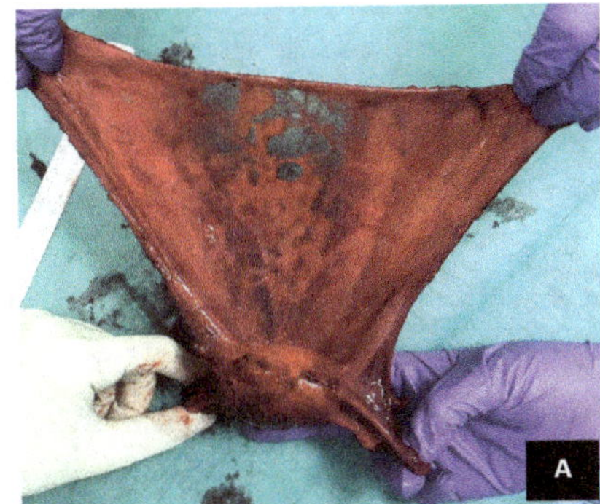

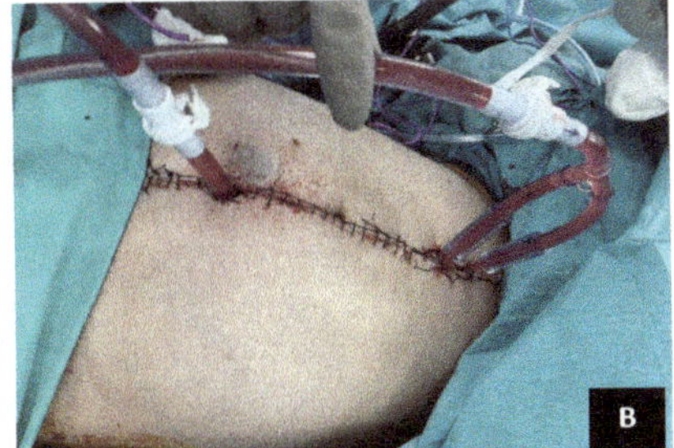

Q1.28

These are 2 different patients with metastatic disease.

1. What is seen in over the umbilicus?

2. What is seen in the surgical photo?

3. What is the management?

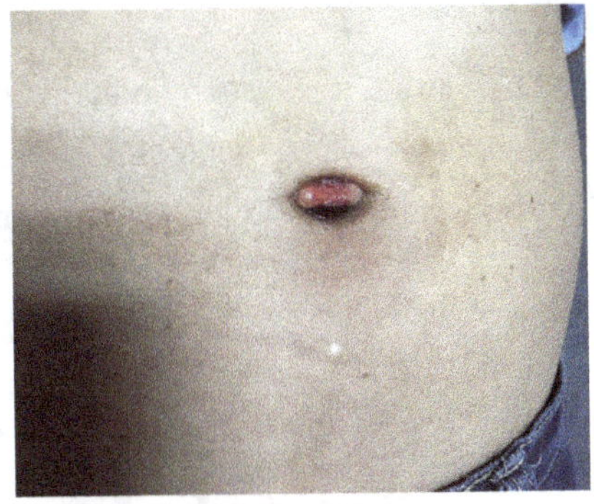

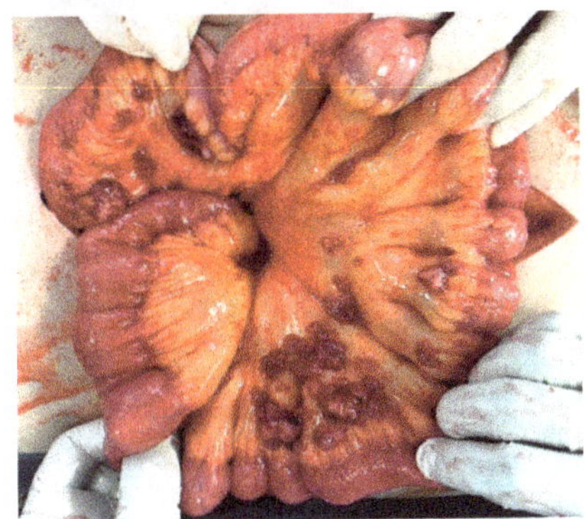

A1.27

1. Peritonectomy has been performed. The peritoneum is displayed superiorly. Inferiorly is the uterus with its fallopian tubes.

2. The abdominal cavity is closed with large bore tubes inserted into the abdominal cavity.

3. Cytoreduction surgery (CRS) combined with hyperthermic intraperitoneal chemotherapy (HIPEC).

4. Gastric, colorectal and ovarian carcinoma with peritoneal metastases and mesothelioma. Studies have shown that successful surgery can prolong survival.

5. It is associated with morbidity and mortality of approximately 30% and 3%, respectively.
   Complications include:
   Toxicity from the HIPEC — liver, blood and renal.
   Visceral organs — intestinal atony, fistula formation, bowel perforation.

A1.28

1. There is a Sister Joseph nodule at the umbilicus.

2. There are multiple nodules on the peritoneum of the small bowel mesentery.

3. Metastatic cancer is stage 4 disease.
   The management is often palliative, unless the patient responds very well to systemic therapy (chemotherapy, immunotherapy or other modalities).

Q1.29

This is a 40-year-old male.

1. What abnormality is seen in the CT scan?

2. What is seen in the surgical specimen?

3. What is the diagnosis?

4. What is the clinical presentation?

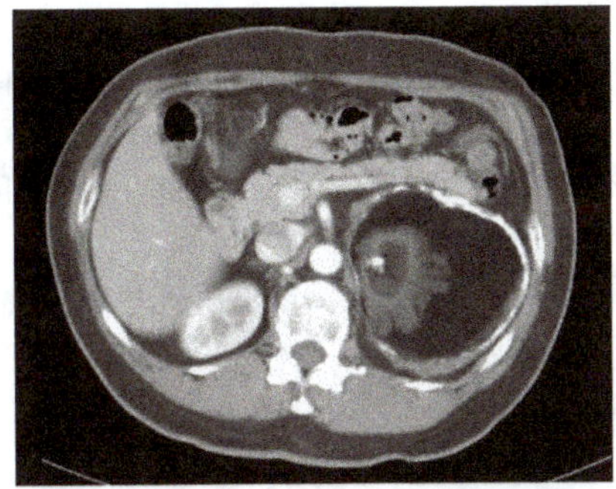

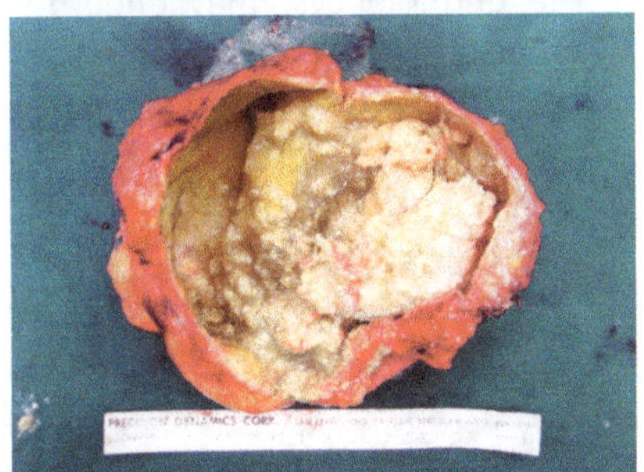

Q1.30

This is a 40-year-old female who has been on follow-up for a large ovarian cyst. Emergency surgery was performed on her.

1. What is the diagnosis?

2. What is the likely clinical presentation?

3. What investigations may be useful for diagnosis?

4. What was performed at surgery?

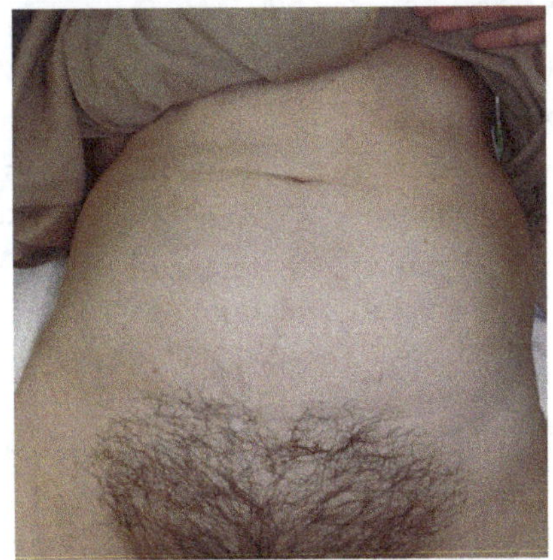

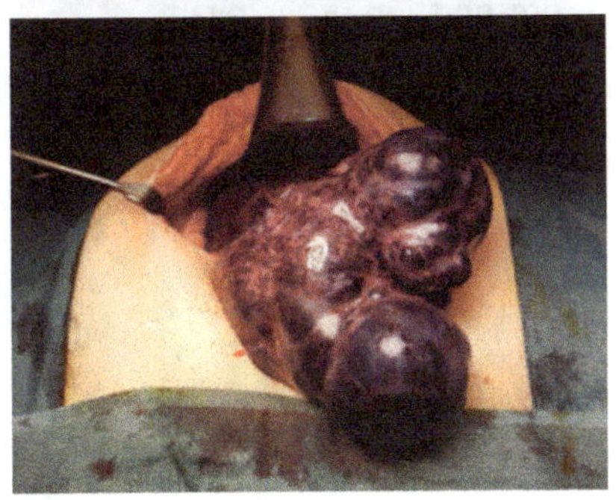

A1.29

1. There is a large, well-defined mass posterior to the tail of the pancreas. It has areas of fluid and soft tissue density with a focus of calcification.

2. There is a 15 × 15 cm large cystic lesion filled with yellow-white sebaceous material.

3. Dermoid cyst, also known as mature cystic teratoma. They are benign tumours of embryonic origin consisting of two or three germ cell layers.

4. They are often asymptomatic and detected on routine imaging for other pathologies.
   The dermoid cyst may undergo complications such as torsion, rupture, adhesions, infections or malignant transformation.

A1.30

1. Torsion of the ovarian cyst. The cyst looks swollen and necrotic.

2. The patient may complain of lower abdominal pain that may be sharp or dull depending on whether the ovary is twisting or untwisting.
   The patient may also have associated nausea and vomiting.

3. Ultrasound with doppler: transvaginal or pelvic.
   CT can be useful to rule out other causes for an acute abdomen.
   The definitive diagnosis of ovarian torsion is made by direct visualization during surgery.

4. The twisted ovary is visualized and untwisted to evaluate if it is potentially viable. If the ovary is unsalvageable, a salpingo-oophorectomy needs to be performed. If the ovary is salvageable, the cyst can be excised with preservation of the ovary.

Q1.31

This is a 60-year-old male who had a previous laparotomy with a creation of an ileostomy 3 years ago.

1. What is seen in the CT scan?
2. What is seen at the stoma site?
3. What is the diagnosis?
4. What is the management?

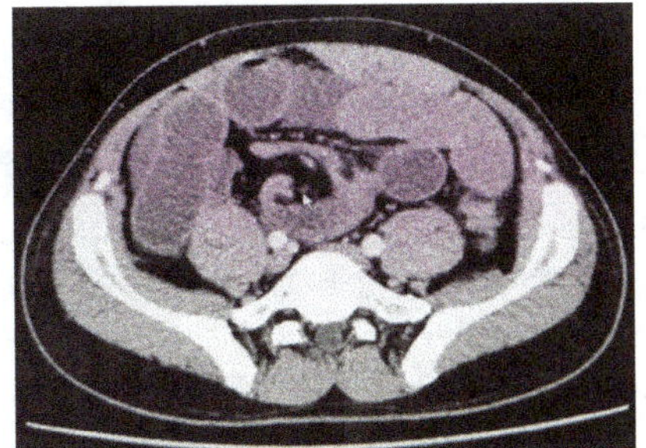

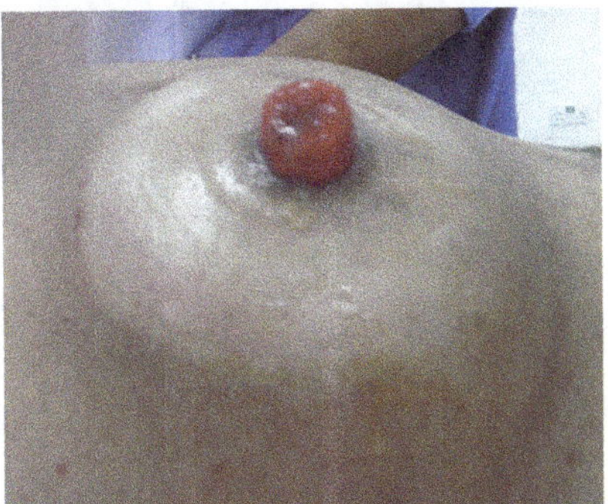

Q1.32

This is an 8-year-old boy who presents with central abdominal pain migrating to the left iliac fossa pain and fever.

1. What are the unusual findings on the X-ray?
2. What is the likely diagnosis?
3. What challenges does it pose in management of these patients?

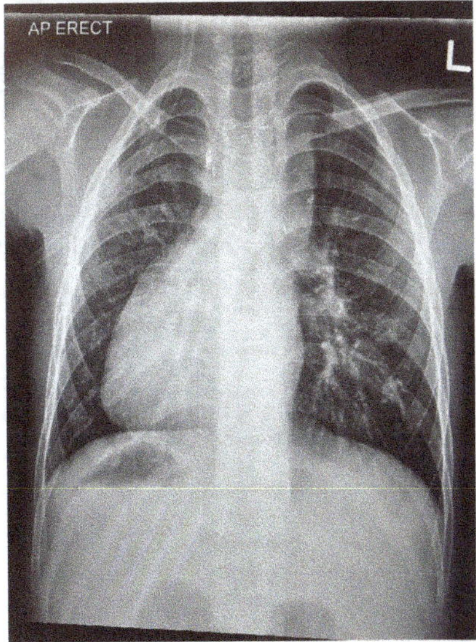

A1.31

1. There are dilated loops of fluid-filled small bowel.

2. There is a "mount-like" swelling around a viable stoma.

3. Parastomal herniation causing intestinal obstruction. The intestines have protruded through the abdominal wall defect created during stoma formation.

4. Surgical intervention is needed to address the intestinal obstruction and prevent a recurrence. Options include repair of the hernia in situ and keeping the stoma, or direct repair of the hernia with stoma re-siting.

A1.32

1. Situs inversus. There is dextrocardia and gastric bubble is beneath the right hemidiaphragm, suggesting that the liver is on the left.

2. Acute appendicitis.

3. Situs inversus is the mirror-image transposition of the organs. Achieving diagnoses of pathologies is the first challenge. The second challenge is the orientation of the anatomy during surgery. Thirdly, as most surgeons are right-handed, the operations can cause difficulties:

Q1.33

This is a 40-year-old male.

1. What abnormality is seen in the CT scan?

2. What will be evident on clinical examination?

3. What surgery was performed?

4. What is a likely indication for surgery?

5. What are patients susceptible to after surgery?

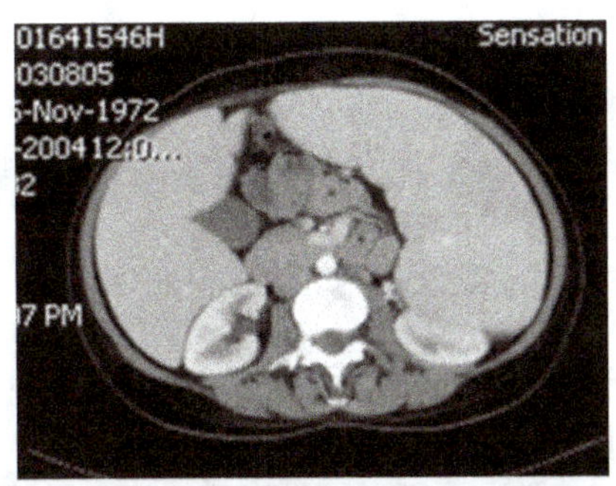

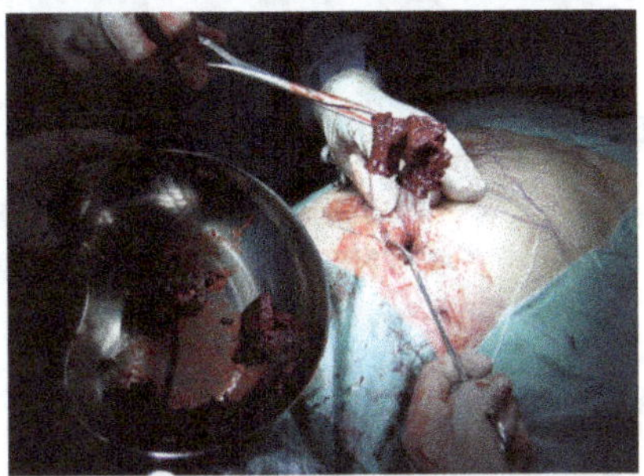

Q1.34

This is a 40-year-old female with left abdominal wall discomfort.

1. What abnormality is seen in the CT scan?

2. What is seen in the surgical picture?

3. What is the likely diagnosis?

4. What medical conditions are associated with this pathology?

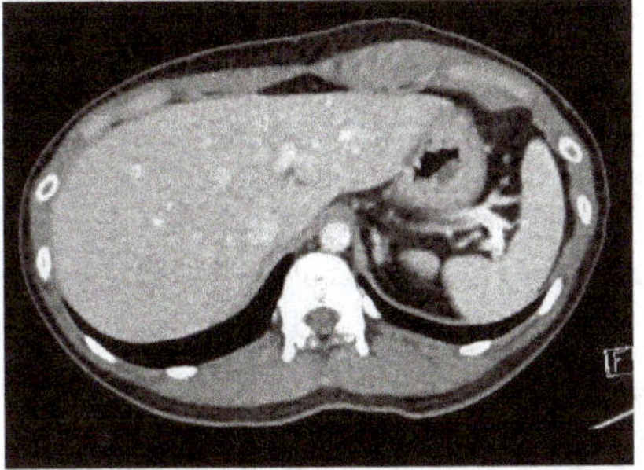

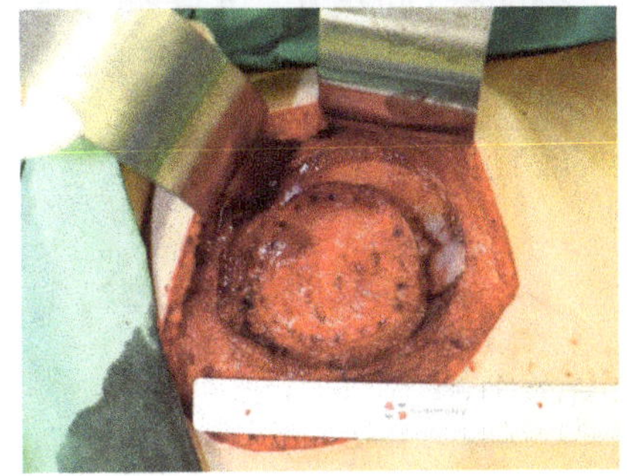

A1.33

1. Splenomegaly.

2. There will be a large palpable mass arising from beneath the left costal margin.

3. Laparoscopic splenectomy. The spleen was mosselated into smaller pieces to ensure the specimen is delivered though a small surgical scar. The enlarged spleen is seen on the pre-op markings on the patient's abdominal wall.

4. Idiopathic thrombocytopenia purpura.
   Splenectomy removes the primary site of platelet clearance and autoantibody production and offers the highest rate of sustained response.

5. Patients who undergo splenectomy are at increased risk of infections secondary to encapsulated organisms such as Haemophilus influenzae, Streptococcus pneumoniae, and Neisseria meningitidis. Vaccinations against these organisms are highly recommended in post-splenectomy patients.

A1.34

1. There is an enlargement in the left anterior rectus abdominis muscle as compared to the right.

2. Surgical resection of the tumour in the anterior rectus abdominis muscle.

3. Desmoid tumour (DT). They commonly occur in the rectus abdominis muscle, head and neck region, pelvis, and in the extremities.

4. They are known to occur in association with pregnancy and with the use of oral contraceptive pills. Patients with Familial Adenomatous Polyposis are at a much higher risk of developing DT (Up to 25% higher than the general population).

2

Trauma and ICU

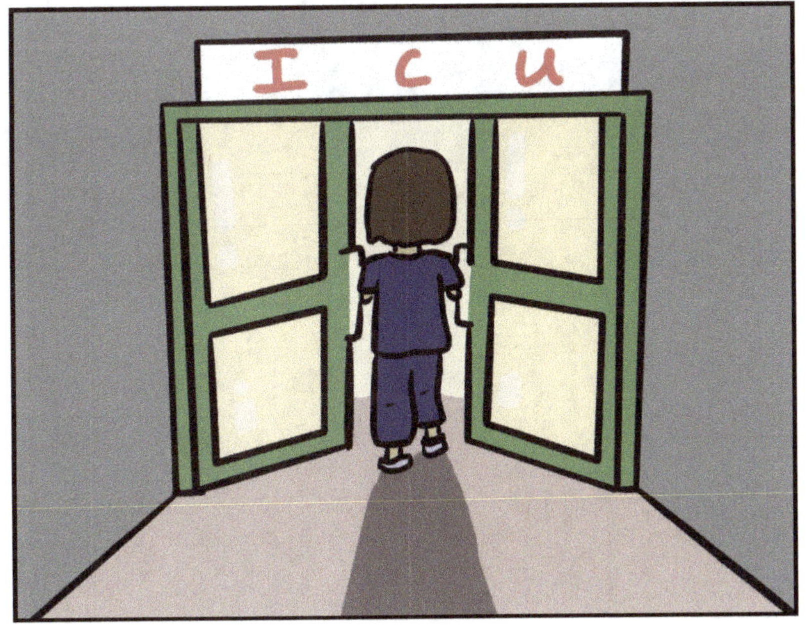

Q2.1

This 30-year-old male is haemodynamically unstable in the intensive care unit (ICU) after being involved in a road traffic accident.

1. What device is shown in the picture?

2. What are the sites through which this device can be inserted?

3. What information can this device provide?

4. What are the potential complications with the use of this device?

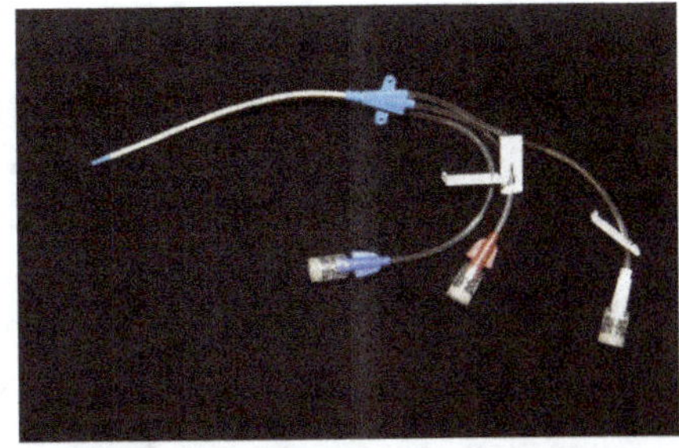

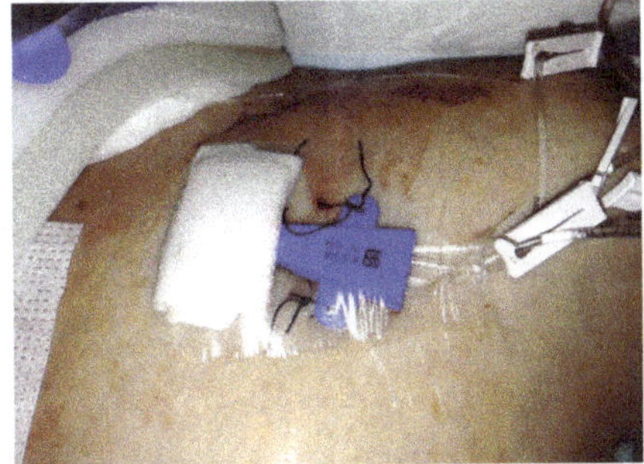

Q2.2

This patient is on mechanical ventilation after sustaining traumatic brain injury. This device was inserted on day 8 of ICU stay.

1. What is the device shown (arrowed)?

2. What are the advantages of this device over the conventional endotracheal tube?

3. How can this device be inserted?

4. What are the complications associated with its use?

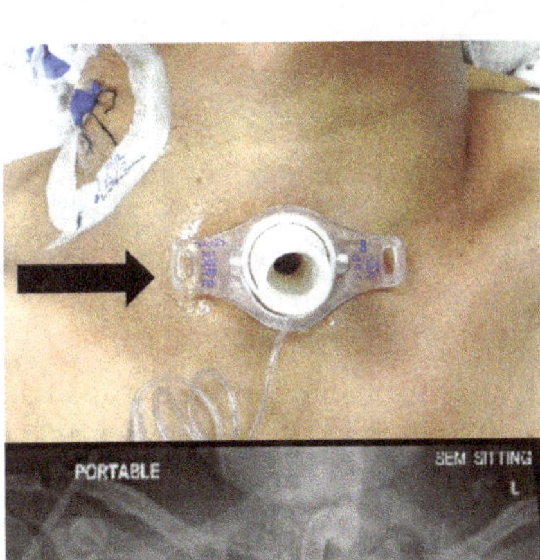

A2.1

1. Central Venous Catheter.

2. Internal and external jugular, subclavian and femoral veins.

3. The central venous pressure (CVP) obtained can be used to assess the preload of the right ventricle which will guide fluid administration.
   Central Venous Oxygen Saturation (ScVO2) measured can be used to assess the adequacy of tissue perfusion.

4. Infection
   Arrhythmia
   Air embolism
   Pneumothorax, haemothorax, pleural effusion
   Pericardial effusion/tamponade
   Vascular injuries

A2.2

1. Tracheostomy tube.

2. It allows prolonged tracheal intubation with reduced risk of laryngeal complications.
   Tracheal toilet (suctioning/cleaning) of the tube is easier.
   Patients tolerate it better, can breathe spontaneously with less breathing effort and speak with the use of a fenestrated tube.

3. Open approach: surgical dissection from the skin to the trachea.
   Percutaneous approach: a needle puncture followed by a guide wire and a dilator.

4. Accidental dislodgement of a tracheostomy tube may result in loss of airway patency.
   Subcutaneous emphysema.
   Stoma site: infection, haemorrhage and erosion.

Q2.3

This patient presented with acute shortness of breath.

1. Name the apparatus shown in the picture.

2. What are 2 common indications for this intervention?

3. What are the contraindications for this intervention?

4. What are the advantages of this intervention?

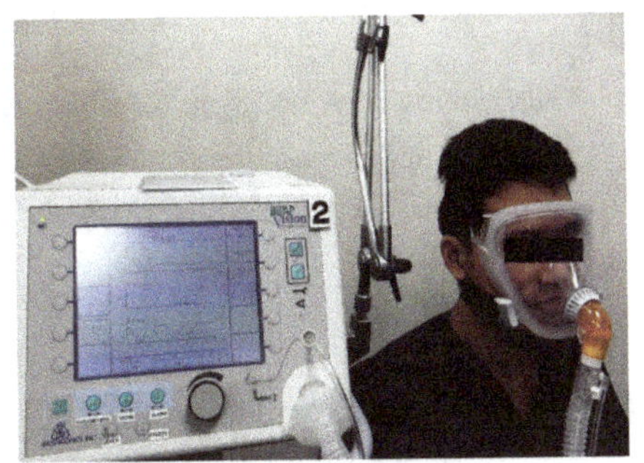

Q2.4

This monitoring device was used in a patient with septic shock.

1. Name the device shown in the picture.

2. What are the uses of this monitoring device?

3. Where are the appropriate sites for insertion?

4. What are the potential complications with its use?

5. What are the limitations of this monitoring device?

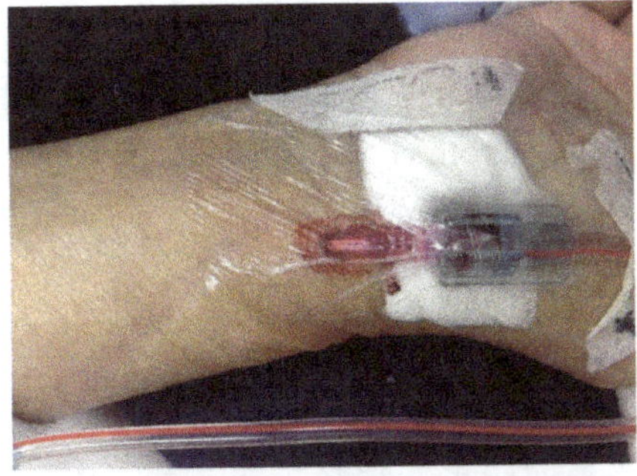

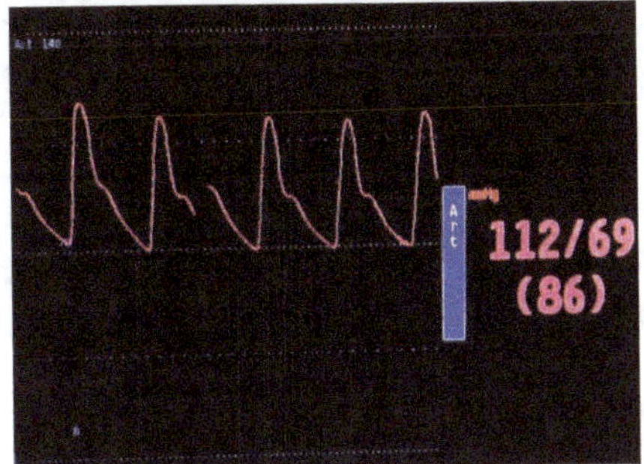

A2.3

1. Non-invasive ventilation (NIV).

2. Congestive cardiac failure.
   Chronic obstructive pulmonary disease exacerbation.

3. Respiratory arrest.
   Depressed conscious state.
   Aspiration risk.
   Haemodynamic instability.
   Uncooperative patient.
   Excessive secretions.
   Recent upper gastrointestinal surgery.

4. Tracheal tube is not required.
   Better patient tolerance.
   Allows patient to speak and communicate.

A2.4

1. Intra-arterial (IA) line blood pressure monitor.

2. Accurate and real-time monitoring of the blood pressure.
   Allows frequent arterial blood gas and other types of blood sampling.
   It can be connected to a sensor to measure the cardiac output.

3. Radial, brachial, femoral and dorsalis pedis artery.

4. Cannula infections, arterial thrombosis and arterial wall injuries (pseudoaneurysms and punctures).

5. Regular calibration is required.
   The sensor must be at the level of the heart for accurate readings.
   Amplification or dampening of the blood pressure readings can occur.

Q2.5

This monitoring device is used routinely for patients.

1. Identify the device shown.

2. What parameters can this device monitor?

3. What are the limitations associated with the use of this device?

4. How can one validate the reading of this device if false measurements are suspected?

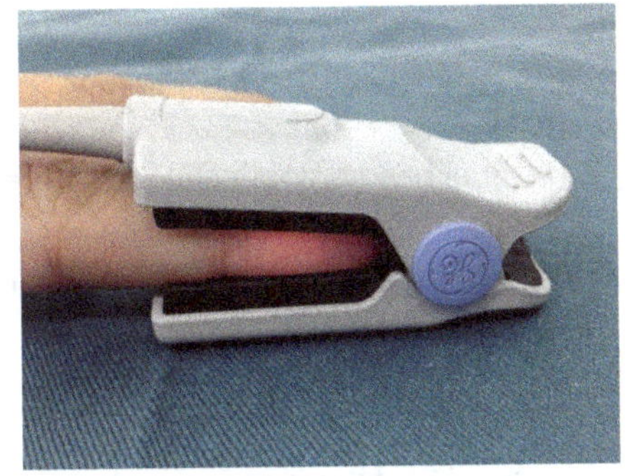

Q2.6

This equipment is often used in the ICU.

1. What supportive management does this machine provide?

2. What type of patients will need this intervention?

3. What are the disadvantages of this intervention?

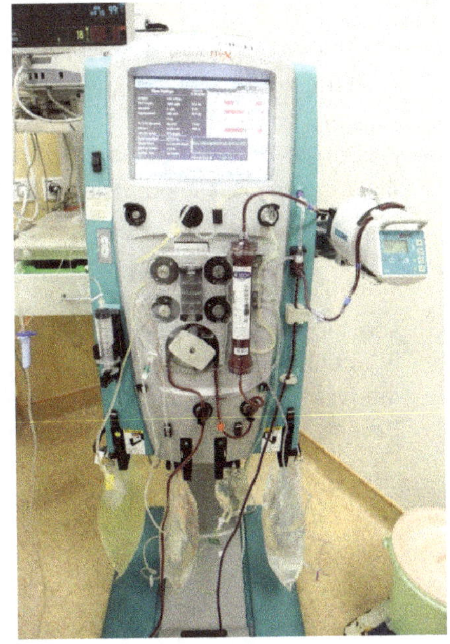

A2.5

1. Pulse oximeter.

2. Pulse rate.
   Arterial haemoglobin oxygen saturation (SpO2).

3. Motion artefacts and excessive light can result in false readings.
   The pulse oximeter may not detect the SpO2 when the patient is in a low perfusion state.
   Presence of carboxyhaemoglobin and methaemoglobin will affect the measurement of SpO2.

4. Arterial blood gas measurement.

A2.6

1. Continuous renal replacement therapy (CRRT).

2. Unstable ICU patients who require renal replacement therapy for "AEIOU" reasons.
   Acidosis,
   Electrolytes (usually potassium)
   Ingestion of poison
   Overloaded with fluids
   Uraemia

3. Logistics: a prolonged period of time during which patient is immobilized. It is labour intensive and costly.
   Intervention: Anticoagulation, vascular access-related issues.
   Patient: haemodynamic instability during the CRRT.

Q2.7

This device can be used for patients in circulatory shock.

1. Name the device shown in the picture.

2. What parameters can this device measure?

3. What parameters can be calculated from the measurements?

4. How can this device aid in the resuscitation of a patient in shock?

5. What alternative device/method can be used to provide similar patient parameters?

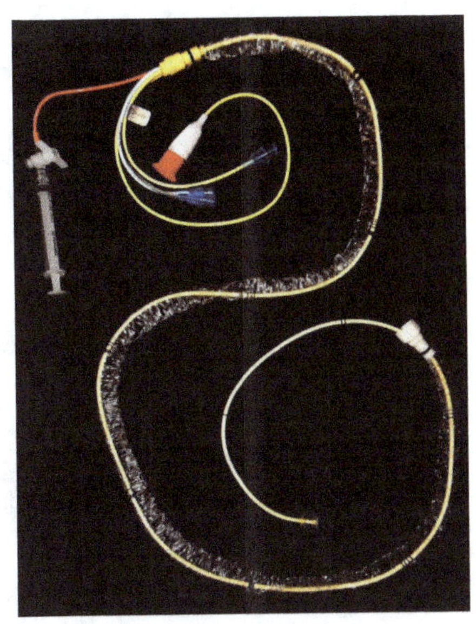

Q2.8

This arterial blood gas sample was taken from a patient who was ventilated and treated for hypoxaemia secondary to congestive heart failure. Loop diuretics have been administered.

1. Describe the acid-base disorder shown in the picture.

2. What are the possible causes of the disorder?

3. How will this disorder affect the patient?

4. What can be done to rectify the disorder?

Blood Gases,Art POCT

Description	Results	Ref.Ranges
pH, POCT	7.52	7.35 - 7.45
pCO2, POCT	30.6	35.0 - 45.0
pO2, POCT	79.0	75.0 - 100.0
Base Excess, POCT	2.3	-2.0 - 2.0
Bicarbonate, POCT	24.7	23.0 - 33.0
Standard Bicarb,POCT	26.5	21.0 - 27.0
O2 Saturation(calc)	96.9	96.0 - 100.0

A2.7

1. Pulmonary Artery Catheter (PAC)/Swan Ganz Catheter.

2. Cardiac Output
   Venous Oxygen Saturation
   Pulmonary Capillary Wedge Pressure/Pulmonary Artery Occlusion Pressure
   Pulmonary Blood Pressure

3. Cardiac output index
   Cardiac stroke volume
   Pulmonary vascular resistance (PVR)/pulmonary vascular resistance index (PVRI)
   Systemic vascular resistance (SVR)/systemic vascular resistance index (SVRI)

4. Aids in the diagnosis of the nature of shock.
   Guides the rate and volume of fluids to be administered.
   Guides the choice and dose of vasopressors and inotropes.

5. Bedside cardiac 2D-echography.

A2.8

1. Mixed metabolic and respiratory alkalosis.

2. Inappropriate ventilator settings resulting in hyperventilation.
   Use of loop diuretics has resulted in metabolic alkalosis.

3. The patient will have difficulty weaning off ventilator support.

4. The ventilator settings should be adjusted to allow permissive hypercarbia but titrated according to the pH of the arterial blood gas.
   Loop diuretics should be changed to other alternatives.

Q2.9

This is a 30-year-old male who was admitted to the ICU for cardiac arrhythmias after sustaining multiple long bone fractures.

1. What is the abnormality seen in the renal panel?

2. What is seen in the urine bag?

3. What is the likely cause?

4. What is the management?

Renal Panel (w/Glu)

Sodium	146	H	mmol/L	135 - 145
Potassium	7.1	HH	mmol/L	3.5 - 5.0
Chloride	111	H	mmol/L	95 - 110
Carbon Dioxide	< 10	L	mmol/L	22 - 31
Creatinine	762	H	umol/L	65 - 125
Urea	21.9	H	mmol/L	2.5 - 7.5
Glucose	5.9	N	mmol/L	4.0 - 7.8
Anion Gap	Invalid			

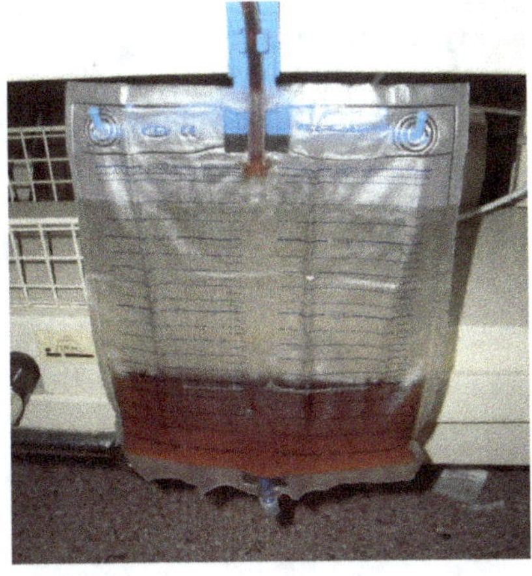

EXTEM

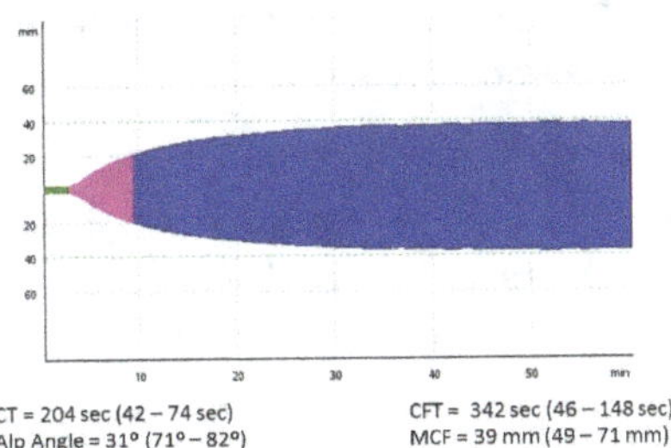

CT = 204 sec (42 – 74 sec)   CFT = 342 sec (46 – 148 sec)
Alp Angle = 31° (71° – 82°)   MCF = 39 mm (49 – 71 mm)

FIBTEM

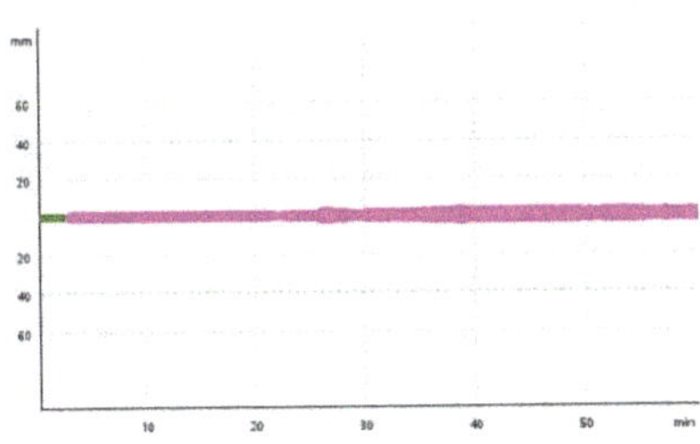

MCF = 5 mm

Q2.10

This test was performed on a patient who had persistent intra-abdominal haemorrhage from liver trauma.

1. Identify the test performed.

2. What information does it provide for patients?

3. What are the advantages of performing this test versus the conventional laboratory coagulation profile?

A2.9

1. Severe hyperkalaemia with raised urea and creatinine.
   Metabolic acidosis.

2. Myoglobinuria. It is characterized by brown to dark-red urine.

3. This is likely due to acute kidney injury secondary to rhabdomyolysis from multi-trauma.

4. **Hyperkalaemia**
   IV Calcium Gluconate to counter the effect of hyperkalaemia on the heart.
   IV Soluble Insulin with Dextrose to shift the potassium into the cells.
   IV Sodium Bicarbonate to correct the acidosis temporarily.
   Polystyrene Sulphonate via enteral route to bind potassium ions in the gut.

   Rhabdomyolysis – mainly supportive.
   Keep patient well hydrated with IV fluids.
   Consider early haemodialysis.

A2.10

1. Rotational Thromboelastometry (ROTEM) which is a type of Viscoelastic Haemostatic Assay.

2. The ROTEM device evaluates the coagulation pathway.

3. It can be performed as a point of care test.
   The result is available quickly, within a short time frame.
   It can detect hyperfibrinolysis, which conventional laboratory tests cannot.

Q2.11

This is a patient receiving nutrition in the ICU.

1. What type of nutrition is this?

2. What are the indications for this?

3. What are the nutritional components?

4. How is it administered?

5. Why is it in a protective dark opaque bag?

6. What are complications associated with its use?

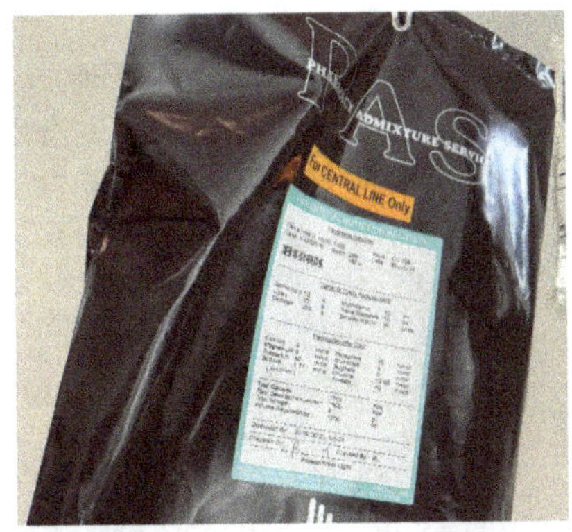

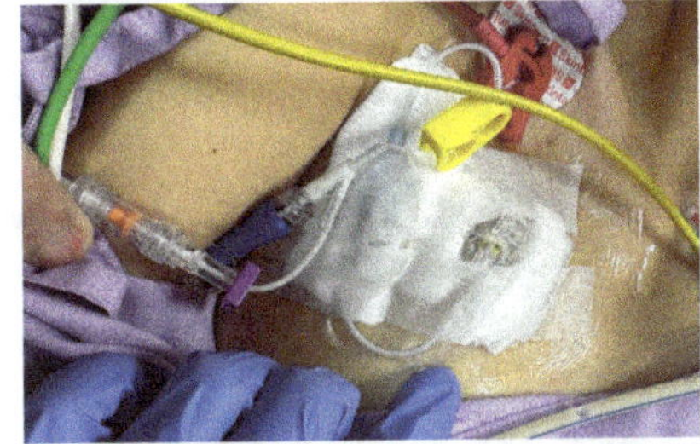

Q2.12

This patient had emergency surgery after a fall from height.

1. What are the principles of trauma surgery?

2. What is damage control surgery?

3. What surgical procedures were performed for this patient as seen in the picture?

4. Why was the abdominal wall not closed?

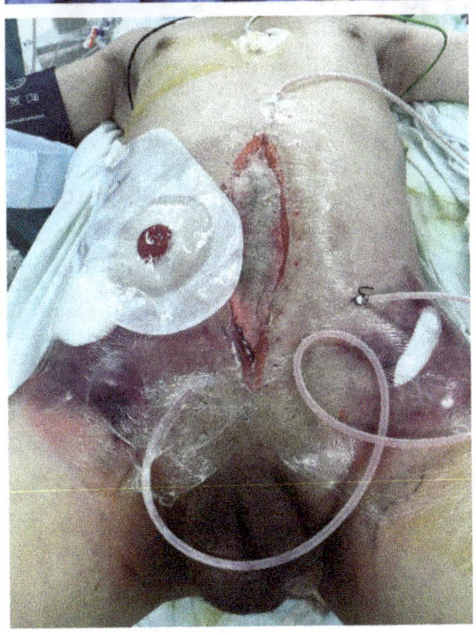

A2.11

1. Total parenteral nutrition (TPN).

2. It is used in patients with impaired gastrointestinal function or contraindications to enteral nutrition.

3. The main three macronutrients are lipid emulsions, proteins, and carbohydrates. The proportion is calculated based on the caloric needs of the patient. Other components include electrolytes, trace elements and vitamins.

4. It is administered through large veins: central venous catheter (CVC), peripheral inserted central catheter (PICC) or an implanted port. Due to its high osmolarity, TPN irritates the smaller peripheral veins.

5. TPN solutions need to be protected from light to prevent photo-degradation and oxidation.

6. Venous access: pneumothorax, air embolism, bleeding and venous thrombosis.
    Catheter site infections.
    Metabolic abnormalities: refeeding syndrome, hyperglycaemia and electrolyte disturbances.

A2.12

1. Control bleeding.
    Identification of injuries
    Control of contamination.

2. It is an abbreviated laparotomy to control intra-abdominal haemorrhage and enteric spill. Further resuscitation is done in the intensive care unit. Staged re-look laparotomies can be scheduled. When the patient has stabilized, definitive repair of all injuries can then be performed.

3. A diverting ileostomy has been performed and the abdominal wall has not been sutured closed. Drains were left in the abdominal cavity.

4. Closure of the abdominal wall might lead to abdominal compartment syndrome. The patient might be scheduled for a re-look laparotomy.

Q2.13

This is a 30-year-old male who fell from height and landed on the left side of his abdomen.

1. What is seen in the CT scan?

2. What is the initial management?

3. What surgery was performed?

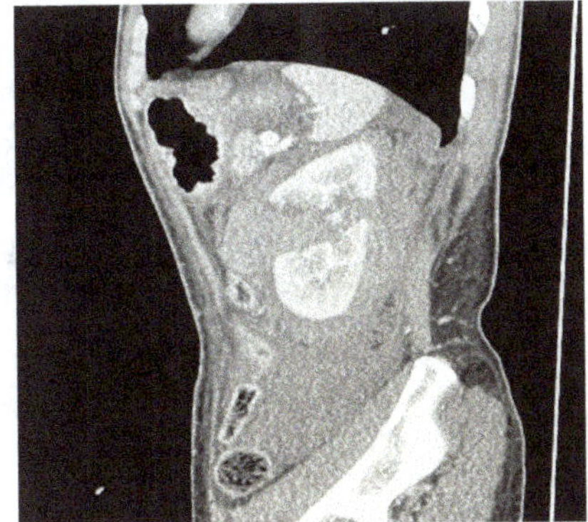

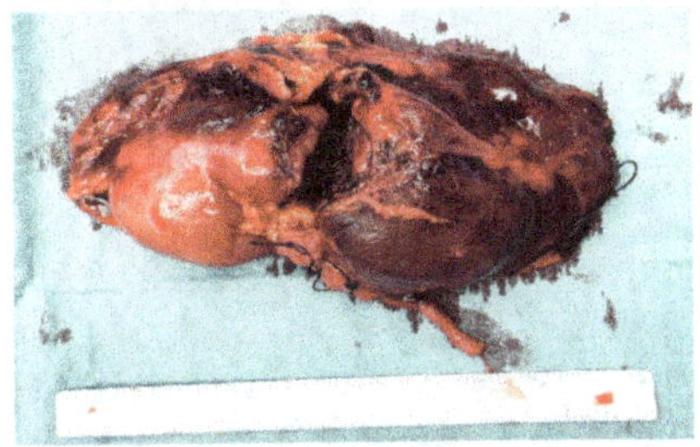

Q2.14

An alcohol intoxicated 65-year-old male is brought into the emergency unit after having a fight in the bar. He was stomped on his neck and now complains of difficulty breathing.

1. What are the principles of management of this patient?

2. What abnormal findings are seen in the CT scan?

3. What other injuries need to be excluded?

4. What is the management?

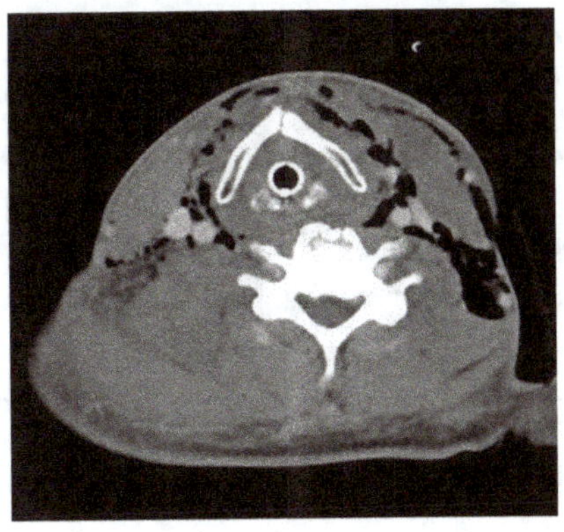

A2.13

1. There is a complete laceration of the kidney with a surrounding haematoma.

2. The patient needs to be haemodynamically stabilized. Non-operative management can be attempted initially. It entails supportive care in the ICU, serial clinical examinations and regular haemoglobin checks. Transfusion of blood products may be needed. Angioembolization may be an option.

3. An emergency nephrectomy. The specimen shows a viable half and the other necrotic half of the kidney. Surgery is necessary if the patient is haemodynamically unstable or has failed trial of non-operative management.

A2.14

1. Check airway, breathing and circulation (ABC).

2. There is subcutaneous and para-laryngeal emphysema with a fractured thyroid cartilage. The soft tissue on the right side is more swollen than the left.

3. Vascular, tracheal and oesophageal injuries.

4. The airway must be secured. This is done initially with endotracheal intubation or tracheostomy. Once ABC is secured, the laryngeal fracture must be repaired.

Q2.15

This is an 82-year-old female with previous spine surgery, who slipped and fell on her left hip.

1. What is the diagnosis as seen on the x-ray?

2. What is likely to be detected on clinical inspection of her lower limbs?

3. What is the management of the patient?

4. What device has been placed on her calves?

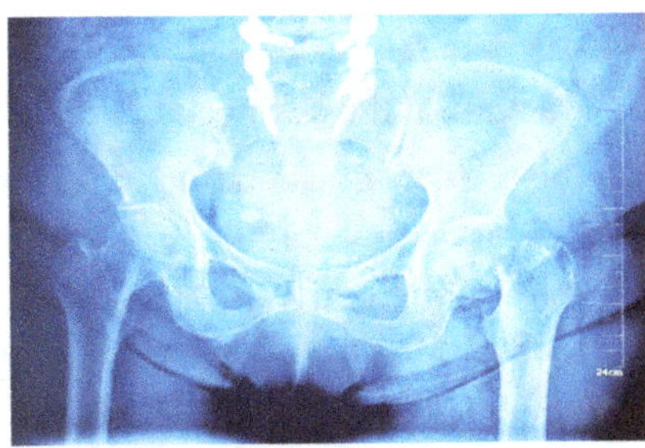

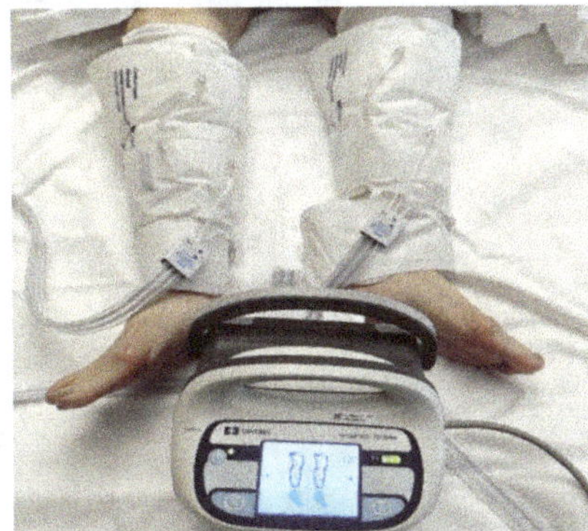

Q2.16

This is a 23-year-old male who suffered blunt abdominal trauma.

1. What bedside procedure is being done?

2. What anatomical regions are assessed?

3. What does it detect?

4. What abnormality is seen in Morrison's pouch?

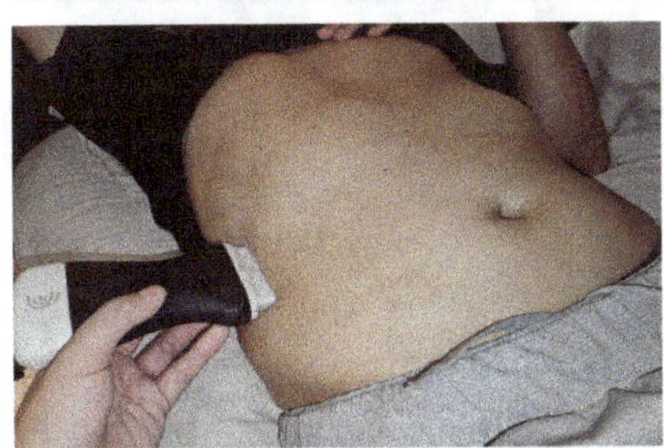

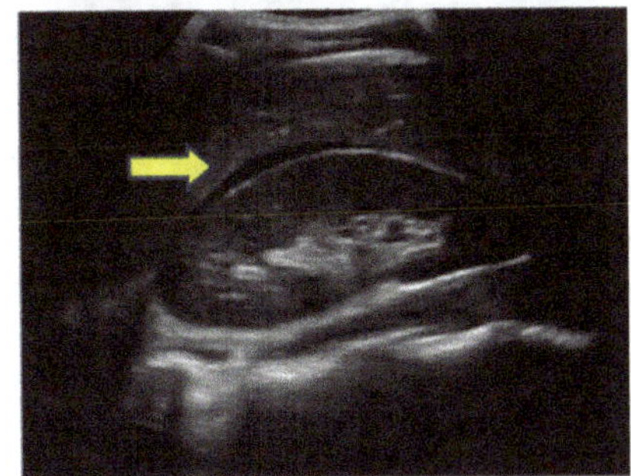

A2.15

1. Fracture of the left neck of femur (NOF).

2. The classic presentation of patients with displaced NOF fractures is a shortened and externally rotated lower limb.

3. The head for femur is likely to be de-vascularised due to the severely displaced fracture. Conservative management is likely to fail. Hemiarthroplasty is the management of choice.

4. Intermittent pneumatic compressions to prevent deep vein thrombosis.

A2.16

1. Focused assessment with sonography in trauma (FAST).

2. Hepatorenal recess (Morrison's pouch), perisplenic area, subxiphoid pericardial window and suprapubic window (Douglas pouch).

3. It is an ultrasound protocol used to assess for hemoperitoneum and hemopericardium.

4. There is a small amount of free fluid between the liver and kidney.

Q2.17

This is a 30-year-old female who was involved in a road traffic accident.

1. What is the initial management of this patient?

2. When is a CT scan indicated?

3. What is seen in the CT scan?

4. If the patient is stable and does not need emergent surgery, what other investigation is needed?

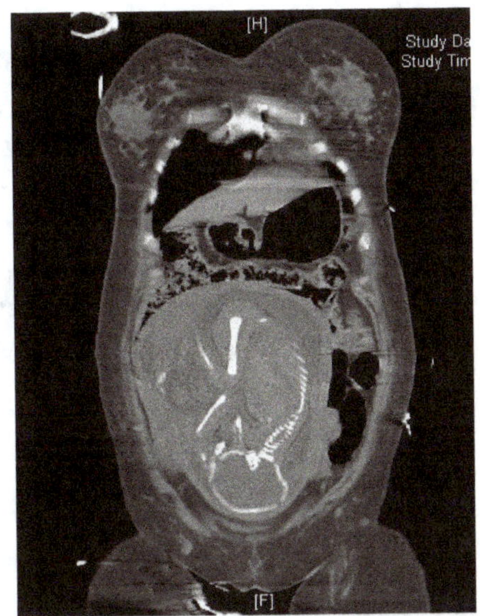

Q2.18

This 19-year-old girl was involved in a road traffic accident and sustained a blunt left flank injury.

1. Comment on her kidneys as seen on the CT scan.

2. What are the treatment options?

3. What are the known complications if left alone?

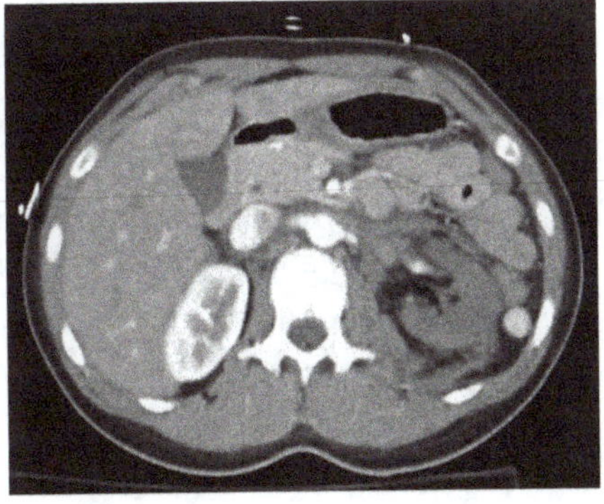

A2.17

1. Check airway, breathing and circulation.

2. It is used for rapid evaluation and accurate diagnosis of known and unknown injuries, if the patient is haemodynamically stable. Urgent laparotomy is necessary without the CT scan if the patient is unstable.

3. There is a foetus in the womb.

4. Obstetric ultrasonogram to confirm the wellbeing of the child. Foetal or late decelerations may be due to maternal hypovolemia, maternal hypoxia, abruptio placentae, or uterine rupture.

A2.18

1. There is a Grade V renal injury with no contrast uptake in the left kidney. The right kidney is well vascularised.

2. In early presentations with delays of under an hour, revascularisation by endovascular stents can be attempted.
    In late presentations, the kidney is necrotic. A nephrectomy is needed.

3. In cases where the kidney has been preserved, hypertension is a common complication because of relative hyperaldosteronism.

Q2.19

This is a 50-year-old male who had previous pelvic surgery one week ago. The patient now presents with shortness of breath.

1. What abnormality is seen in the CT scan?

2. What other investigations would be useful to confirm the diagnosis?

3. What is the management?

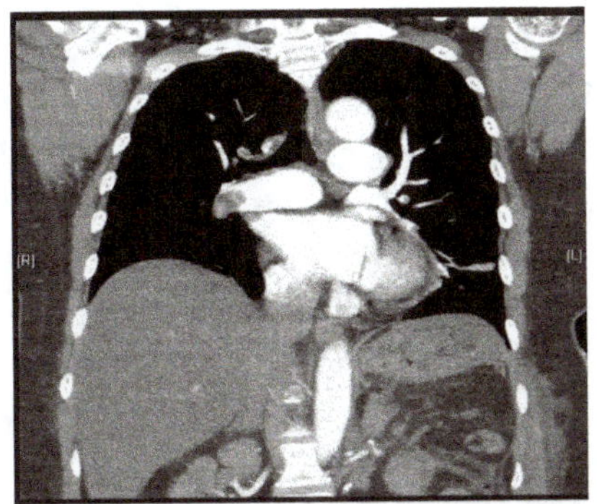

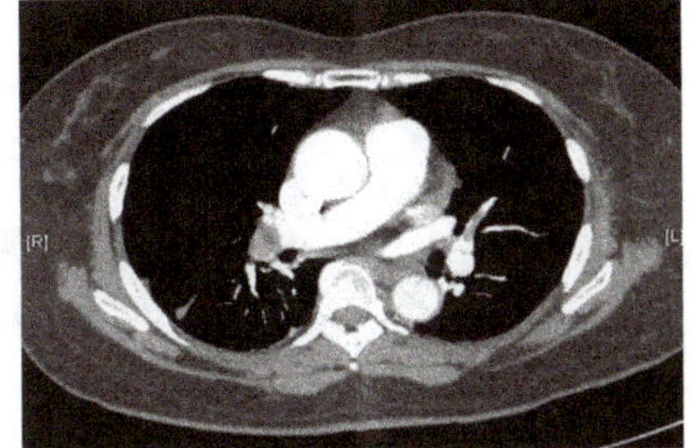

Q2.20

This is a 40-year-old male who had emergency surgery performed for a ruptured aortic aneurysm.

1. What is seen displayed on the floor of the operating theatre?

2. What is the definition of a massive blood transfusion?

3. What are complications of massive blood transfusion?

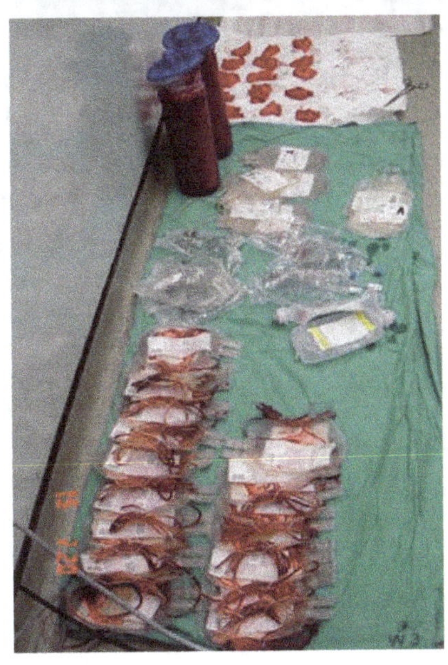

A2.19

1. Coronal and axial images show a filling defect in the right pulmonary artery, consistent with a pulmonary embolism.

2. Arterial blood gas analysis, Brain natriuretic peptide (BNP), Troponin and D-dimer.

3. Stable patients: anticoagulation.
   Unstable patient: thrombolysis or surgical embolectomy.

A2.20

1. The number of blood products and fluids used during the surgery to keep the patient haemodynamically stable.

2. A massive transfusion involves the administration of 10 units or more of whole blood or packed red blood cells (PRBCs) within 24 hours.

3. Coagulopathy: arises from clotting factor consumption, reduced clotting factor activity due to dilution, prolonged shock, hypoxia-induced acidosis, and hypothermia.
   Metabolic abnormalities: metabolic alkalosis and hypocalcemia, which is due to sodium citrate and citric acid added to blood products during storage to prevent coagulation.
   Hypothermia: When stored at 4°C, the rapid infusion of cold blood can induce a drop in core body temperature.
   Transfusion-Related Acute Lung Injury (TRALI).
   Transfusion-Associated Circulatory Overload (TACO).

3 Upper GI

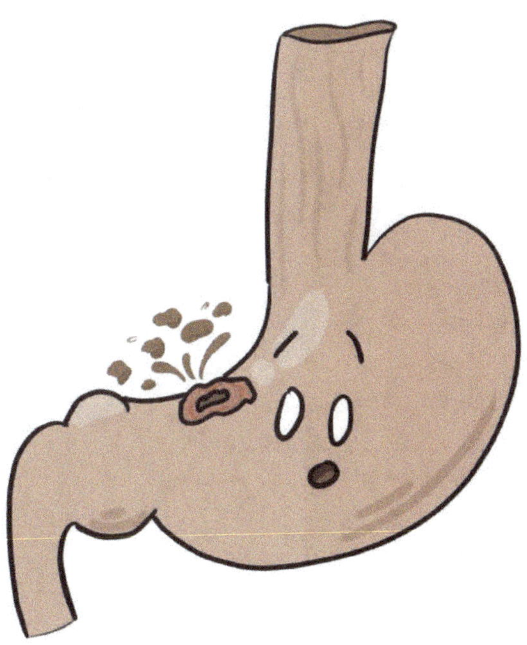

Q3.1

This is a 40-year-old male with oesophageal motility issues.

1. What radiological study was performed in picture A and what abnormality does it demonstrate?

2. What is the investigative study seen in picture B?

3. What is the diagnosis?

4. What is the likely clinical presentation of this patient?

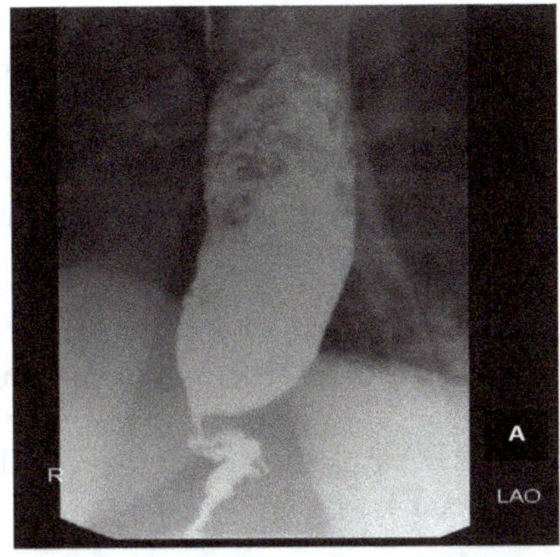

Q3.2

This 50-year-old male presents with dysphagia.

1. What abnormality is seen in the oesophagus at endoscopy?

2. What is seen in the CT scan?

3. What is the diagnosis?

4. What is the pathogenesis?

5. What is the management?

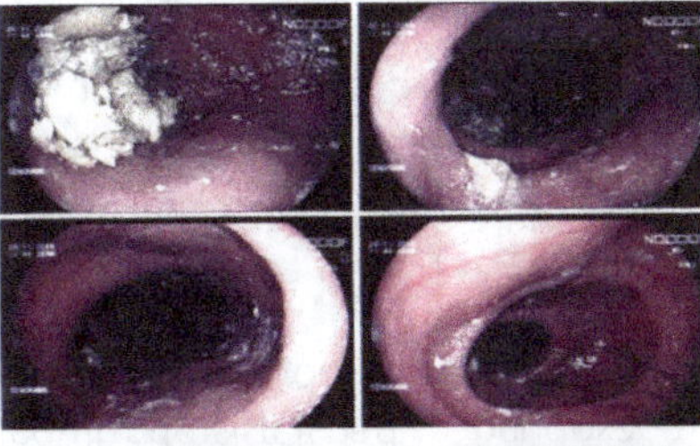

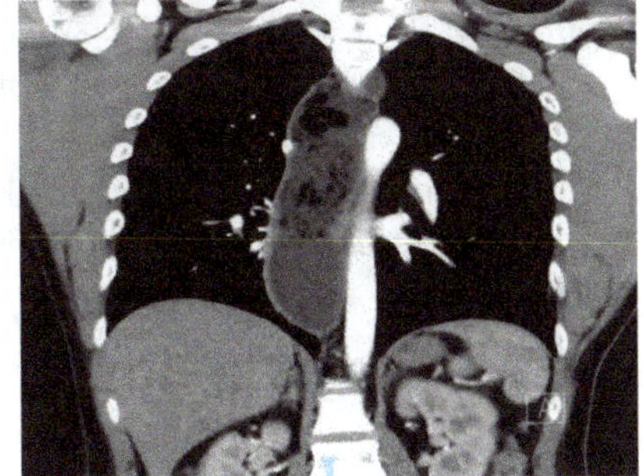

A3.1

1. The barium contrast study shows dilatation of the esophagus with smooth tapering of the distal end ("bird's beak" appearance). There will be lack of peristalsis of the oesophagus.

2. Oesophageal manometry. It measures the motility and function of the oesophagus and the sphincter.

3. Achalasia.

4. Dysphagia and regurgitation are the common presenting symptoms. As the disease progresses, patients may have symptoms of regurgitation with possible aspiration, nocturnal cough, heartburn, and weight loss from eating difficulties.

A3.2

1. The oesophagus is dilated with food debris in it. There should be no food in a fasted patient's stomach prior to a gastroscopy.

2. The entire oseophagus is dilated with a smooth narrowing distally.

3. Achalasia.

4. It is a primary esophageal motility disorder characterized by the absence of oesophageal peristalsis and impaired relaxation of the lower oesophageal sphincter (LES) in response to swallowing. The LES is hypertensive in 50% of patients. These abnormalities cause a functional obstruction at the gastroesophageal junction (GEJ).

5. Non-surgical options: pharmacotherapy (calcium channel blockers and nitrates), endoscopic intrasphincteric botulinum toxin injection, or pneumatic dilatation.
Surgical options: laparoscopic Heller myotomy and peroral endoscopic myotomy.

Q3.3

This is a 50-year-old male with liver cirrhosis.

1. What abnormality is seen in the oesophagus at endoscopy in picture A?

2. What is the pathogenesis?

3. What is the clinical presentation of this pathology?

4. What was performed as seen in picture B?

5. What other problems could this patient develop?

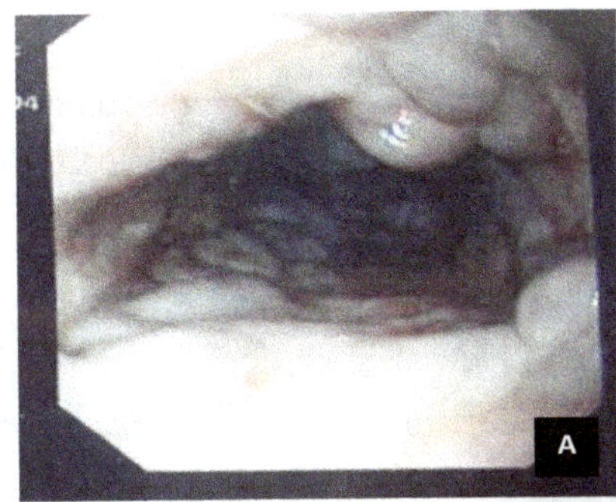

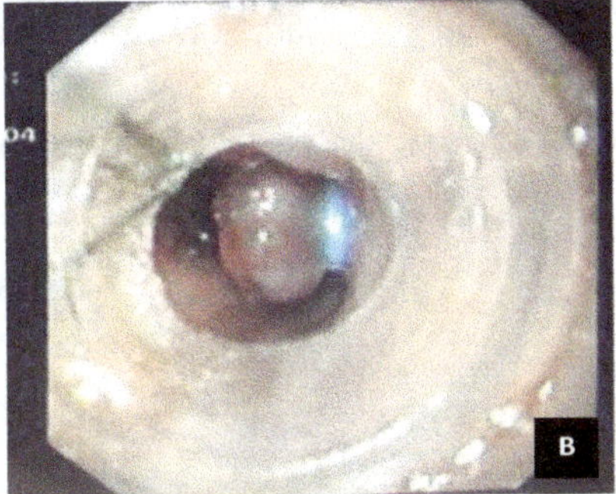

Q3.4

These are pictures of the gastro-oesophageal junction (taken in narrow band imaging) of two different patients.

1. What does picture A show?

2. What does picture B Show?

3. What symptoms will patient B have?

4. What will happen if patient B is left untreated?

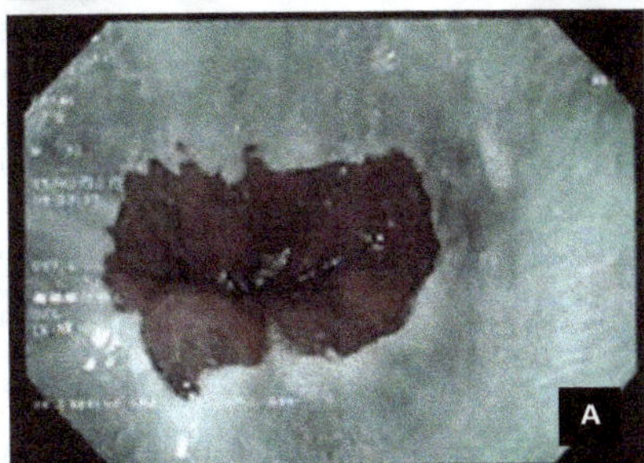

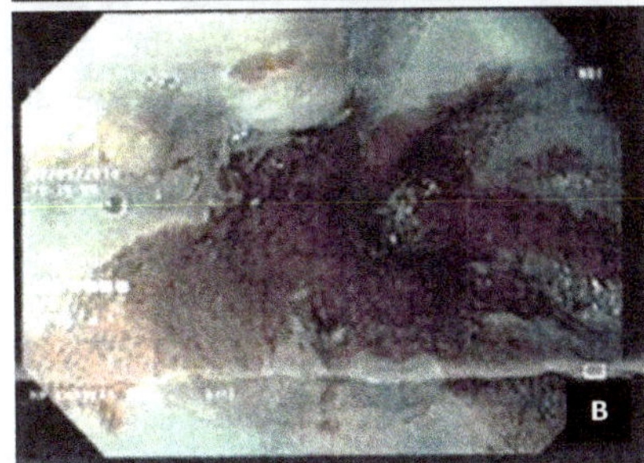

A3.3

1. Varices. They are dilated submucosal distal oesophageal veins connecting the portal and systemic circulations.

2. Varices are due to portal hypertension. Portocaval anastomosis develop to decompress the portal circulation. This occurs when the difference in pressures between the portal venous and inferior vena cava/hepatic vein is too high. Liver cirrhosis is the most common cause.

3. Varices are often asymptomatic or may present with severe gastrointestinal bleeding.

4. Banding of the varices was performed. The blue band seen is constricting the varix.

5. Splenomegaly, ascites, portosystemic encephalopathy and caput-medusae.

A3.4

1. Patient A has a normal gastro-oesophageal junction. The oesophageal mucosa is white whilst the stomach mucosa is pink. The transition between the 2 mucosae is called the Z-line.

2. There are multiple irregularities in the mucosal transition zone between the oesophagus and stomach.

3. Heartburn and acid regurgitation. Symptoms are usually worsened after having large meals and lying down.

4. Patients with symptomatic and persistent reflux can develop Barrett's oesophagus, which is a precursor lesion for adenocarcinoma of the oesophagus.

Q3.5

This is a 60-year-old man who had a gastroscopy.

1. What is seen at endoscopy?
2. What is his likely clinical presentation?
3. What is the diagnosis?
4. What is seen in the PET scan?

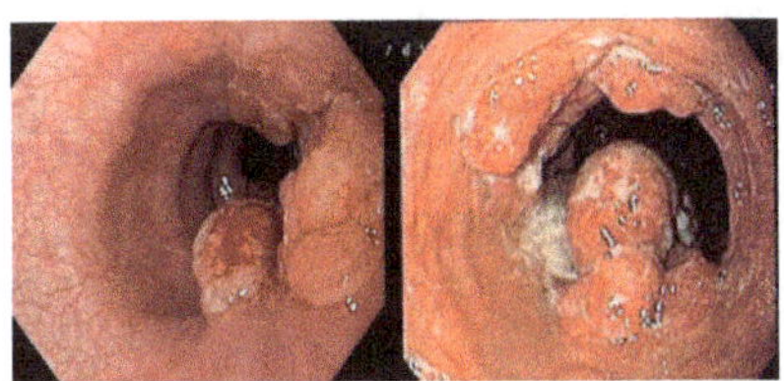

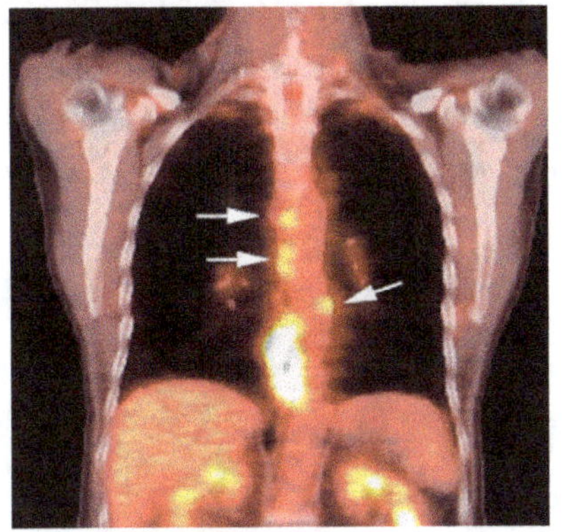

Q3.6

This 60-year-old man had surgery for oesophageal cancer.

1. What surgery was performed?
2. How do we prepare patients for this surgery?
3. What are complications of this surgery?
4. What does the post-surgical CT scan demonstrate?

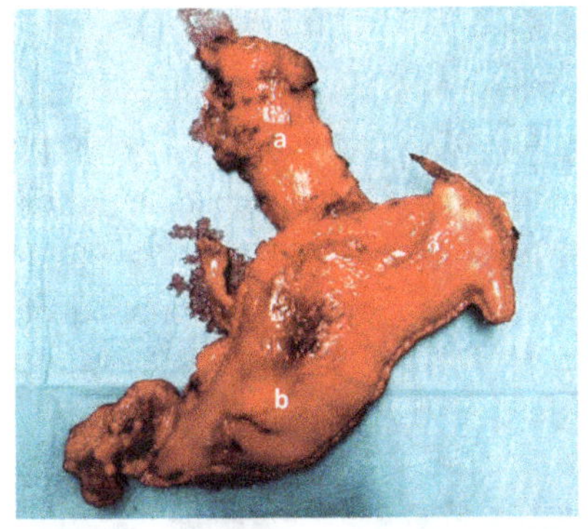

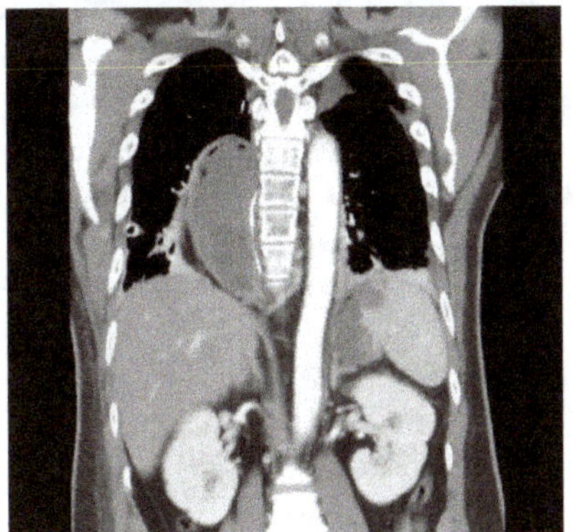

A3.5

1. There is an ulcerative tumour in his oesophagus.

2. Progressive dysphagia from solid to liquid food. This can lead to weight loss. Less commonly, they may present with hematemesis, melaena or occult gastrointestinal bleeding.

3. Oesophageal cancer. Squamous cell or adenocarcinoma.

4. The cancer is in the lower third of the oesophagus. There are metastastic mediastinal lymph nodes.

A3.6

1. Ivor Lewis oesophagectomy. The surgical specimen comprises of the lower half of the oesophagus (a) and proximal portion of the stomach (b).

2. Patients with oesophageal pathology are often undernourished because of progressive dysphagia. Pre-operative nutrition needs to be boosted.

3. Complications from oesophagectomy occur in 40% of patients.
   - Respiratory — Atelectasis, pleural effusion, and pneumonia.
   - Cardiac — Cardiac arrhythmias and myocardial infarction.
   - Sepsis — Wound infection, anastomotic and chyle leak and pneumonia.

4. The stomach is "pulled up" into the thorax. It is essential to confirm the integrity of the anastomosis before oral feeding of the patient is commenced.

Q3.7

This is a 75-year-old man.

1. What is seen in the PET CT scan?
2. What procedure is being performed for him?
3. What are the indications for this modality of treatment?
4. What are potential side effects of this treatment?

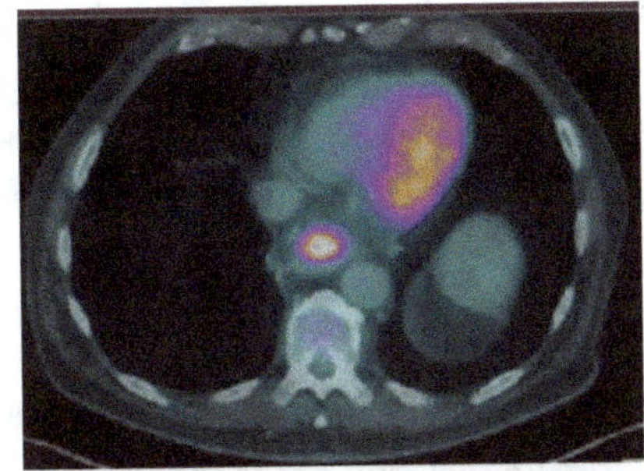

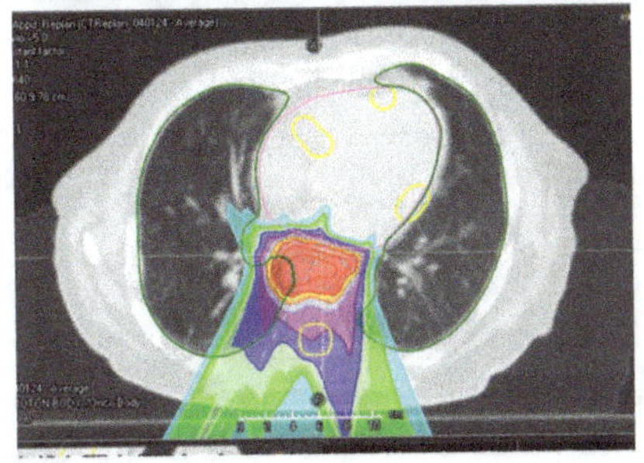

Q3.8

This is a 45-year-old man.

1. What pathology is detected on the contrast study of the oesophagus?
2. What is seen on gastroscopy?
3. What is the likely diagnosis?
4. What is the clinical presentation?
5. What is the management?

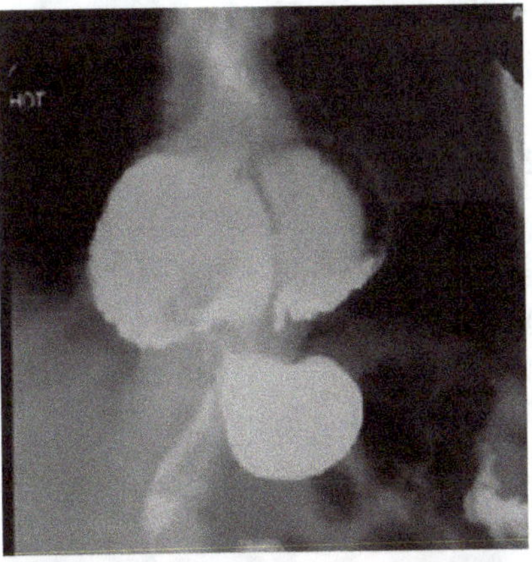

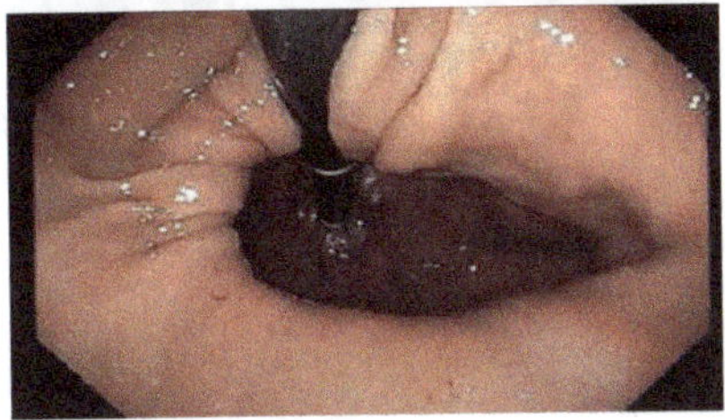

A3.7

1. The lower thoracic oesophagus is thickened and uptake-avid.
2. Proton beam radiotherapy. It exploits the finite range of protons to spare heart and lungs from unnecessary radiation exposure, hence reducing toxicity.
3. Patients with squamous cell carcinoma of the oesophagus who are unfit for surgery or have inoperable tumours.
    Preoperative(neoadjuvant) treatment to "downsize" the tumour.
4. Acute radiation oesophagitis with dysphagia.
    Radiation dermatitis.
    Radiation pneumonitis.

A3.8

1. There is a large bulbous lesion filled with contrast in the lower mediastinum. The contrast flows into the intra-abdominal stomach.
2. The aperture of the gastro-oesophageal junction is enlarged instead of the usual tight lower oesophageal sphincter.
3. Para-oesophageal hiatus hernia.
4. They may experience heartburn and regurgitation.
5. Initial treatment is with proton pump inhibitors. This large hernia will benefit from surgical fundoplication.

Q3.9

This is a 74-year-old man who presented with epigastric discomfort.

1. What is seen at gastroscopy?
2. What are the risk factors for developing this pathology?
3. What is the management?
4. What complications can occur if the pathology persists?

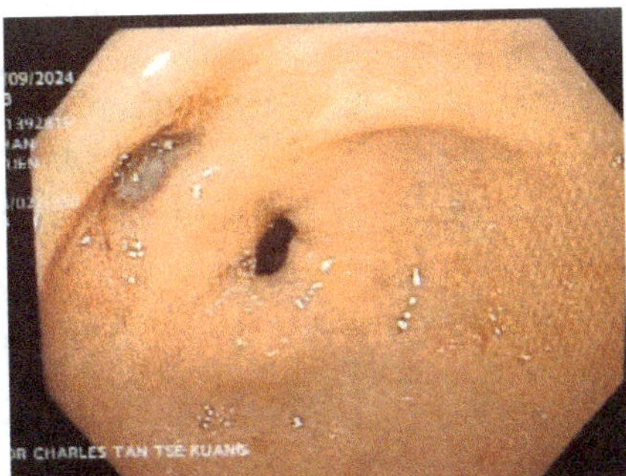

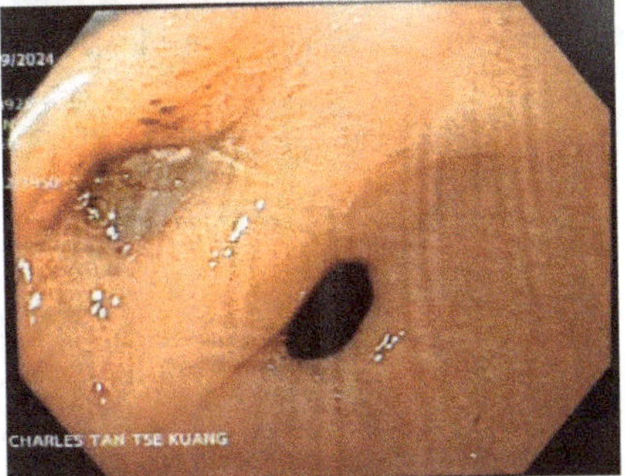

Q3.10

An emergency gastroscopy was performed for this 50-year-old man who had a gastric mucosa biopsy 2 days ago.

1. What is seen in picture A?
2. What is the likely clinical presentation?
3. What was performed in picture B?
4. What are other endoscopic modalities for haemostasis?

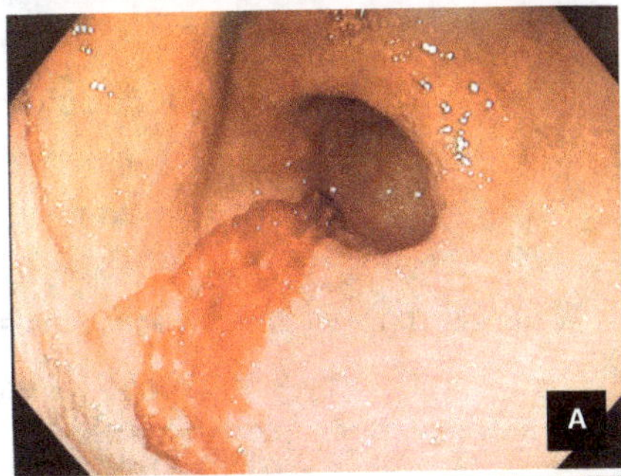

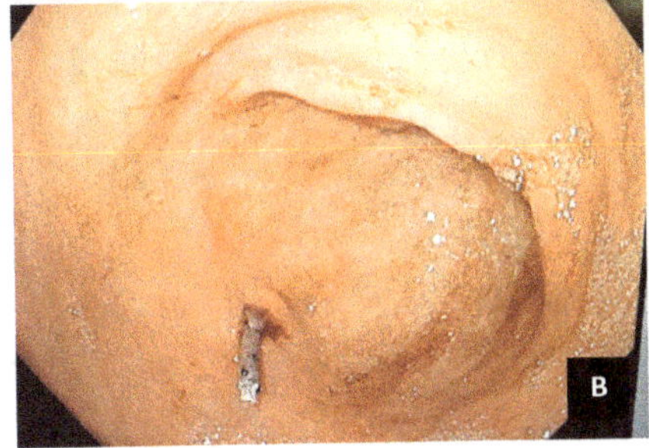

A3.9

1. There is an ulcer in the antrum at the 10 o'clock position with respect to the pylorus. There is slough in the base of the ulcer with no active bleeding.

2. Helicobacter pylori infection, non-steroidal anti-inflammatory drugs (NSAID) and smoking.

3. Biopsy at endoscopy to exclude a gastric carcinoma.
   Triple therapy medication (2 antibiotics and a proton pump inhibitor).
   Gastroscopy 6 weeks later to ensure healing of the ulcer.

4. Bleeding and perforation of the gastric ulcer. Gastric cancer needs to be excluded in a persistent ulcer.

A3.10

1. There is active bleeding in the stomach.

2. He presented with melaena. Because it was a slow bleed, he was haemodynamically stable and did not present with haematemesis or in hypovolaemic shock.

3. A metal clip was applied at the bleeding point.

4. Injection therapy with diluted adrenaline or with absolute alcohol.
   Thermal endoscopic therapy with a heater or bipolar probe.

Q3.11

This is a 40-year-old man with a history of peptic ulcer disease who had emergency laparotomy.

1. What is seen in this large basin?
2. What would he have presented with?
3. What is seen in the surgical picture (duodenotomy)?

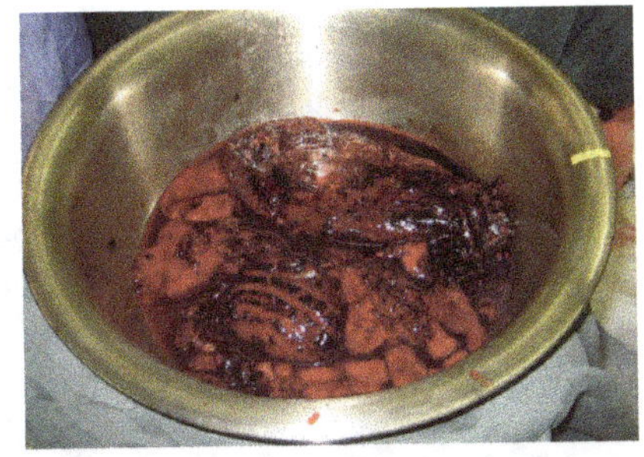

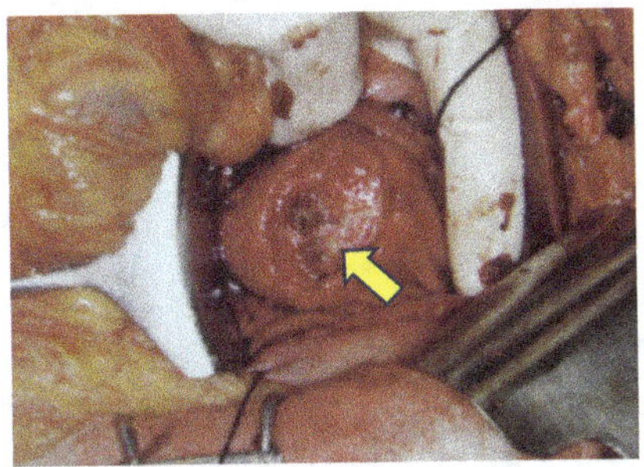

Q3.12

This is a 60-year-old man.

1. What is seen in the x-ray?
2. What is seen in the CT scan?
3. What is the diagnosis?
4. What will be detected on physical examination?
5. What is the most likely cause for this problem?

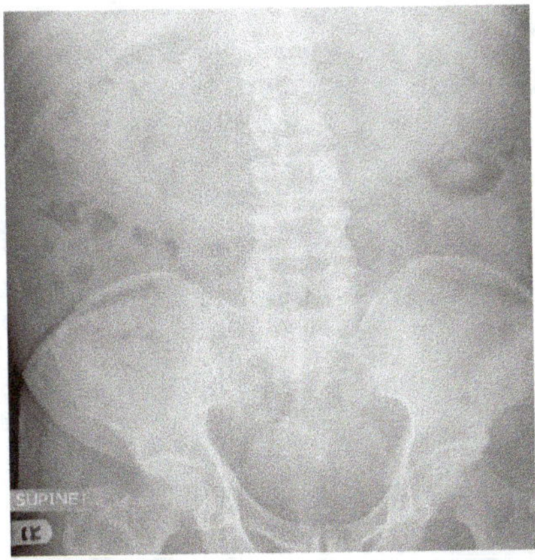

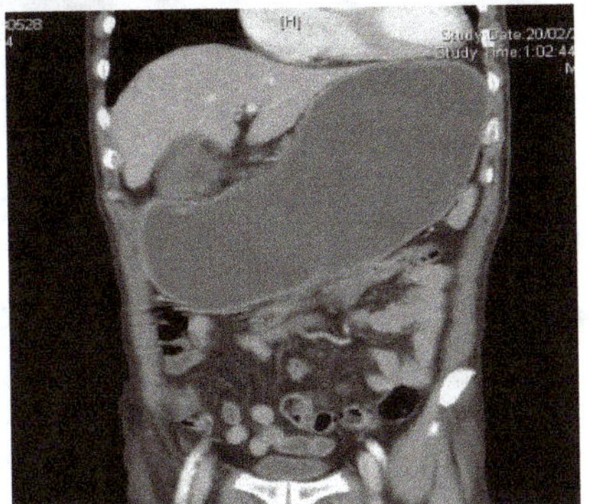

A3.11

1. There is a large amount of fresh blood and clots.

2. Haematemesis and melaena with circulatory haemodynamic shock.

3. The duodenum is opened (duodenotomy) and the arrow shows a posterior duodenal ulcer which has eroded posteriorly into the gastroduodenal artery causing severe haemorrhage into the gastrointestinal tract.

A3.12

1. There is paucity of bowel shadows in the upper abdomen. The radiolucent transverse colon has been "pushed" down.

2. There is a grossly dilated stomach which is filled with fluid.

3. Gastric outlet obstruction (GOO).

4. A large non-tender mass in the upper abdomen. If there is air and fluid in the dilated stomach, we may elicit a succussion splash.

5. Peptic ulcer disease or malignancy near the pylorus causing a stenosis.

Q3.13

This 40-year-old female presented with acute abdominal pain.

1. What is seen in the CT scan?
2. What would be detected on physical examination?
3. What is seen in the surgical picture?
4. What is the management?

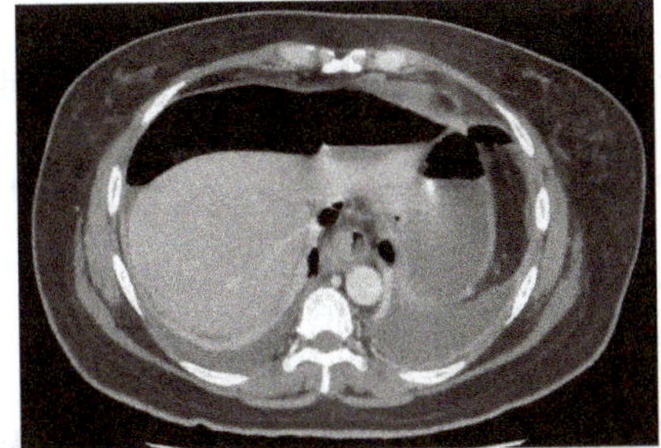

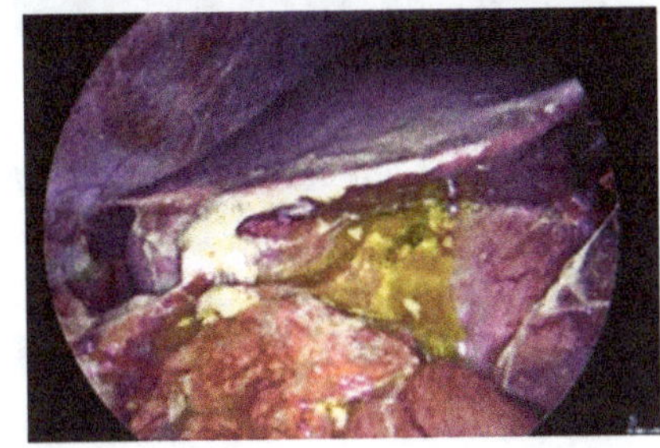

Q3.14

This is a 60-year-old chronic smoker, who had emergency surgery performed on him.

1. What is seen in picture A as indicated by the arrow?
2. What is the most likely cause for this?
3. What is seen in picture B?
4. What is seen in picture C?

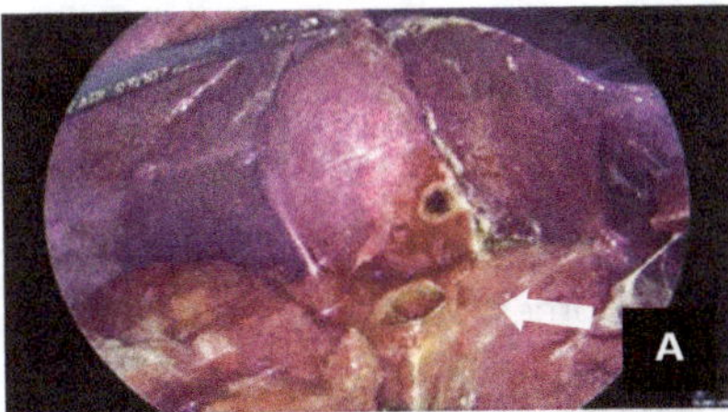

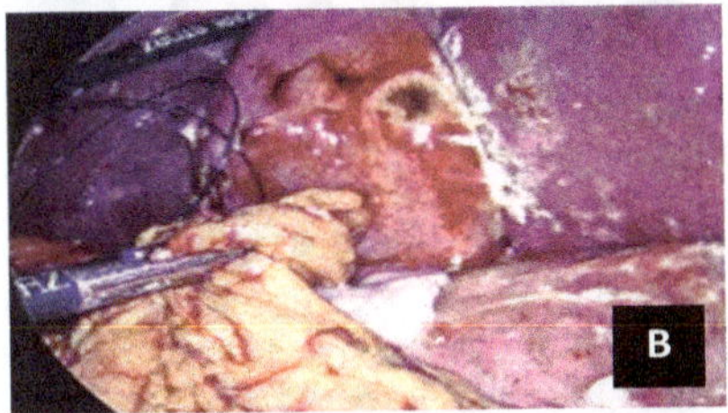

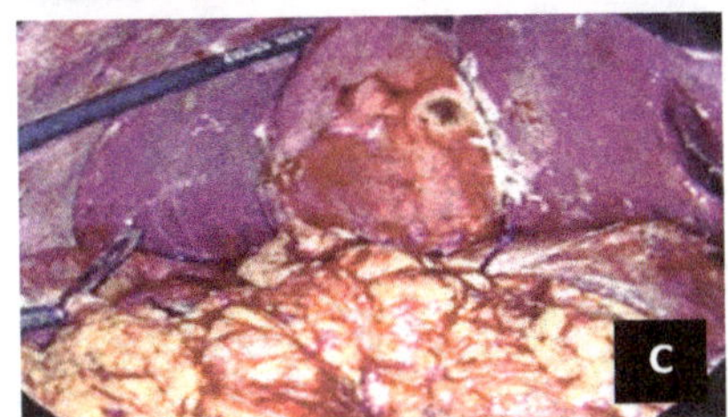

A3.13

1. The CT scan shows intraperitoneal "free gas". The gas is not within the visceral organs.

2. She would be septic with a painful, tender and distended abdomen due to generalized peritonitis.

3. Yellow bile-stained bowel contents have spilled out just under the right lobe of the liver around the duodenum.

4. Emergency surgery to identify the perforation and to seal it so as to prevent further spillage of bowel contents.
   The soilage in the peritoneal cavity has to be cleared by suction and copious irrigation lavage.
   Intravenous antibiotics have to be administered to treat the systemic sepsis.

A3.14

1. There is a perforated viscus. Taking reference from the liver and gallbladder superiorly, the perforation is in the duodenum.

2. Peptic ulcer disease. Smoking is his risk factor.

3. The omentum has been mobilized.

4. The perforation has been sealed with an omentum patch stitched to it.

Q3.15

This is a 50-year-old Japanese man.

1. What is seen at gastroscopy?

2. What can be used to assess the depth of invasion of the lesion?

3. What procedure was performed for the lesion?

4. What is the diagnosis?

5. What are some possible complications from the procedure?

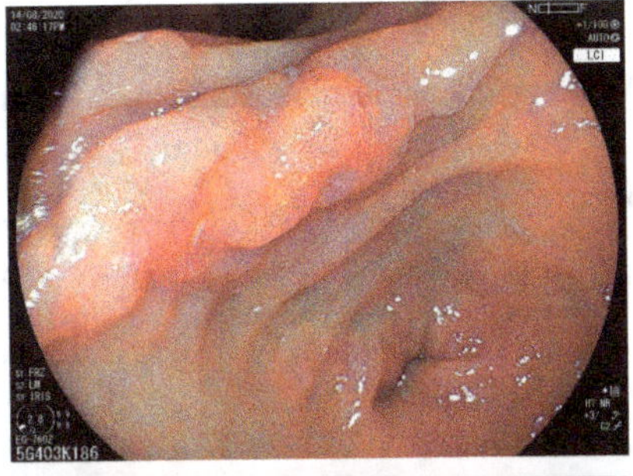

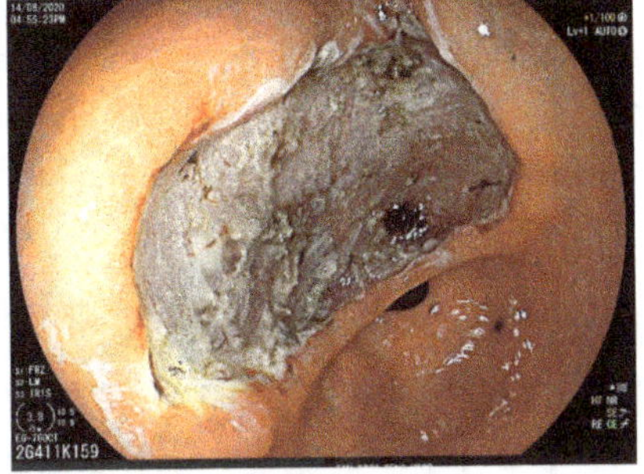

Q3.16

This is a 60-year-old man.

1. What surgery was performed?

2. What is the pathology seen?

3. What is the indication for this surgery?

4. What is the role of lymph node dissection in this surgery?

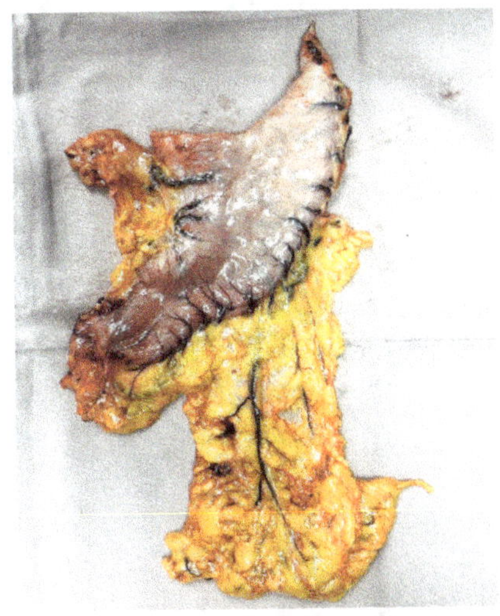

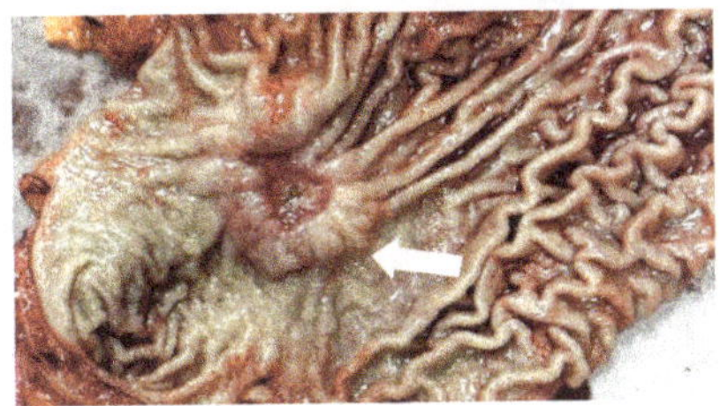

A3.15

1. There is a multilobulated lesion arising from the mucosa/submucosa at the lesser curve.

2. Endo-ultrasonography (EUS).

3. Endoscopic mucosal resection (EMR) or endoscopic submucosal dissection (ESD).

4. Early gastric cancer (EGC). It is an invasive carcinoma involving only the stomach mucosa or submucosa, independently of lymph node status. EGC represents 50% of cases in Japan and in South Korea, and 20% of all newly diagnosed gastric cancers in Western countries.

5. Bleeding and perforation.

A3.16

1. Subtotal gastrectomy with lymph node dissection and omentectomy.

2. Malignant gastric ulcer.

3. Subtotal gastrectomy is the treatment for gastric cancer located in the distal third of the stomach.

4. Lymph node (LN) dissection was initially classified as D1 to D4, depending on the extent and removal of each LN station according to the primary tumor location. The Japanese Gastric Cancer Association recommends a D2 LN (more than 25 nodes) dissection in most gastric cancers.

Q3.17

This surgical specimen was removed from a 65-year-old male who presented with vomiting, early satiety, weight loss and anaemia.

1. What is the pathological condition?

2. What are the associated risk factors?

3. How does the tumour spread?

4. What are some sequelae specific to this surgical procedure?

5. What is seen in the radiology study and why is it performed after surgery?

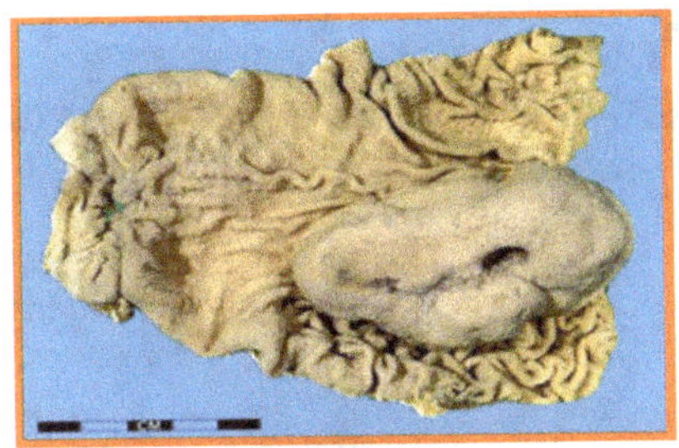

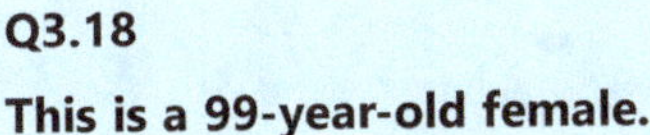

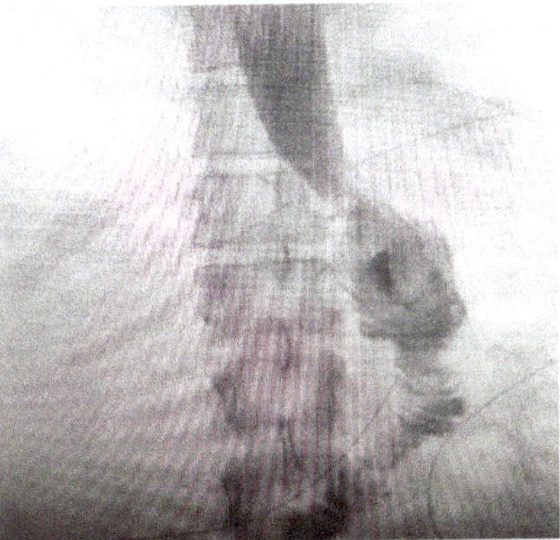

Q3.18

This is a 99-year-old female.

1. What surgery was performed for her?

2. What are indications for this procedure?

3. What are the surgical approaches for the tube placement?

4. What are complications associated with this?

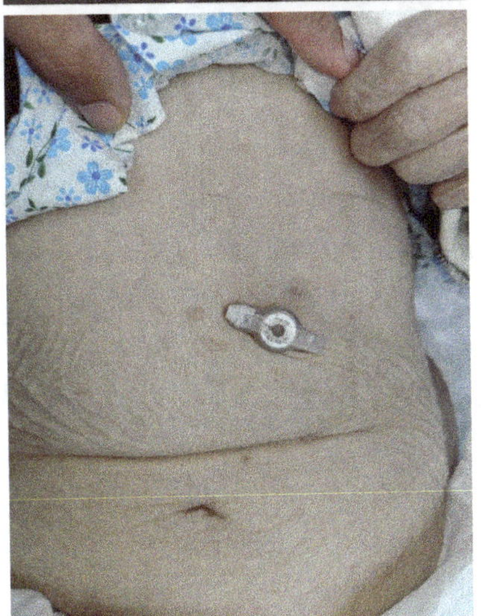

A3.17

1. Gastric Carcinoma.

2. Smoking, alcohol, preserved food, atrophic gastritis and Helicobacter pylori infection.

3. Direct invasion: to adjacent organs.
   Nodal spread: Tumour node metastasis (TNM) system is the standard staging system. Remote lymphatic spread to left supraclavicular nodes (Virchow).
   Transperitoneal: to the surface of the ovaries (Krukenburg tumours) or "drop metastases" in the pouch of Douglas.

4. Post-gastrectomy syndromes include small capacity, dumping syndrome, bile gastritis, afferent loop syndrome, efferent loop syndrome, anemia, and metabolic bone disease.

5. The contrast study shows the oesophageal-jejunal anastomosis. It is performed to confirm the integrity of the anastomosis by no (absence of contrast leakage).

A3.18

1. There is a gastrostomy tube inserted into the stomach.

2. Patients who are unable to tolerate oral feeding.
   Neurological: stroke, cerebral tumors and prolonged coma.
   Obstruction: Neck and oesophageal malignancy, previous radiotherapy.

3. Open surgery or endoscopic percutaneous approach.

4. Early: infection, haemorrhage, bowel injury.
   Late: tube blockage or migration.

Q3.19

This 40-year-old patient has a gastrointestinal stromal tumour (GIST) in the stomach.

1. What is seen at endoscopy?

2. What is the difference in the endoscopic findings between an adenocarcinoma and a GIST?

3. What are differential diagnoses?

4. What further investigation can be performed at gastroscopy?

5. What was performed for the lesion?

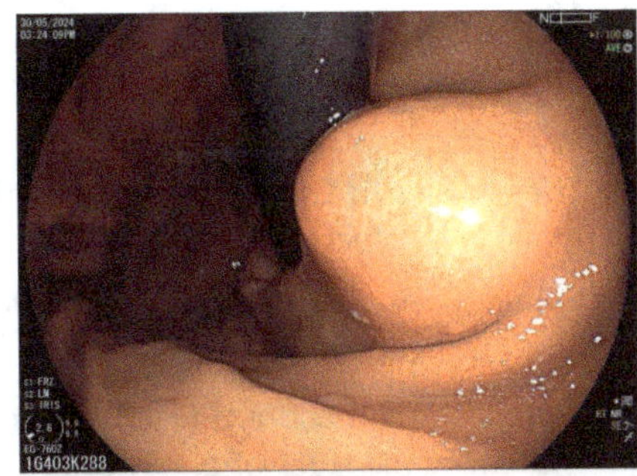

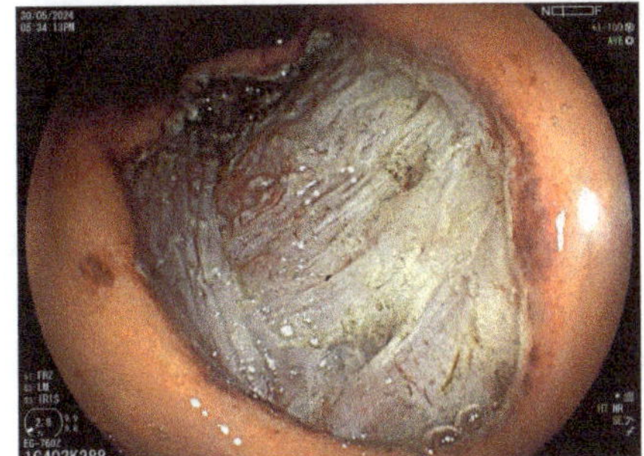

Q3.20

This is a 40-year-old female patient who had surgery.

1. Describe the findings in picture A.

2. What is the likely diagnosis?

3. What is the likely clinical presentation?

4. What surgery was performed in picture B?

5. If there is evidence of metastatic disease, what would be the treatment?

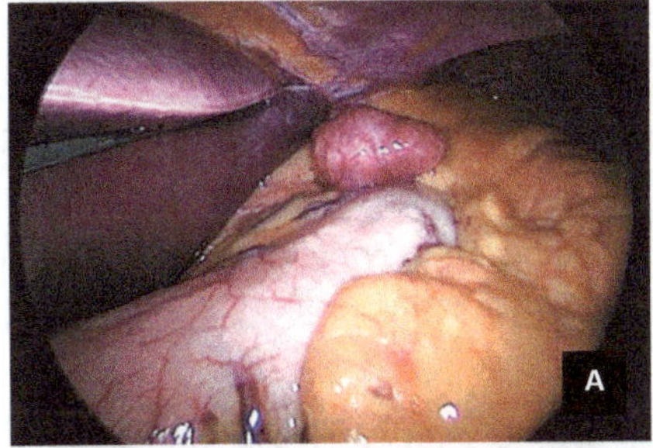

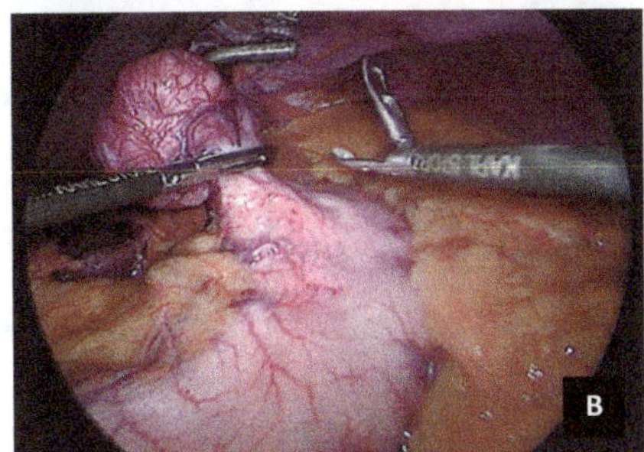

A3.19

1. There is a submucosal lesion in the cardia of the stomach. It is submucosal because the mucosa is preserved.

2. The mucosa of an adenocarcinoma will be ulcerated/distorted. In a GIST, the mucosa is intact.

3. Other submucosal lesions include lipoma, lymphangioma, cyst, leiomyoma and carcinoid tumour.

4. Endoscopic ultrasound (EUS) to ascertain the size, depth and possibly the mesenchymal layer of origin of the tumour.
   A superficial biopsy of the mucosa is futile. A deeper biopsy of the tumour can be achieved under EUS guidance.

5. En-bloc endosopic resection of the tumour.

A3.20

1. An exophytic pedunculated mass at the anterior wall of the stomach.

2. Gastrointestinal stromal tumours (GIST). They occur throughout the entirety of the GI tract, but most commonly present in the stomach (60%).

3. Being an exophytic lesion, the patient was asymptomatic. The tumour was an incidental finding on imaging.

4. The tumour was resected at the base.

5. In metastatic disease, the patients would be treated with tyrosine kinase inhibitors (e.g. imatinib).

Q3.21

This 50-year-old man had intra-abdominal surgery.

1. What surgery was performed?

2. What is the aim of the surgery?

3. What are some complications of the surgery?

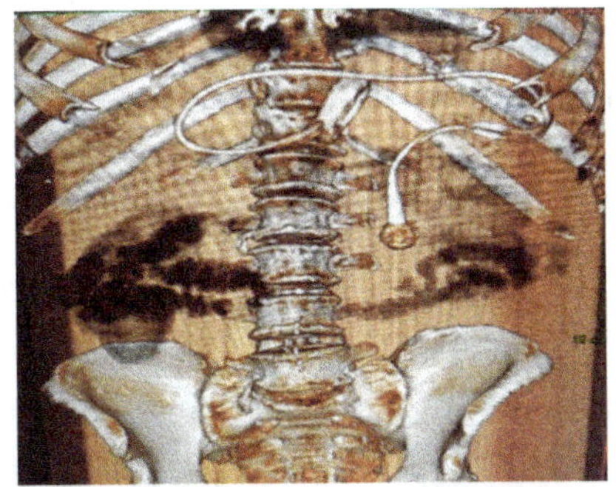

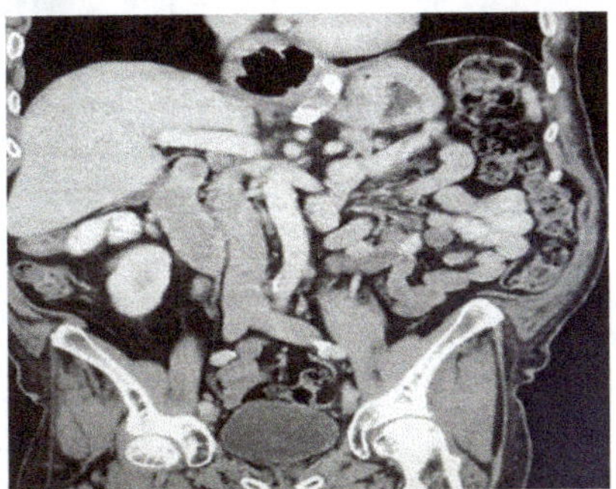

Q3.22

This is a 40-year-old obese patient who had surgery.

1. What surgery was performed?

2. What are other bariatric surgical procedures?

3. What are indications for this surgery?

4. What are complications of this surgery?

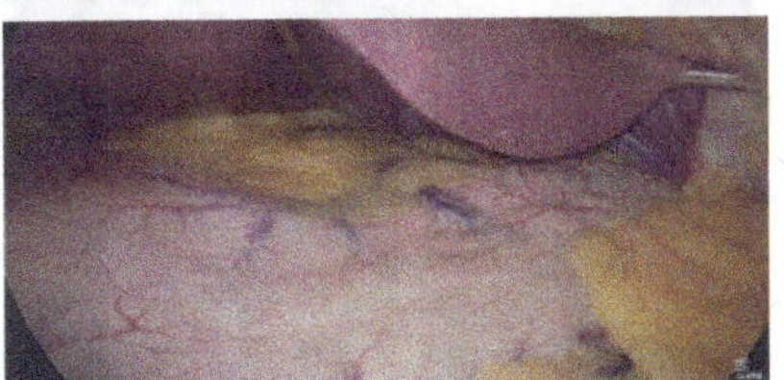

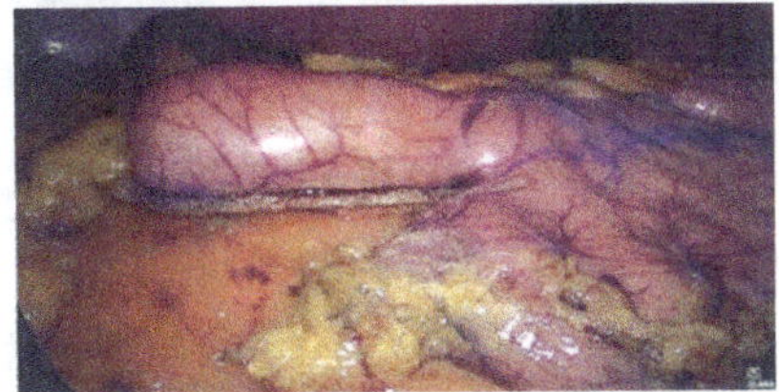

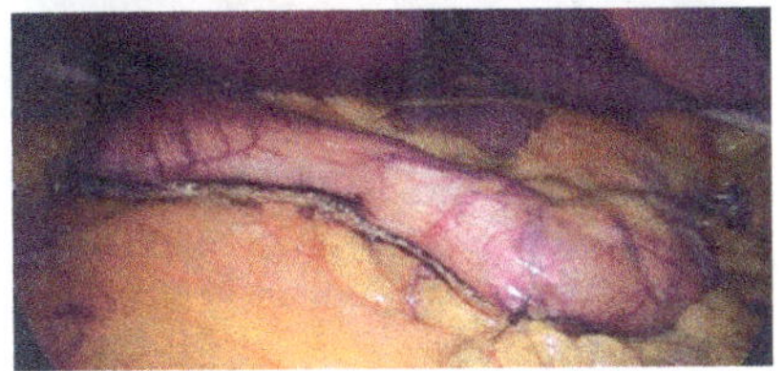

A3.21

1. Gastric banding of the stomach. It is a restrictive type of surgery in which a silicone band is placed around the top portion of the stomach.

2. The band generates a small pouch with limited volume which will provide an early and prolonged feeling of satiety. The band slows the passage of food from the pouch to the lower part of the stomach, thus leading to decreased food intake and subsequent weight loss.

3. Band erosion, band slippage and oesophageal dilatation. This patient has a paraoesophageal hiatus hernia due to the surgery (as seen in the CT scan).

A3.22

1. Sleeve gastrectomy. It has become the most popular weight loss surgical procedure. The lower portion of the stomach is divided and removed from the patient. The new smaller stomach or "sleeve," forces the patient to eat smaller portions.

2. Laparoscopic Roux-en-Y gastric bypass or gastric banding (least popular).

3. BMI greater than 35, uncontrollable type 2 diabetes or metabolic syndrome.

4. Early: haemorrhage or leak at the staple line.
   Late: stricture, gastroesophageal reflux and nutritional deficiencies.

4 Colon

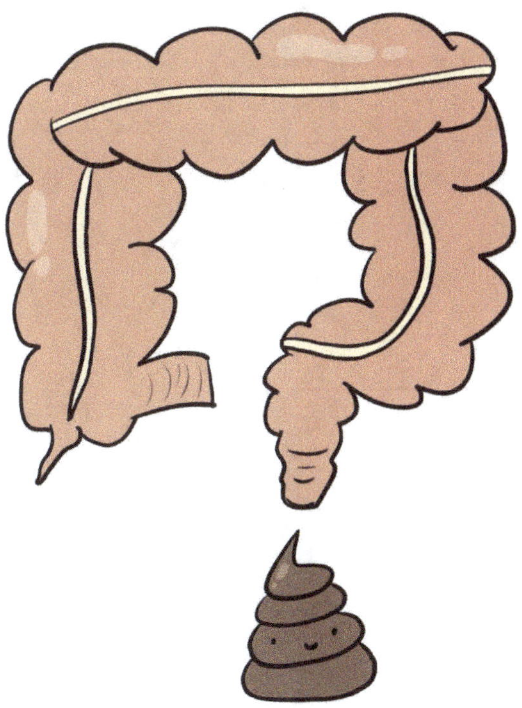

Q4.1

This is a 30-year-old male.

1. What is the pathology around his anus?
2. What is the diagnosis?
3. What is the presenting complaint?
4. What is the management?

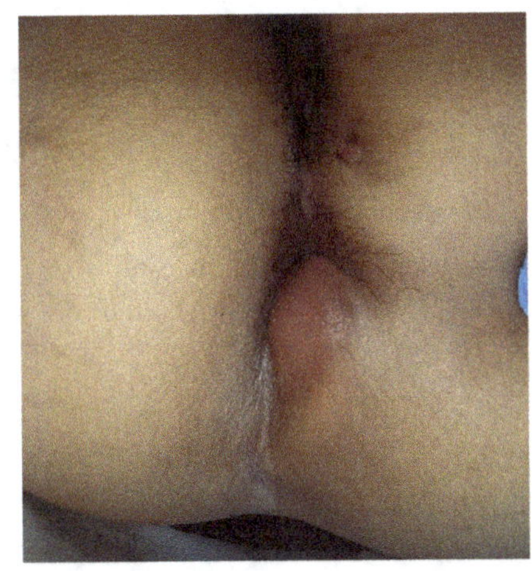

Q4.2

Surgery was performed for these two different patients with similar pathology.

1. What is the diagnosis?
2. What procedure was performed in picture A?
3. What procedure was performed in picture B?
4. What symptoms could the patients be experiencing?
5. What investigations can be done prior to surgery?
6. What morbidity must be avoided during surgery?

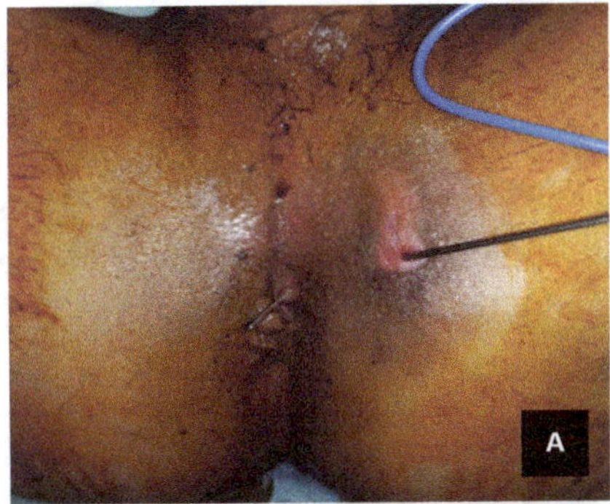

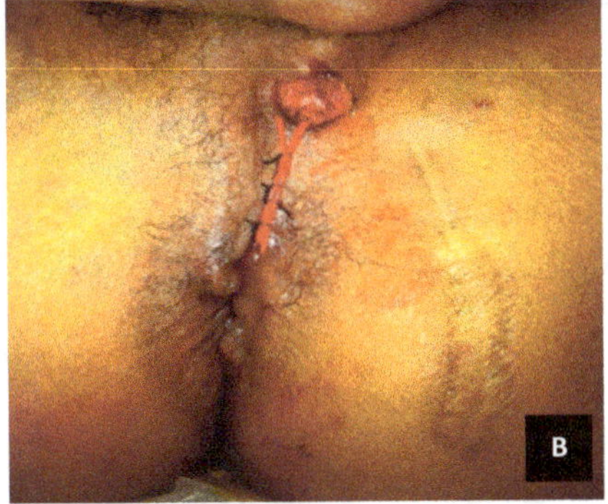

A4.1

1. There is an inflamed swelling at the 3–6 o'clock position around the anus.
2. Perianal abscess.
3. Severely painful lump around the anus, worse with pressure (sitting and defaecating).
4. The abscess needs incision and drainage of the pus. 1/3 of patients will subsequently develop a perianal fistula.

A4.2

1. Anal fistula.
2. Probing a low anal fistula tract with excision of the fistula tract.
3. Seton placement in a high anal fistula tract.
4. Chronic perianal pain and tenderness accompanied by persistent discharge from the fistula opening.
5. Endoanal ultrasound or MRI to identify the presence of multiple tracts and their relationship to the anal sphincter.
6. Damage to the anal sphincters will result in faecal incontinence.

Q4.3

These are pictures of two different patients.

1. What is the diagnosis?
2. What is the likely clinical presentation?
3. What are the predisposing factors?
4. How can we manage the problem?
5. What complications may arise after surgery?

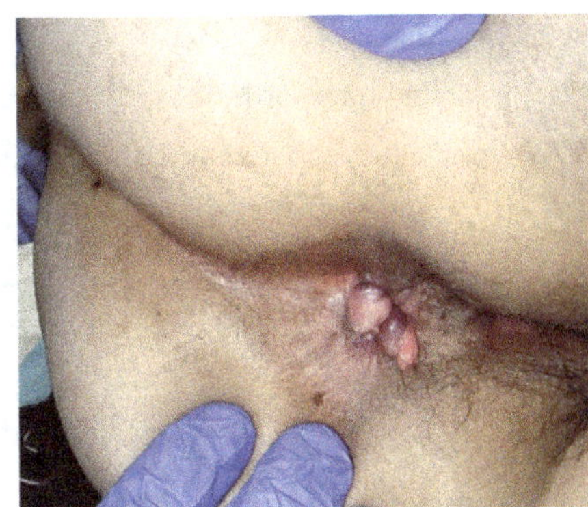

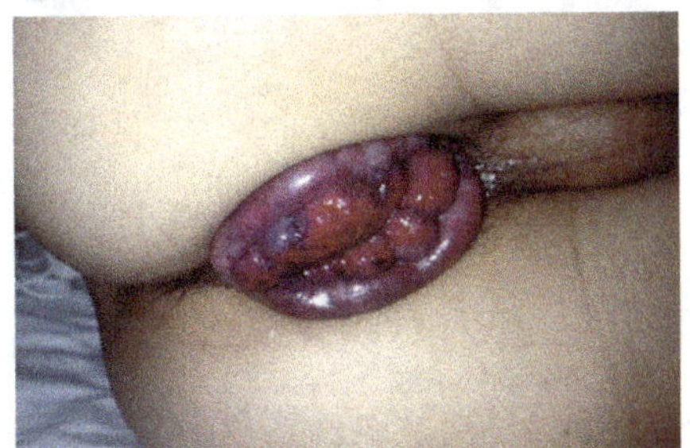

Q4.4

These are pictures of two different female patients.

1. What is the diagnosis?
2. What is the likely clinical presentation?
3. What investigations may be helpful?
4. What is the management?

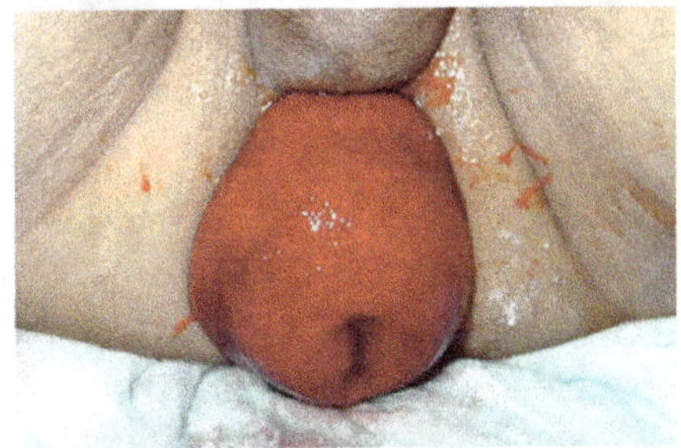

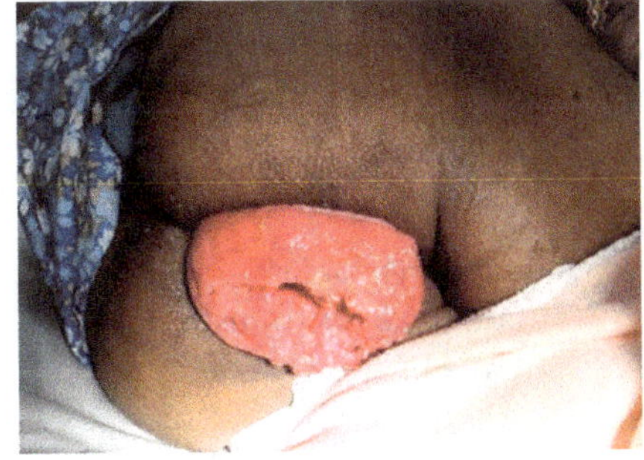

A4.3

1. Prolapsed haemorrhoids.

2. Pain, bleeding, perianal mass and pruritus.

3. Prolonged sitting on the toilet bowl, constipation, straining at defecation and pregnancy.

4. Reducible: patients are advised to address the predisposing factors.
    Irreducible: surgical removal.

5. Early: Bleeding, infection and pain causing acute retention of urine.
    Late: Faecal incontinence if the anal sphincter has been damaged or anal stricture due to scarring from circumferential excision of the piles.

A4.4

1. Rectal prolapse.

2. The mass protrudes initially upon straining, but later prolapses spontaneously without effort. The mass may initially spontaneously reduce, but later need manual reduction. Patients may experience incontinence.

3. Barium enema or CT to look for redundancy of colon.
    Colonoscopy to exclude other colonic lesions.
    Video defecography to distinguish rectal prolapse from mucosal prolapse.

4. Abdominal:
    Anterior resection — redundant colon is resected.
    Rectopexy — A mesh is fixed to the presacral fascia, wrapping the rectum to keep it in position.
    Perineal:
    Anal encirclement — a nonabsorbable band is placed subcutaneously around the anus to restrict the size.
    Delorme mucosal sleeve resection.

Q4.5

This is a 30-year-old male who presents with a lump over his sacral region.

1. What is the diagnosis in picture A?

2. What is the pathophysiology?

3. What is the clinical presentation?

4. How was the pathology managed as seen in picture B?

5. How was the pathology managed as seen in picture C?

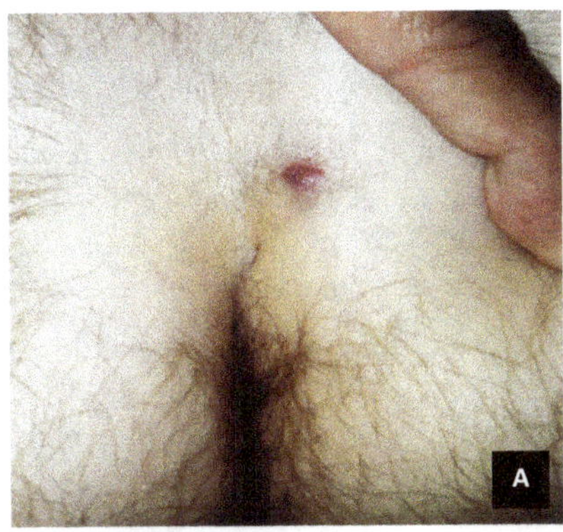

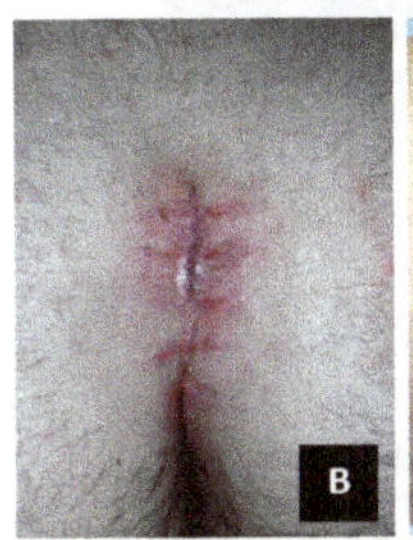

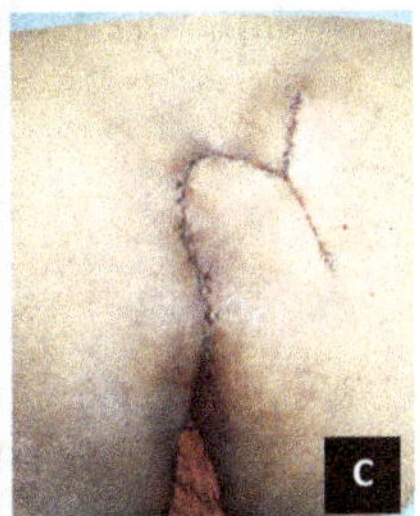

Q4.6

This patient presented with anal pain after a bout of constipation 3 months ago.

1. What can be seen in picture A?

2. What is seen in picture B?

3. What is the pathogenesis?

4. What is the management?

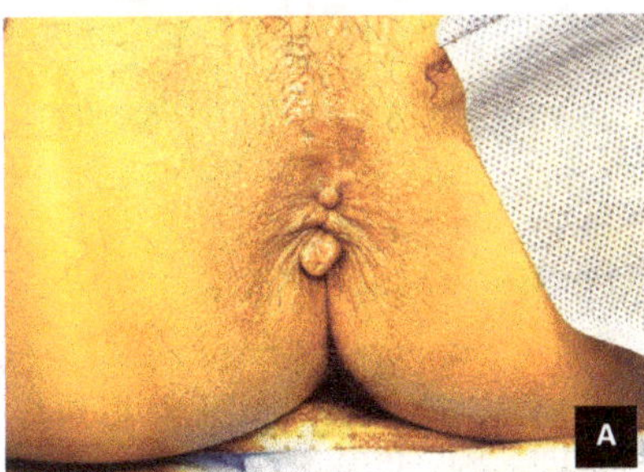

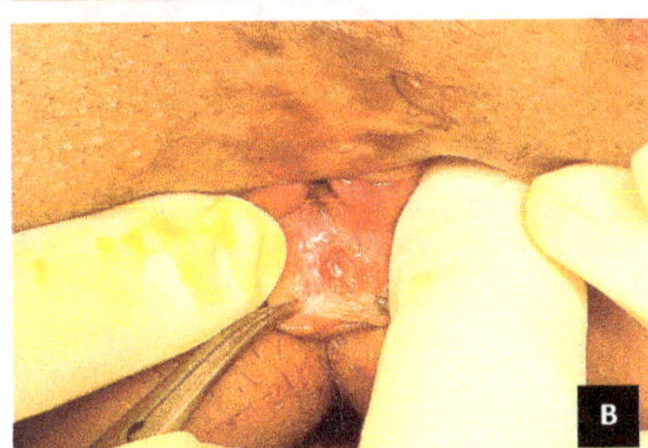

A4.5

1. Pilonidal sinus.

2. Folliculitis develops, which produces oedema and follicle occlusion. The infected follicle extends and ruptures into the subcutaneous tissue, forming a pilonidal abscess. This results in a sinus tract that leads to a deep subcutaneous cavity.

3. They often present as a painful lump that discharges. The condition can be chronic.
   Loose hair may be seen projecting from the site.

4. The pilonidal sinus was excised with primary closure.

5. A flap-based procedure was performed. This is for complex or recurrent disease.

A4.6

1. A sentinel pile at the 6 o'clock position.

2. Anal fissure/tear at the 6 o'clock position.
   It is a split in the anoderm at the dentate line. 80–90% of these are located in the posterior midline.

3. Once a fissure has formed, a cycle of repeated tears results from defaecation, preventing healing by secondary intention. Patients often have increased anal sphincter tone.

4. Initially conservative: stool softeners and reduction of anal sphincter tone with topical nitrates or calcium channel blockers.
   If conservative management fails: the anal sphincter tone can be reduced either with "chemical sphincterotomy" using botulinum toxin injections, or surgical lateral internal sphincterotomy.

Q4.7

This is a 70-year-old male.

1. What is seen in the AXR?
2. What is the diagnosis?
3. What is his clinical presentation?
4. What is the management?
5. What is seen in picture B?

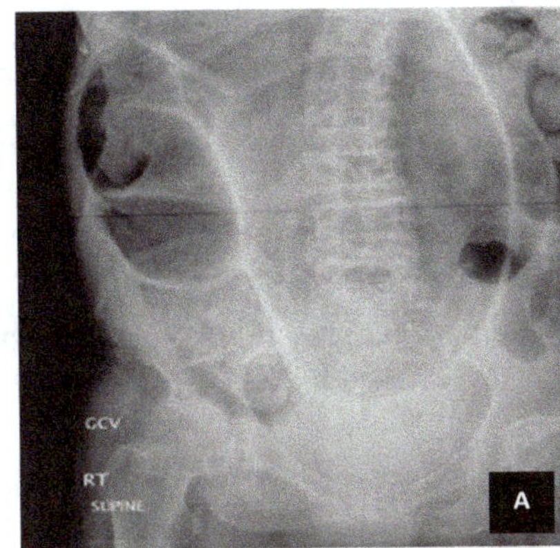

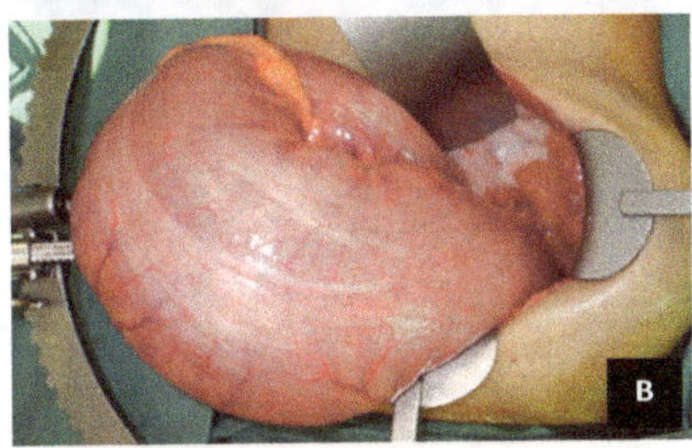

Q4.8

This is a 50-year-old male who underwent colonoscopy.

1. What pathology was detected during colonoscopy?
2. How is this pathology classified based on histology?
3. How was the pathology managed?
4. Why is this procedure in (3) necessary?

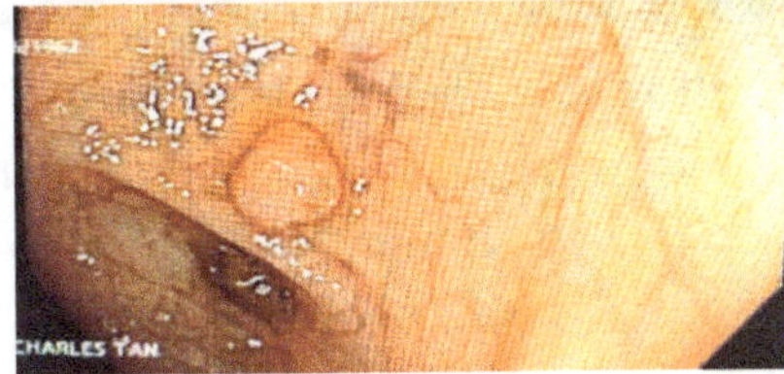

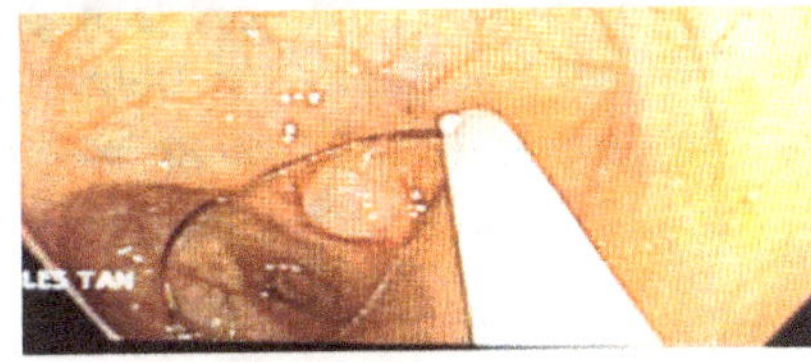

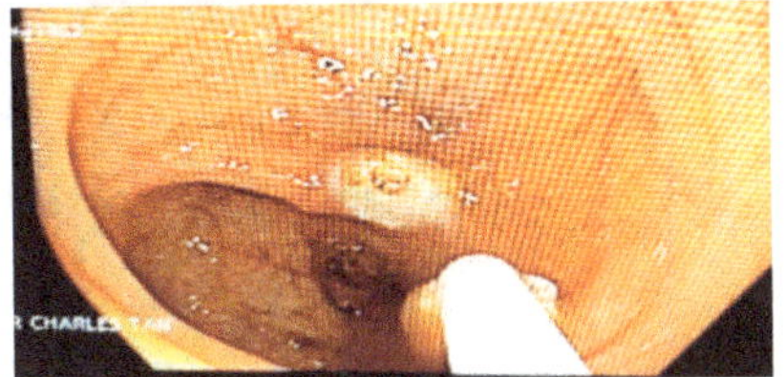

A4.7

1. There is a dilated loop of large bowel in the shape of a coffee bean that nearly occupies the entire abdominal cavity.

2. Sigmoid volvulus.

3. He will experience abdominal pain, distention and constipation. Clinical examination will reveal abdominal distention and tenderness.

4. Endoscopic decompression and detorsion is the first line of treatment. Surgical options include detorsion with sigmoidopexy or sigmoid resection with primary anastomosis.

5. A dilated sigmoid colon volvulus during open surgery.

A4.8

1. There was a pedunculated polyp. Polyps can be flat or sessile.

2. Adenomatous: tubular (80%), tubulovillous and villous.
   Non-neoplastic: hyperplastic or juvenile.

3. Snare polypectomy.

4. Colorectal cancer develops from polyp adenomas. The adenoma-carcinoma sequence is a stepwise pattern of mutational activation of oncogenes and inactivation of tumour suppressor genes that results in cancer.

Q4.9

This is a patient who had a long course of oral antibiotics.

1. What is seen at colonoscopy?

2. What is the likely diagnosis?

3. What is the likely clinical presentation?

4. What is the pathophysiology?

5. What is the management?

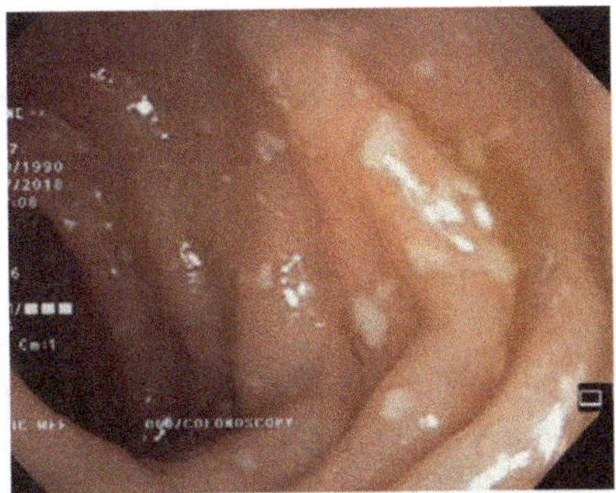

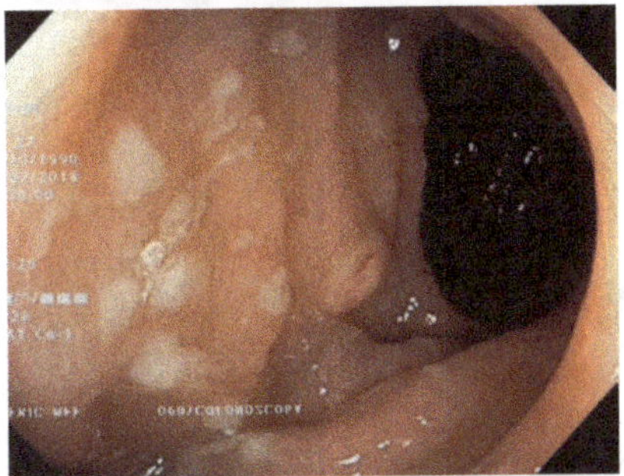

Q4.10

This is a 60-year-old male. He is not septic.

1. What is seen on the AXR and CT scan?

2. What are the clinical symptoms and signs?

3. What are some possible causes?

4. How can we manage the patient?

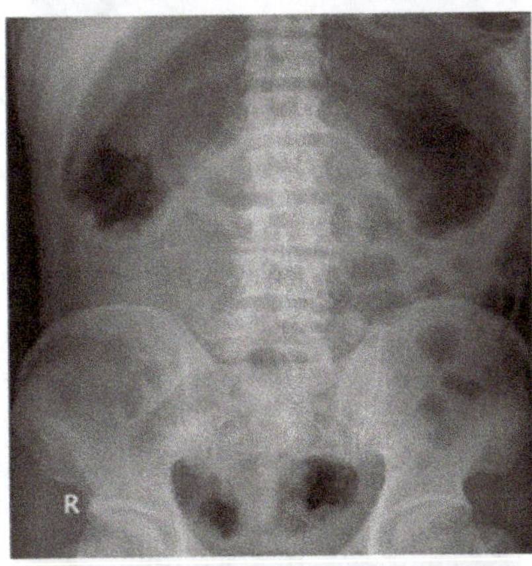

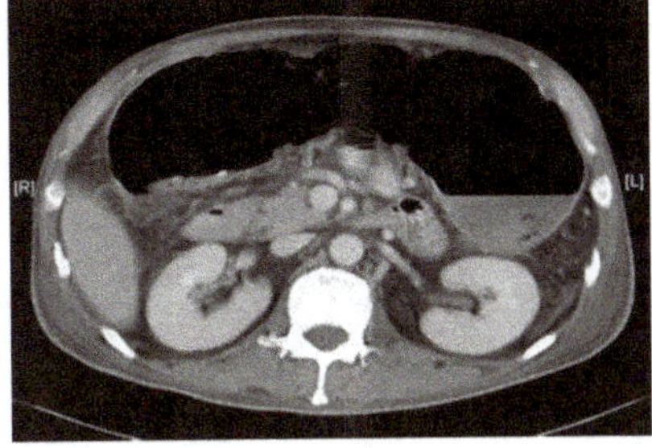

A4.9

1. There are raised yellowish nodules or plaques with pseudomembranes on the surface of the colonic mucosa.

2. Pseudomembranous colitis.

3. Patients commonly experience diarrhoea, fever, abdominal cramping, and full blood count may reveal leukocytosis.

4. The administration of antibiotics disrupts the normal colonic biome, which allows for Clostridium difficile (CD) colonization. CD induces colitis via exotoxin production, which causes inflammation, colonic cell cytoskeleton disruption, and cellular death.

5. Oral therapy with metronidazole is the recommended first-line therapy. Vancomycin is an effective alternative.

A4.10

1. Megacolon of the transverse colon.
   The dilation is often accompanied by a paralysis of the peristaltic movements of the affected bowel.

2. The patient will experience constipation and abdominal bloating. On clinical examination, there will be a distended tympanic abdomen.

3. Neurological: Parkinson's disease, diabetic neuropathy, spinal cord injury.
   Systemic disease: Scleroderma, dermatomyositis, systemic lupus erythematosus.
   Metabolic diseases: Hypothyroidism, hypokalaemia.
   Medication: e.g. Risperidone, anti-psychotic medications.

4. Exclude toxic megacolon.
   Conservative management would involve fluid resuscitation and to treat any sepsis. Next is to identify and address the cause.
   In an unstable patient with signs of impending perforation, surgical resection may be necessary.

Q4.11

This is a 60-year-old male who had a colonoscopy.

1. What is detected on the endoscopy in picture A?
2. What problems can it cause?
3. What is the pathophysiology?
4. What is the management?
5. What is seen at endoscopy in picture B?

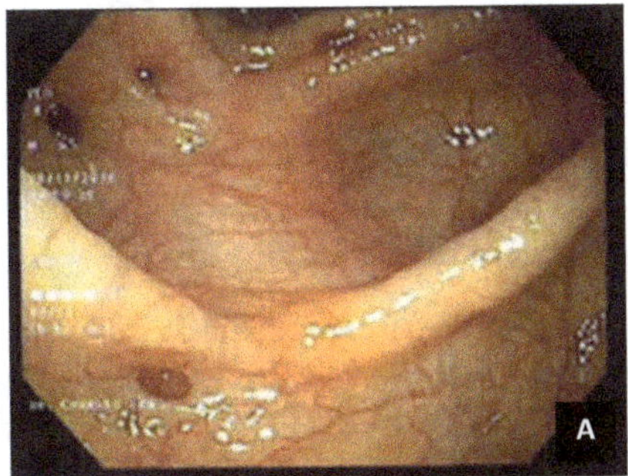

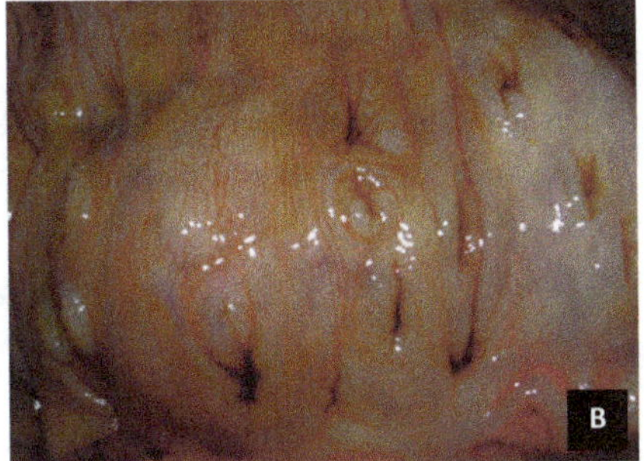

Q4.12

This is a 60-year-old male.

1. What is seen in his rectum on endoscopy?
2. What is seen in the CT scan?
3. What would his symptoms be?
4. What are differential diagnoses?
5. How can we obtain the diagnosis?

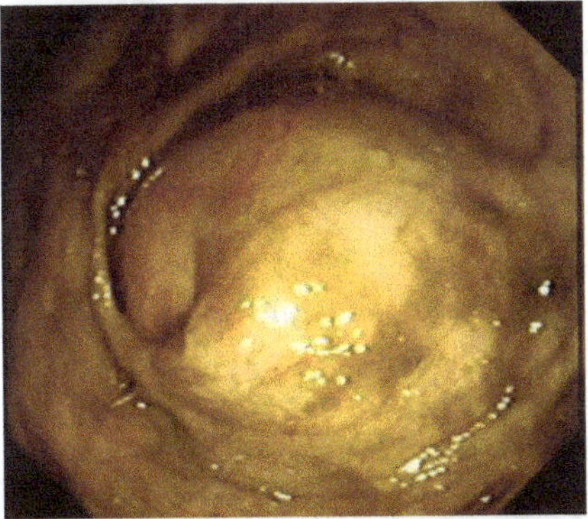

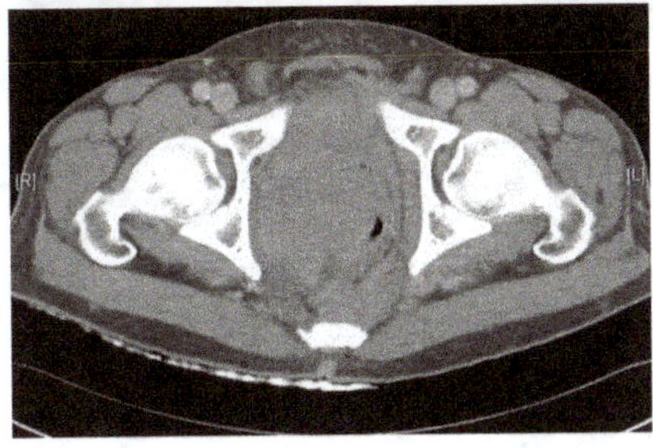

A4.11

1. Diverticular disease of the colon.

2. Diverticular disease is often asymptomatic.
   Symptomatic diverticular disease may present with bleeding and inflammation.

3. An acquired diverticulum is a mucosal protrusion through the intestinal wall that occurs along natural areas of weakness. Diverticula typically occur at sites where the vasa recta penetrate the circular layer, between the taeniae in the colon.

4. Asymptomatic, no treatment is needed.
   Diverticulitis: initial treatment is with intravenous antibiotics.
   Diverticular bleeding: 80% of bleeds stop spontaneously.
   Surgical intervention is needed if the bleeding or infection persists.

5. Active diverticular bleeding in the colon. It is difficult to identify the exact source of bleeding.

A4.12

1. There is a large growth in the rectum. The mucosa is preserved.

2. There is a large mass in the pelvis causing narrowing of the rectal lumen.

3. Tenesmus (the feeling of incomplete defaecation).

4. As the mucosa is preserved, the tumour arises from the mesenchymal layer. Differential diagnoses include gastrointestinal tumours and lymphoma.

5. Obtain histology via a deep biopsy beyond the mucosal layer.

Q4.13

This is a 50-year-old male with endoscopic pictures of his rectum and sigmoid.

1. What is seen in the pictures?

2. What is the likely diagnosis?

3. What is the likely clinical presentation?

4. What other systemic manifestations might he have?

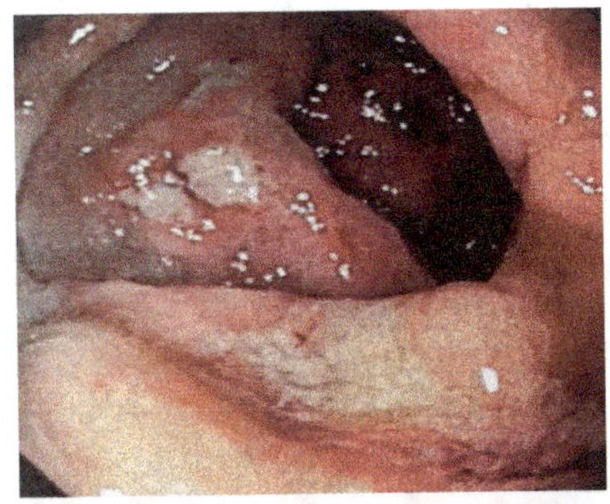

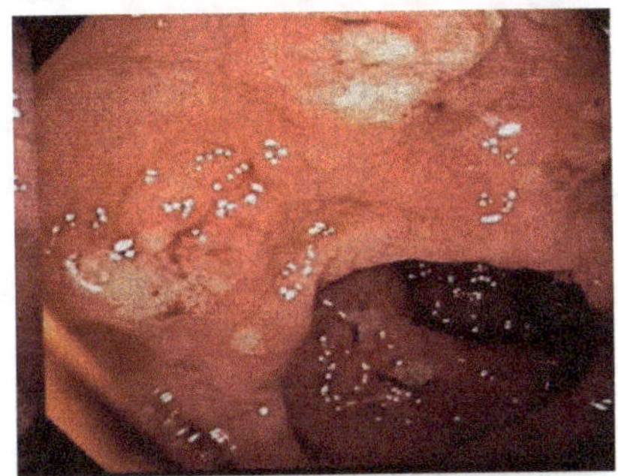

Q4.14

This is a 22-year-old male.

1. What surgery was performed?

2. What is the diagnosis?

3. What is the indication for this surgery?

4. What is the genetic inheritance?

5. What other pathology is he at risk of developing?

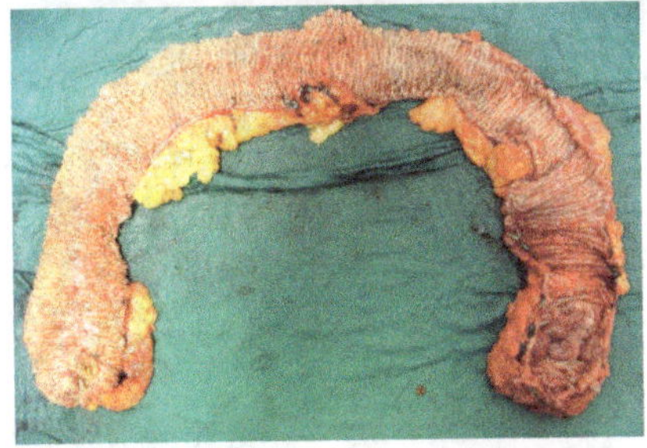

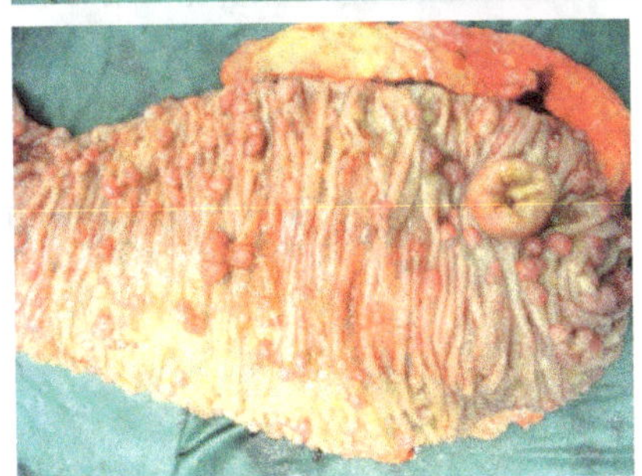

A4.13

1. There are multiple ulcerative lesions in the sigmoid and rectum.

2. Inflammatory bowel disease. Ulcerative Colitis.

3. Bloody diarrhoea, with or without mucus. Associated symptoms include urgency or tenesmus, abdominal pain, malaise, weight loss, and fever, depending on the extent and severity of the disease.

4. Extraintestinal manifestations affect 30% of patients with ulcerative colitis. They include episcleritis, scleritis, uveitis, peripheral arthropathies, erythema nodosum, and pyoderma gangrenosum.

A4.14

1. Total colectomy.

2. Familial adenomatous polyposis (FAP). There are multiple polyps in the colon.

3. FAP ultimately results in an almost 100% lifetime risk of colorectal cancer, typically occurring by age 40. Colectomy is recommended to reduce the risk of developing colorectal cancer.

4. FAP results from mutations in the APC gene, a tumour suppressor gene located on chromosome 5. The disease is inherited in an autosomal dominant manner.

5. He is at risk of developing other malignancies, such as desmoid tumours and adenocarcinoma of the duodenum and the papilla of Vater.

Q4.15

This is a 60-year-old male.

1. Describe the contents, abdominal wall position and exterior "construction" of the stoma.
2. What stoma is it?
3. What are common indications for this stoma?
4. What are complications associated with this stoma?

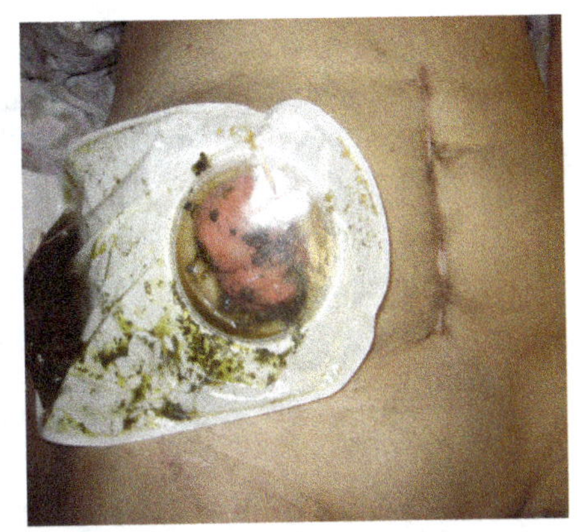

Q4.16

This is a 70-year-old male.

1. Describe the contents, abdominal wall position and exterior "construction" of the stoma.
2. What stoma is it?
3. What are possible indications for this stoma?
4. What are possible complications?

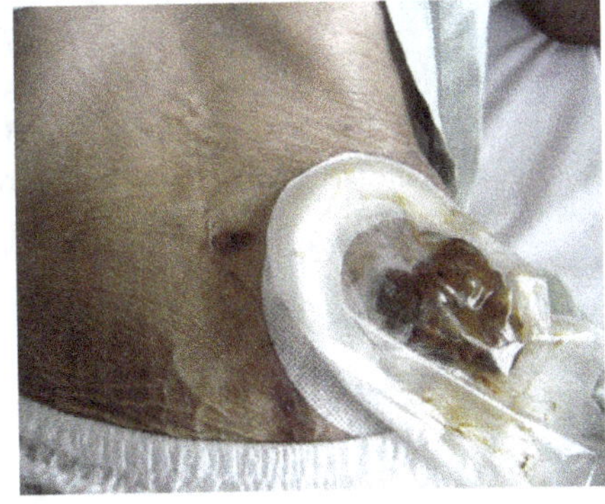

A4.15

1. Contents: greenish small bowel contents.
   Position: right side of abdominal wall.
   "Construction": spouting (to allow a good seal with the stoma bag).

2. An ileostomy (end or loop).

3. To divert stool away from the colon.
   - Protect a distal colon anastomosis by reducing the risk of an anastomotic leak.
   - Evacuate stool if the entire colon has been removed.
   - Emergency relief of bowel obstruction.

4. Electrolyte imbalance and fluid loss due to the high output from the ileostomy.

A4.16

1. Contents: formed faeces.
   Position: left side of abdominal wall.
   "Construction": flushed with the abdominal wall (does not need a good seal with the bag).

2. Colostomy.

3. Perforated sigmoid diverticulitis.
   Abdominoperineal resection.

4. Stoma prolapse, retraction, parastomal herniation and bleeding.

Q4.17

This is a 68-year-old male who presented with a rectal mass that was palpable on digital rectal examination.

1. What abnormality is seen in the rectum at endoscopy in picture A?

2. What are his likely clinical symptoms?

3. What is the likely diagnosis?

4. What was seen in the transverse colon of the same patient?

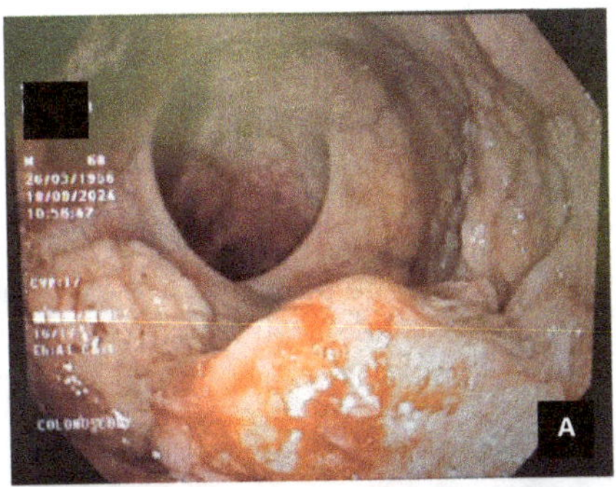

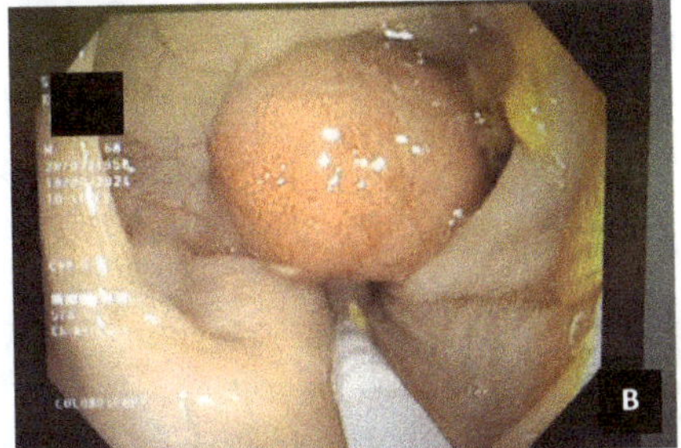

Q4.18

This is a 70-year-old female with a caecal carcinoma awaiting surgical resection. She complains of right-sided abdominal pain with fever for 1 week.

1. What problems can a caecal cancer cause?

2. What can be seen in the CT scan?

3. What is the most likely cause for the abdominal pain?

4. What surgery was performed for her?

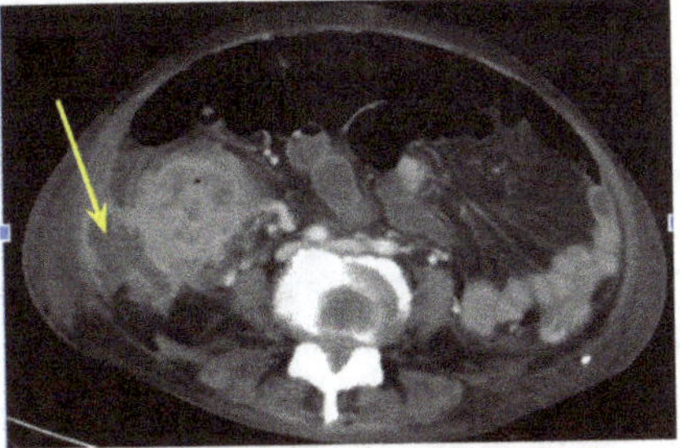

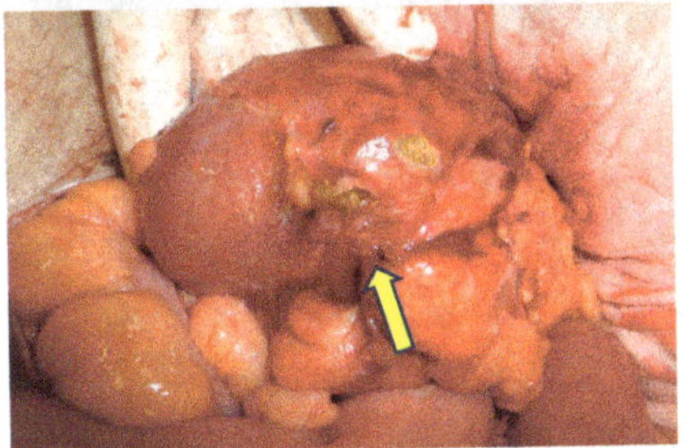

A4.17

1. There is an ulcerative lesion with active bleeding.

2. Fresh per rectal bleeding and tenesmus.

3. Rectal cancer — adenocarcinoma.

4. A large colon polyp. Synchronous lesions may occur in the colon.

A4.18

1. Bleeding presenting as melaena and intestinal obstruction.

2. There is a large mass in the right colon with some fat stranding. There is a small fluid collection (arrowed).

3. Perforation of the caecal cancer has caused inflammation and pus collection in the retroperitoneal flank space.

4. The surgical picture shows the perforation (arrowed) in the caecal cancer. Resection of the tumour was performed.

Q4.19

This 60-year-old male was recently diagnosed with descending colon cancer.

1. What problems can a descending colon cancer cause?

2. What is seen in the CT scan?

3. What are the management options?

4. Based on the surgical picture, what was performed for the patient?

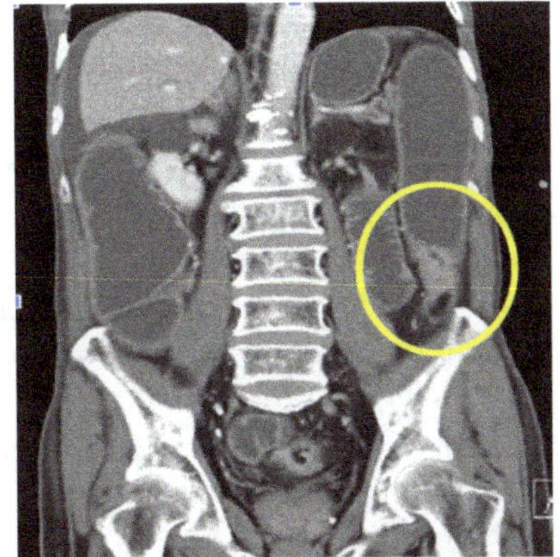

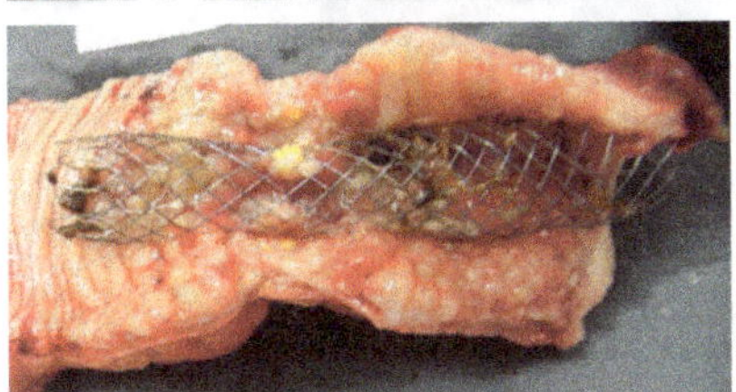

Q4.20

This is a 61-year-old male.

1. What surgery was performed for him as seen in picture A?

2. What is the likely location of the tumour (arrowed) as seen in picture B?

3. What is the likely clinical presentation?

4. What are complications of this surgery?

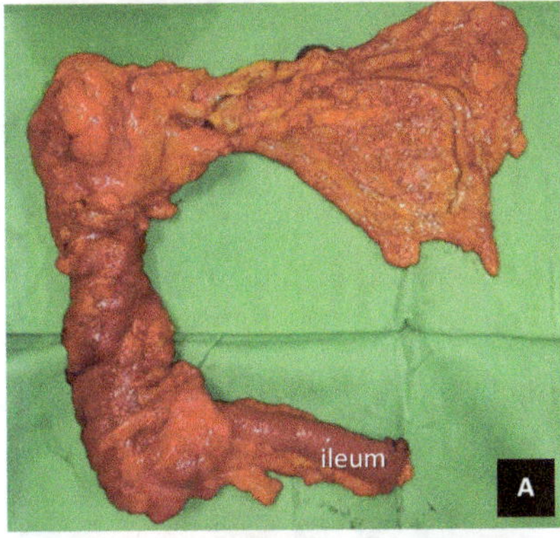

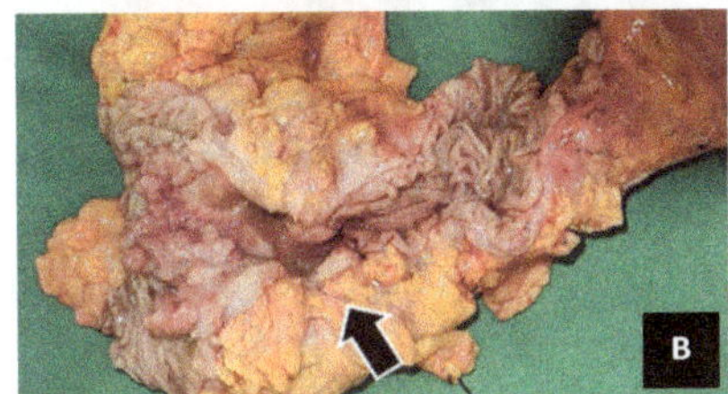

A4.19

1. Bleeding, change in bowel habit and intestinal obstruction.

2. There is an obstructed descending colon cancer with proximal bowel obstruction.

3. An emergency procedure is necessary to relieve the obstruction to avoid bowel perforation with faecal peritonitis.
   - Resection of the tumour with primary anastomosis.
   - Loop colostomy proximal to the obstructed tumour.
   - Stenting.

4. Emergent endoscopic endoluminal stenting. After colonic decompression, resection of the tumour (along with the stent) was performed, with primary colon anastomosis.

A4.20

1. Right hemicolectomy. The distal ileum continues to the ascending and proximal transverse colon, with attached omentum.

2. In the caecum. There are adequate proximal and distal margins to either side of the tumour. Visible to the right of the tumour is ileal mucosa.

3. Anaemia (this patient presented with a haemoglobin of 7g/dL) and bowel obstruction (the tumour caused narrowing of the lumen).

4. Anastomotic leak and right ureteric injury.

Q4.21

This patient underwent a sigmoid resection with primary anastomosis for adenocarcinoma of the sigmoid colon 2 years ago. Colonoscopy was performed during surveillance.

1. What is the likely diagnosis?
2. What are the possible symptoms?
3. What blood test is useful for surveillance?
4. What are the treatment options?

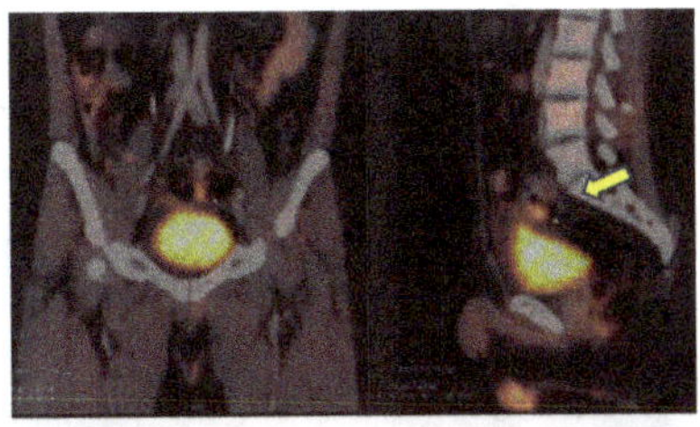

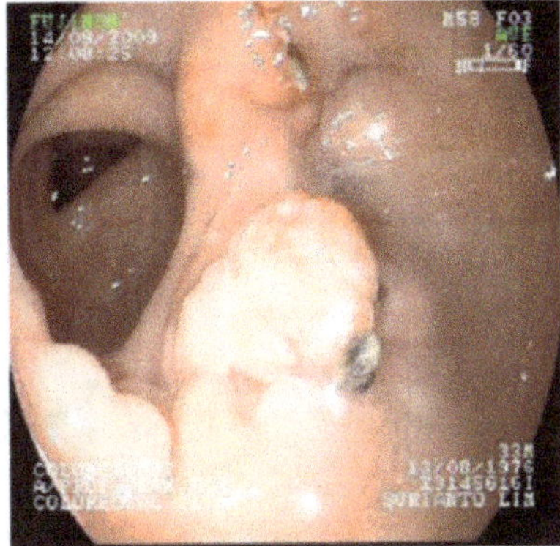

Anastomotic site

Q4.22

This is a 60 year-old male who presented with an obstructed colon cancer.

1. What does the PET scan show?
2. How was the obstruction managed in this patient?
3. What are complications of this procedure?
4. What are alternatives to manage the obstruction?

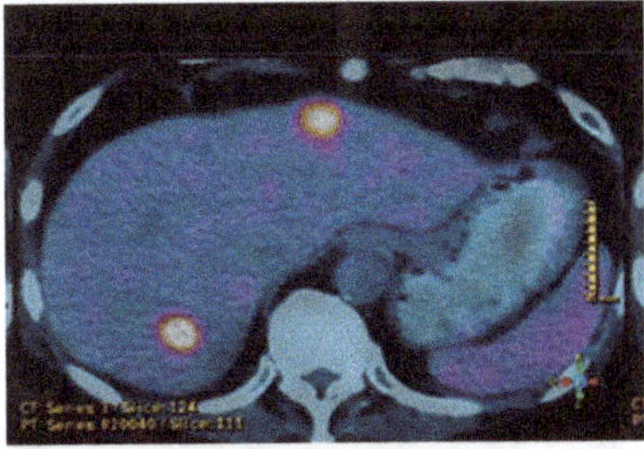

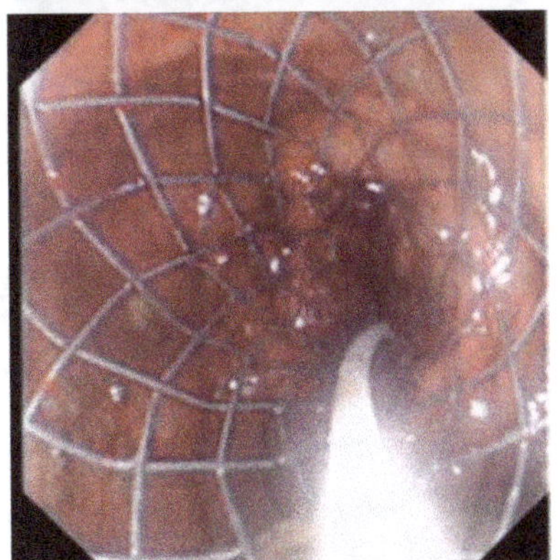

A4.21

1.   Anastomotic recurrence of the colon cancer.

2.   Bleeding per rectum, loss of weight and loss of appetite, decrease in calibre of stools and change in bowel habit.

3.   Carcinoembryonic antigen (CEA).

4.   In the absence of metastatic disease, surgical resection can be considered.

A4.22

1.   There are multiple liver metastases.

2.   Colonic stenting.

3.   Short-term: Failure of procedure and perforation.
     Long-term: Stent dislodgement or migration, perforation, re-obstruction. (the tumour may continue to bleed and grow intra-luminally).

4.   This patient has stage 4 colon cancer. End colostomy or loop colostomy can be performed to alleviate the obstruction.

Q4.23

This is a 50-year-old male who presents with a lump at the anus that is increasing in size.

1. Describe what you see.
2. What further clinical investigation is needed?
3. What is the diagnosis?
4. Which group of patients are at risk of developing this pathology?

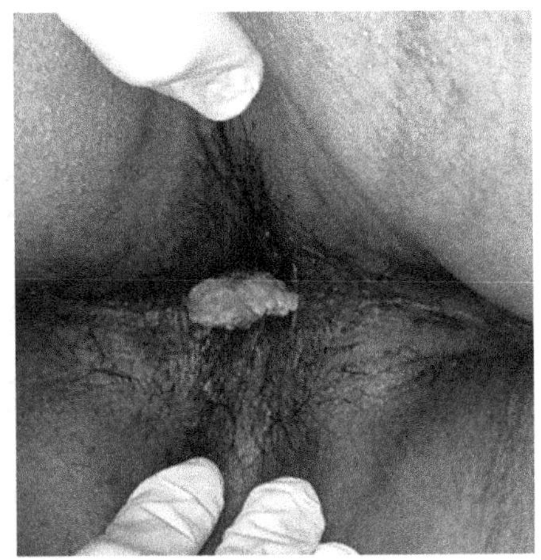

Q4.24

This is a 45-year-old male.

1. Describe the pathology seen in the patient.
2. What is the likely diagnosis?
3. What are the clinical symptoms?
4. What abnormality on the CT scan can be detected on physical examination?
5. How was this patient managed?

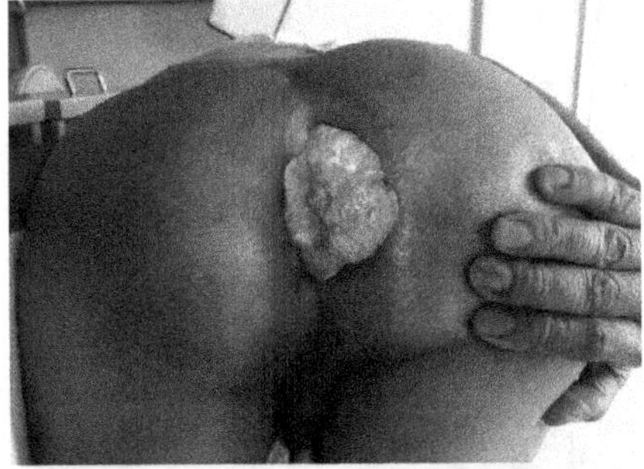

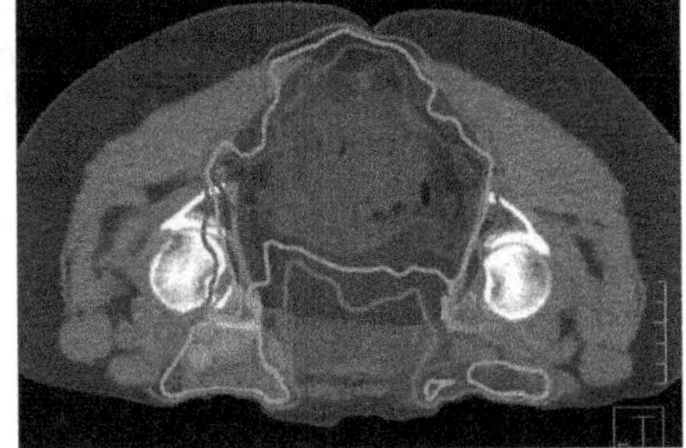

A4.23

1. There is an irregular pink nodule arising at the anus. There is no active bleeding.

2. A per-rectal examination is necessary to check for extension of the lesion into the anal canal. Patient needs to be examined for inguinal lymphadenopathy.

3. Anal squamous cell carcinoma. It develops at the anal squamocolumnar junction and arises from a precancerous lesion called high-grade anal intraepithelial neoplasia (AIN).

4. AIN is common in HIV-positive patients. This group of patients need surveillance by means of high-resolution anoscopy and close follow-up.

A4.24

1. There is a large irregular fungating mass at the anus.

2. Squamous cell carcinoma.

3. Haematochezia, tenesmus, obstruction, narrow calibre stools, incontinence.

4. Palpable inguinal nodes.

5. Being a large tumour, primary surgery would involve sacrificing the anal sphincter and leaving the patient with a permanent colostomy bag. Neoadjuvant treatment was attempted for this patient, with definitive intensity modulated radiotherapy and concurrent chemotherapy. Radiation target includes the anal tumour and its extensions, rectum and perirectal nodes, inguinal nodes, external and internal iliac nodes.

5 Hepatobiliary

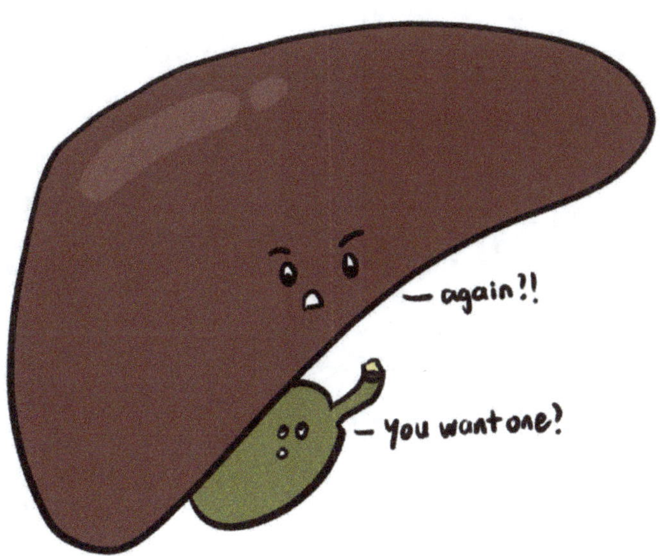

Q5.1

This 40-year-old female with a gallbladder problem was brought to the urgent care centre.

1. What is the pathology seen in the CT scan?

2. What is the likely clinical presentation?

3. What is the management?

4. What complications can occur if the problem is left alone?

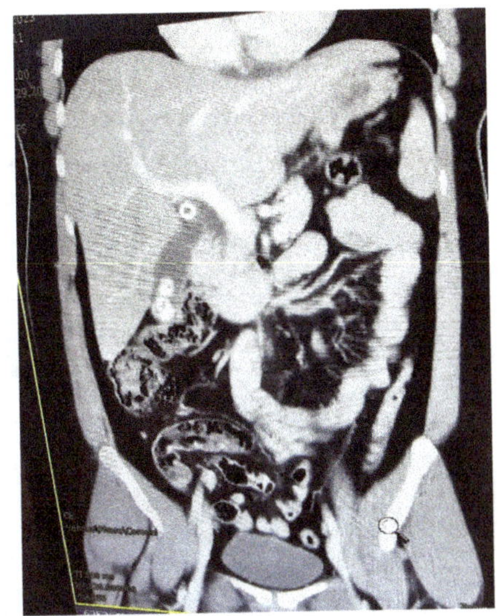

Q5.2

This is a 40-year-old female who had emergency surgery.

1. What is seen in picture A?

2. What is the likely clinical presentation?

3. What is the likely diagnosis?

4. What surgery did this patient have?

5. What is the critical anatomy demonstrated at surgery in Picture B?

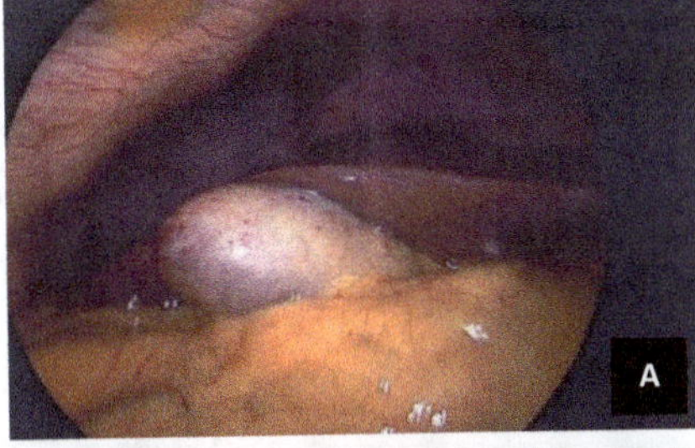

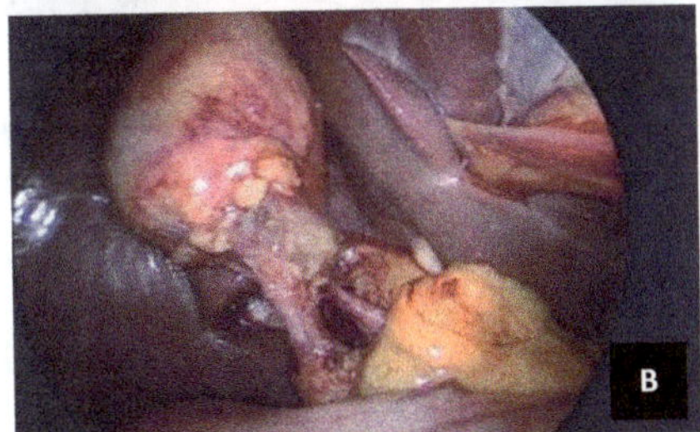

A5.1

1. There are calcified stones in the gallbladder fundus. One stone is impacted at the infundibulum/cystic duct.

2. Biliary colic. Acute right hypochondrial pain radiating to the back.

3. Analgesia and surgical removal of the gallbladder (laparoscopic is the preferred approach).

4. Persistent/recurrent biliary colic, cholecystitis and cholangitis.

A5.2

1. An inflamed swollen gallbladder.

2. The patient will be febrile and experience right hypochondrium pain. There will be localised tenderness and guarding of the right hypochondrium. Murphy's sign may be positive.

3. Acute cholecystitis.

4. Laparoscopic Cholecystectomy.

5. The gallbladder is retracted superolaterally to demonstrate Calot's triangle. The cystic artery and duct are well visualised. Avoiding injury to the common bile duct is critical.

Q5.3

This is a 45-year-old female who had an emergency procedure performed on her common bile duct (CBD).

1. What is the yellow fluid seen coming out from the CBD?

2. What is the diagnosis?

3. What is the likely clinical presentation?

4. What procedure was performed at endoscopy?

5. What is the likely cause?

6. What is seen in the x-ray?

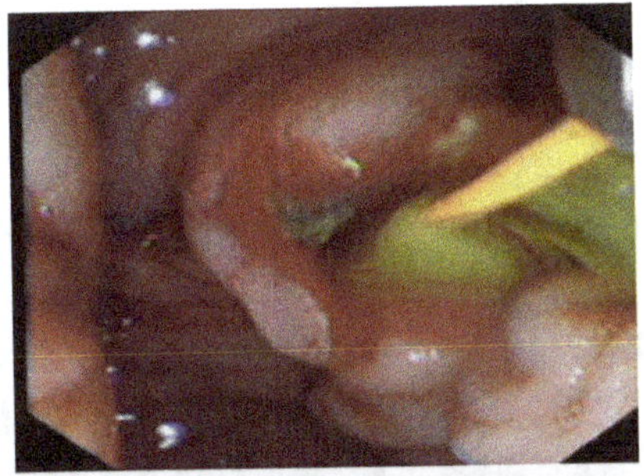

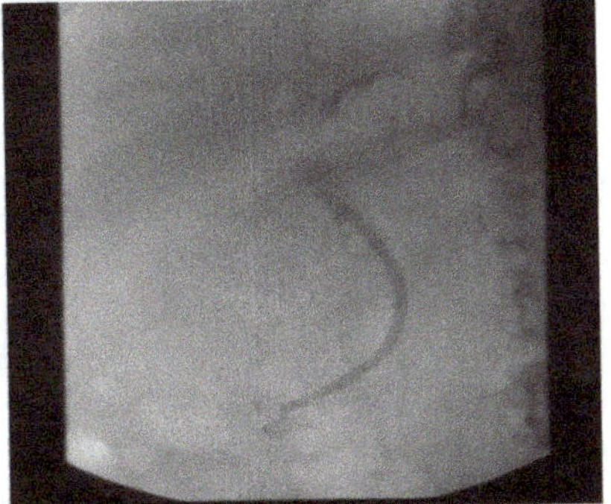

Q5.4

This is a 60-year-old male.

1. What procedure was performed?

2. What is seen in the radiological image?

3. How was the problem managed as seen in the photo?

4. What are some complications of this procedure?

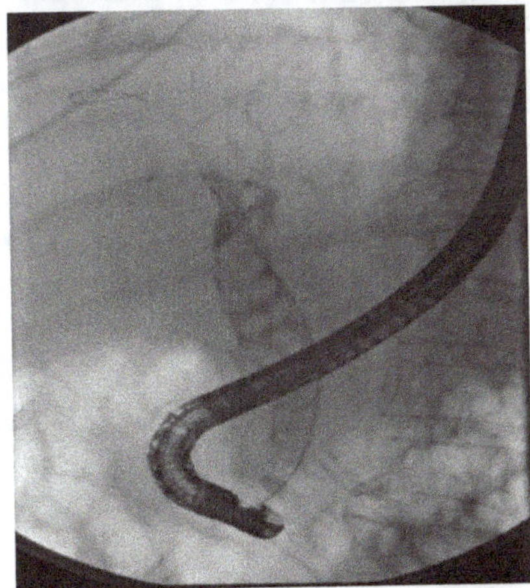

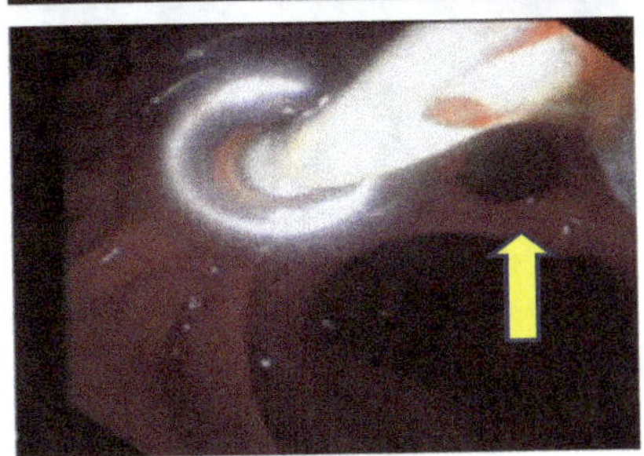

A5.3

1. Pus / Purulent bile.

2. Acute suppurative cholangitis.

3. Charcot's triad. She will have fever and chills, right upper abdominal pain and obstructive jaundice.

4. Cannulation of the ampulla of Vater to decompress the biliary tree. Pus is seen draining out from the common bile duct.

5. It is often due a stone impacted at the ampulla around the sphincter of Oddi.

6. An endobiliary stent is left in place across the ampulla of Vater to maintain constant drainage of the bile into the duodenum.

A5.4

1. Endoscopic retrograde cholangiopancreatogram (ERCP).

2. There are multiple "filling defects" of contrast in the dilated common bile duct (CBD) suggestive of multiple gallstones in it.

3. Successful dredging of the CBD stones with a balloon catheter. The stone (arrowed) is beside the balloon.

4. Perforation of the CBD or duodenum, bleeding post-sphincterotomy or pancreatitis.

Q5.5

A procedure was performed on this 70-year-old female.

1. What procedure was performed under radiological guidance?

2. What are complications of this procedure?

3. What is the likely clinical presentation of this patient?

4. Describe what fluid is collected in the two bags.

5. What serum laboratory studies would be abnormal?

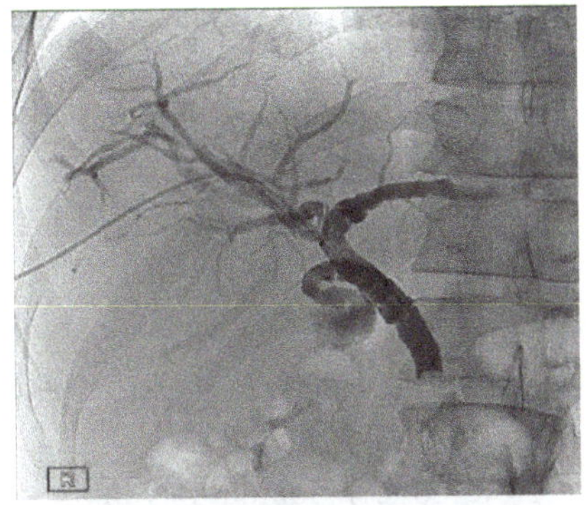

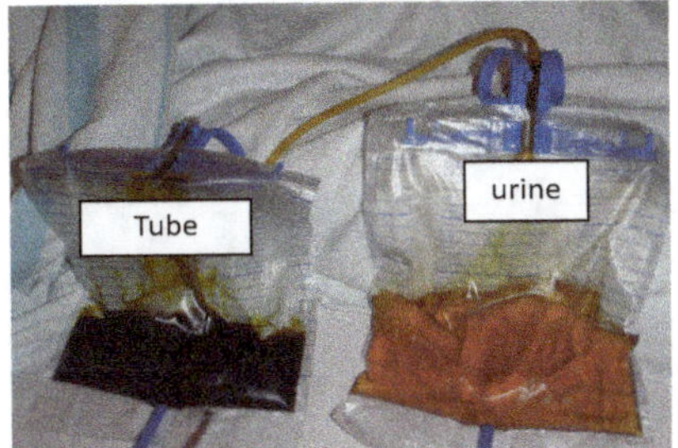

Q5.6

This is a 56-year-old female who had surgery.

1. What abnormality is seen in the MRI?

2. What is the likely clinical presentation?

3. What is Courvoisier's law?

4. Based on the surgical specimen, what surgery was performed?

5. What are complications specific to this surgery?

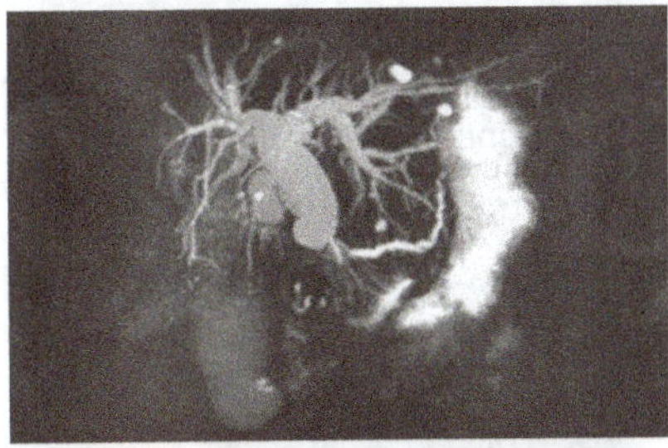

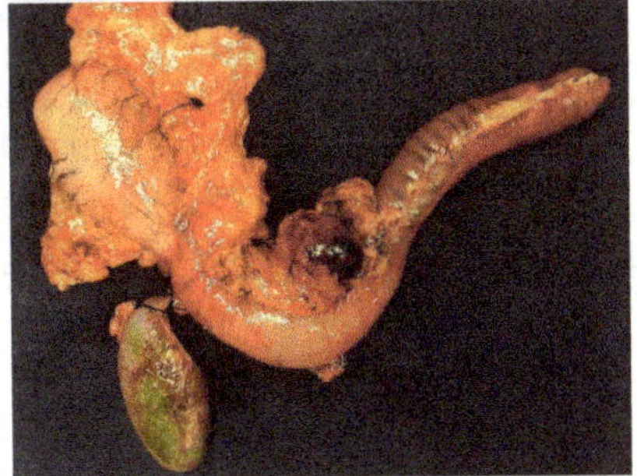

A5.5

1. Percutaneous transhepatic biliary drainage. The liver is punctured to enter the peripheral dilated intrahepatic bile duct system.

2. Complications can occur in 5% of cases. The include bile peritonitis, intraperitoneal haemorrhage, haemobilia, cholangitis, subphrenic abscess, and lung collapse.

3. Progressive obstructive jaundice with pruritis or acute cholangitis.

4. Dark green bile is in seen in the tube drainage bag and tea-coloured urine is seen in the urine bag.

5. Elevated conjugated bilirubin, alkaline phosphatase (ALP) and gamma-glutamyl transpeptidase (GGT).

A5.6

1. The common bile duct (CBD), intra and extra-hepatic bile ducts are dilated. The pancreatic duct is normal.

2. Obstructive jaundice.

3. If the gallbladder is palpable in a jaundiced patient, it is unlikely to be due to gallstones. Gallstones would have given rise to chronic inflammation and subsequent fibrosis of the gallbladder.

4. The Whipple procedure (pancreaticoduodenectomy) was performed. It involves removing the head of the pancreas, gastric antrum, the first part of the small intestine, gallbladder and CBD. Three anastomoses are performed, pancreas to stomach or jejunum (pancreaticojejunostomy), hepaticojejunostomy and gastrojejunostomy.

5. Pancreatic leak causing (gastrointestinal and intraperitoneal) haemorrhage, pancreatic fistulas or anastomotic leaks.

Q5.7

This patient had previous open bile duct surgery one month ago.

1. What imaging is seen here?
2. What is the purpose of the tube?
3. When is the tube removed?

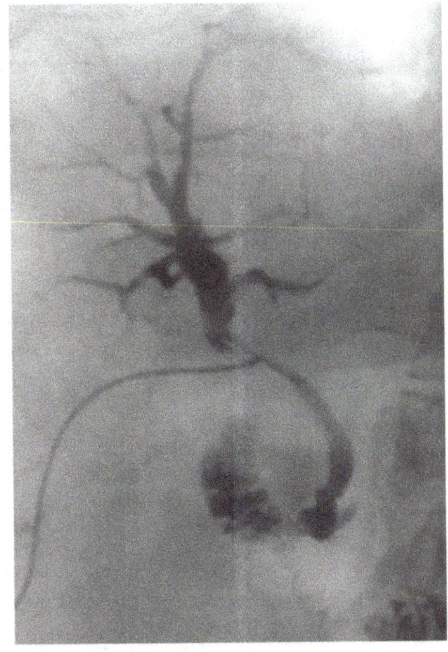

Q5.8

This is a 60-year-old male.

1. What procedure has been performed?
2. What did the patient present with?
3. What is the most likely clinical diagnosis of this patient?
4. What are complications of this procedure?

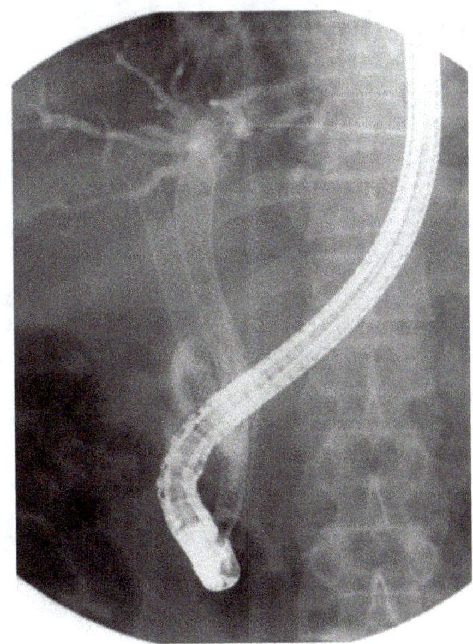

A5.7

1. T-tube cholangiogram. There is flow of contrast from the biliary tree down to the duodenum.

2. The T-Tube is a drainage tube placed in the common bile duct after common bile duct (CBD) exploration through the supra-duodenal choledochotomy. It is utilized to mitigate the risks of CBD stenosis following primary closure of the supra-duodenal choledochotomy. It acts as a controlled fistula by providing an external drainage of bile.

3. T-tubes are made of soft materials like rubber latex. They are removed once the contrast demonstrates good unobstructed flow of bile/contrast from the CBD to the duodenum.

A5.8

1. Endoscopic deployment of a self-expanding biliary metallic stent. (Biliary stents are made of plastic or metal).

2. Obstructive jaundice.

3. Inoperable advanced pancreatic, cholangio or ampullary carcinoma.

4. Luminal blockage by sludge.
   Tumour overgrowth into the stents.
   Dislodgment or migration of the stents.

Q5.9

This is a 70-year-old male who had previous surgery.

1. What abnormality is seen in the CT scans?

2. What are the causes?

3. Can this radiological finding occur without surgical intervention?

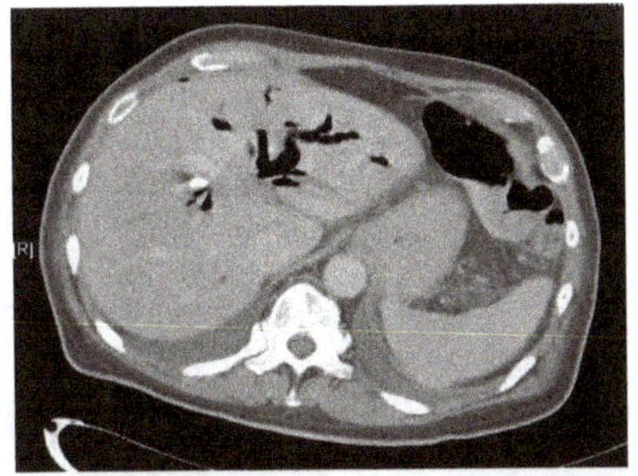

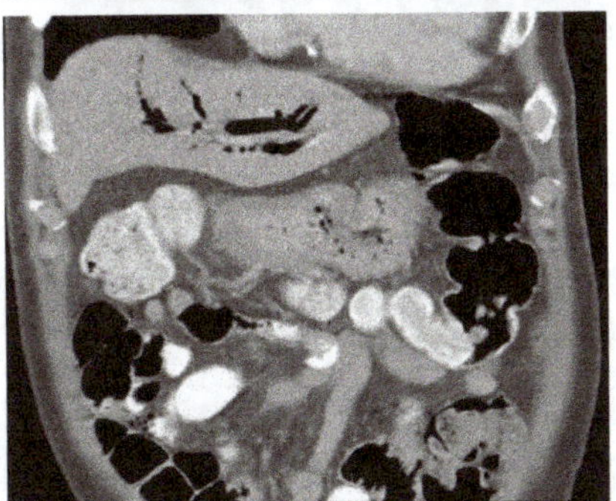

Q5.10

This is a 60-year-old male who had refused surgery to remove a large gallstone. He presents with a distended abdomen.

1. What abnormality is seen in the abdominal x-ray?

2. What does the CT scan show?

3. What is the pathogenesis?

4. What is the likely clinical presentation?

5. What is the management?

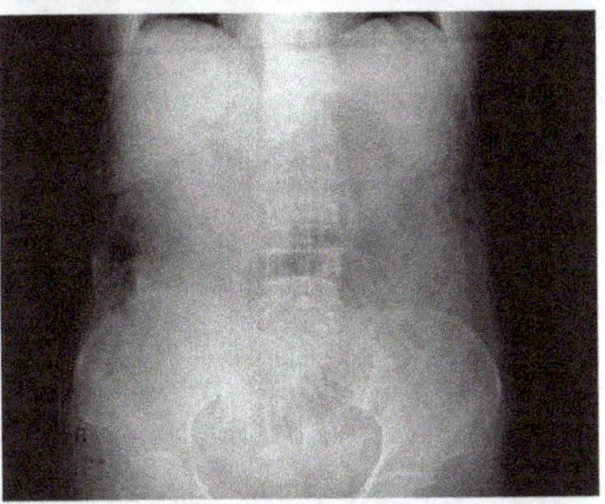

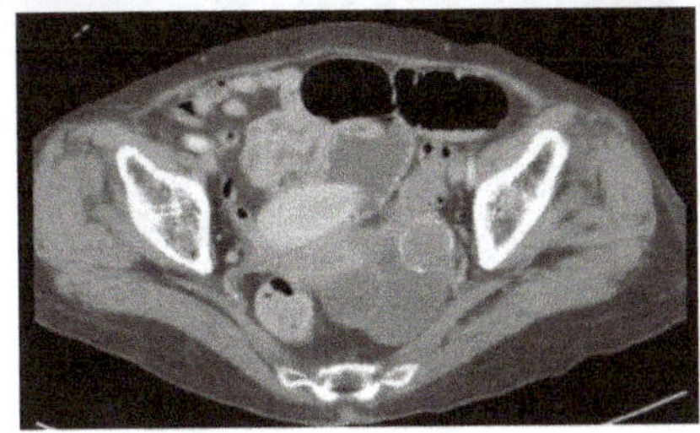

A5.9

1. Pneumobilia/aerobilia. It refers to the presence of air within the biliary system.
   It indicates a possible communication between the biliary system and the gastrointestinal tract.

2. It usually develops after surgical bilio-enteric anastomosis, percutaneous or endoscopic biliary interventions. The most common cause is previous diverting surgery for biliary obstruction, such as choledochojejunostomy or choledochoduodenostomy.

3. The aerobilia could be caused by gas-forming bacteria leading to life-threatening sepsis. Other causes include cholecystoduodenal fistula, choledochoenteric fistula and cholecystocolic fistula.

A5.10

1. There is pneumobilia and dilated small bowel.

2. Dilated small bowel with a larger radio-opaque gallstone in it.

3. The large gallstone has fistulated into the small bowel (most often the duodenum) and lodged in the narrowest part (most often the ileocaecal junction).

4. Abdominal colic with abdominal distension due to the mechanical bowel obstruction. Gallstone ileus is a misnomer because it is not an ileus.

5. Removal of the gallstone in the bowel with closure of the fistula.

Q5.11

This is a 60-year-old male.

1. What is seen on the CT scan?
2. What is the diagnosis?
3. What is the likely clinical presentation?
4. What is the management?

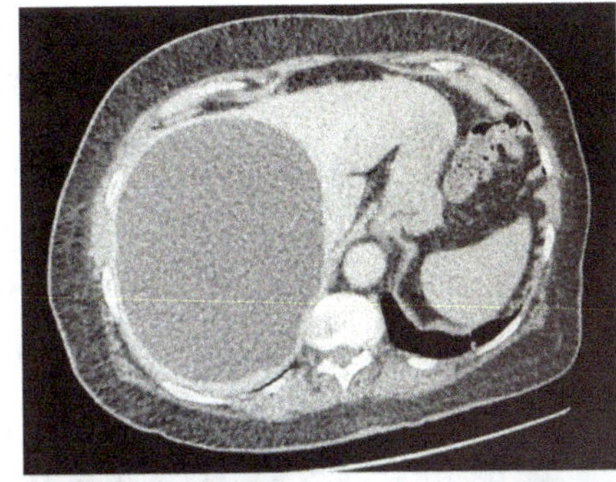

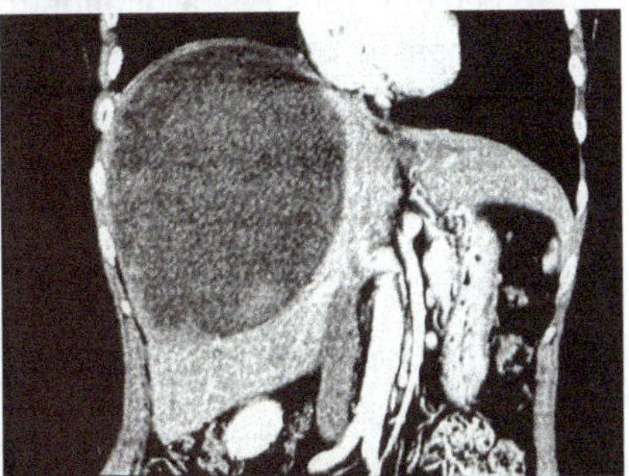

Q5.12

This is a 55-year-old male.

1. How are liver lesions best diagnosed on the CT scan?
2. What are the CT findings of the lesion in the liver?
3. What is the diagnosis?
4. What is the clinical presentation?
5. What is the management?

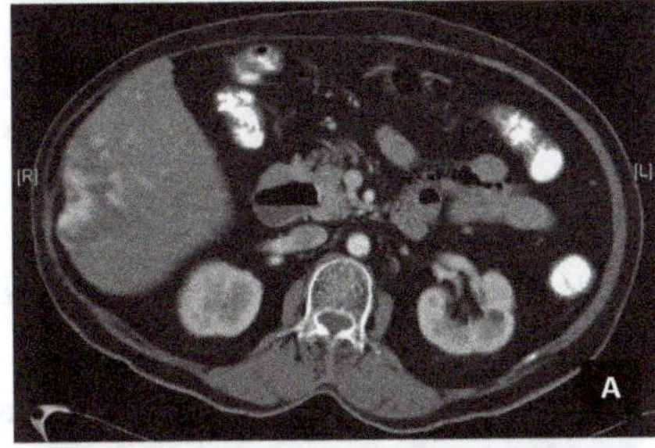

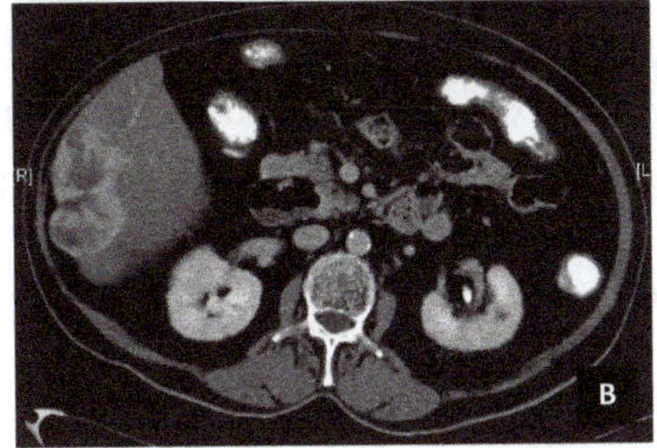

A5.11

1. There is a large homogenous hypodense well-defined lesion in the right hemi-liver.

2. Large simple liver cyst.

3. This large cyst may manifest with dull right quadrant abdominal pain with abdominal distension. There may be a palpable mass in the right upper quadrant.

4. Asymptomatic small cysts can be managed conservatively.
   Management options for symptomatic large ones include
   - Percutaneous cyst aspiration followed by sclerotherapy
   - Laparoscopic cyst fenestration
   - Partial hepatic cystectomy
   - Segmental hepatic resection

A5.12

1. A triphasic liver CT scan protocol is used. The scans are done in a dedicated early arterial, portal venous and late delayed phase.

2. Picture A is the early arterial phase (as seen by the contrast enhanced aorta). There is peripheral, discontinuous, nodular enhancement. Picture B is the delayed phase (kidneys starting to excrete the contrast). There is progressive centripetal enhancement.

3. This is suggestive of a cavernous haemangioma.

4. There are generally asymptomatic and found on imaging studies. Larger ones may cause abdominal discomfort. Bleeding within the lesion can lead to expansion of Glisson's capsule and cause abdominal pain.

5. In asymptomatic patients, surveillance with interval scans is recommended. In symptomatic patients, surgical resection should be considered.

Q5.13

This is a 60-year-old male who presented with fever.

1. What abnormality is seen in the CT scan?
2. What is the most likely diagnosis?
3. What is the pathogenesis?
4. Why is this pathology often detected late?
5. What is the initial management?
6. What surgery was performed for this patient?

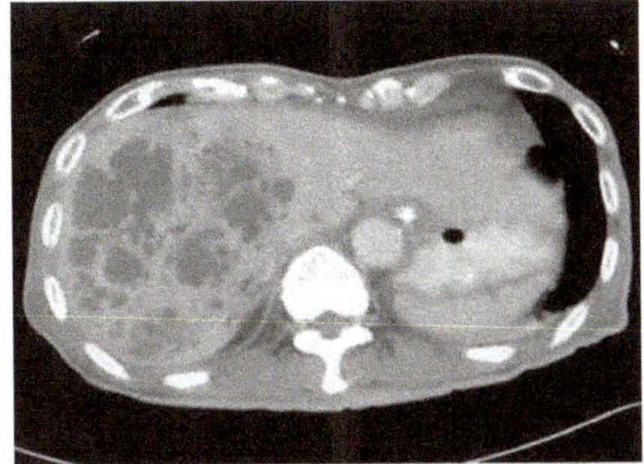

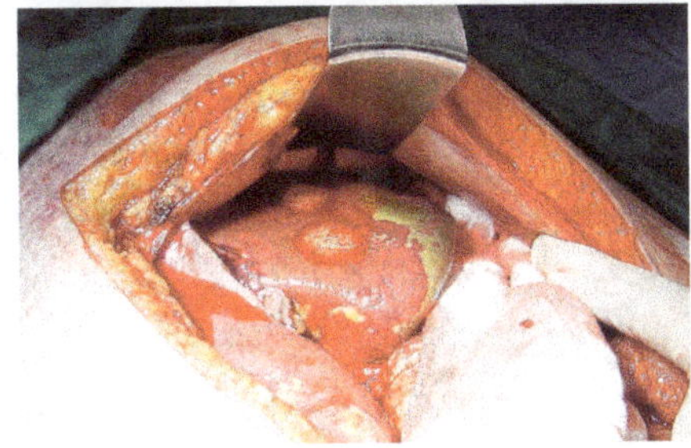

Q5.14

This is a 60-year-old male with hepatitis.

1. What is seen in the CT scans?
2. What is the diagnosis?
3. What are risk factors?
4. What is the clinical presentation of this pathology?
5. How is the diagnosis confirmed?

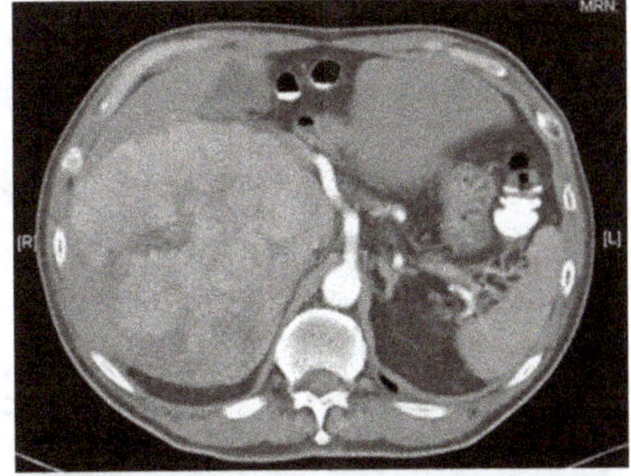

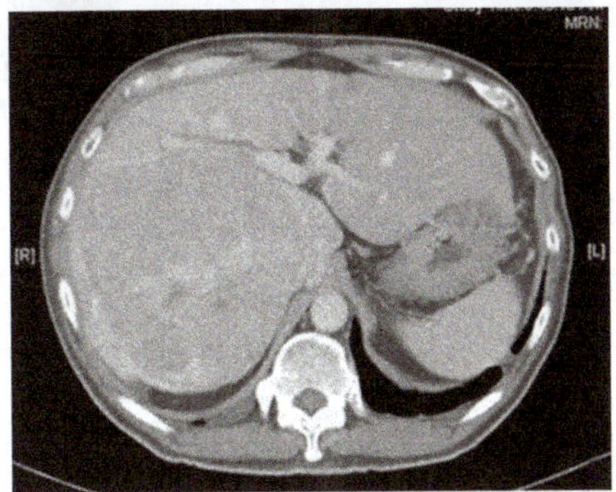

A5.13

1. There are multiple hypodense variegated lesions in the right lobe of the liver.

2. Liver abscess.

3. Majority of abscess are bacterial in aetiology. The common route of bacteria seeding into liver is via:
   a) Arterial: systemic seeding from other areas in the body.
   b) Portal vein: diverticulitis, appendicitis, enteritis.
   c) Biliary tract: ascending cholangitis and cholecystitis.

4. History and abdominal signs are minimal.
   The liver abscess is tender, but as the liver is under the ribcage, abdominal examination would be negative for tenderness on palpation.

5. Intravenous antibiotics and percutaneous drainage.

6. Surgical drainage. It is performed after unsuccessful initial conservative management.

A5.14

1. There is a large mass in the right lobe of the liver. It is hyperdense (enhances) in the arterial phase (the aorta is bright) but hypodense in the portal-venous phase.

2. Hepatocellular carcinoma (HCC).

3. Hepatitis B and hepatitis C strongly predispose to the development of chronic liver disease and subsequent development of HCC. There is an increased association with non-alcoholic fatty liver disease (NAFLD) and non-alcoholic steatohepatitis (NASH).

4. Patients are often asymptomatic. HCC is increasingly detected during routine screening of patients with cirrhosis, using ultrasonography and serum alpha-fetoprotein (AFP) measurements.

5. The diagnosis of HCC can often be established on the basis of non-invasive imaging, without biopsy confirmation.

Q5.15

This is a 60-year-old male who had liver surgery.

1. What pathologies are seen in the intra-op picture?

2. What is seen in the left hand?

3. What are causes for this liver condition?

4. What other problems might the patient develop due to his liver condition?

5. What surgery was performed for this patient?

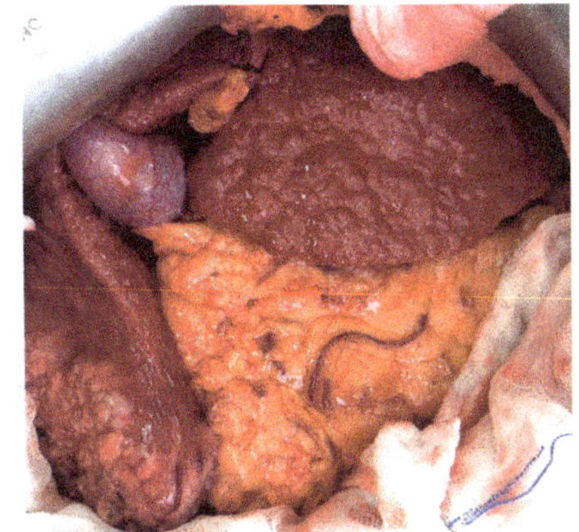

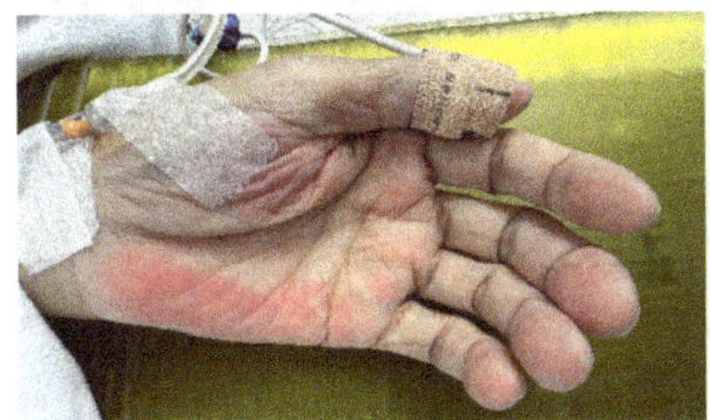

Q5.16

This is a 56-year-old man with hepatitis B who had liver surgery.

1. What does the MRI image show?

2. What surgery has been performed?

3. What is the most likely diagnosis?

4. What are some preoperative assessment/tests needed prior to surgery?

5. What serum tumour marker test might be elevated?

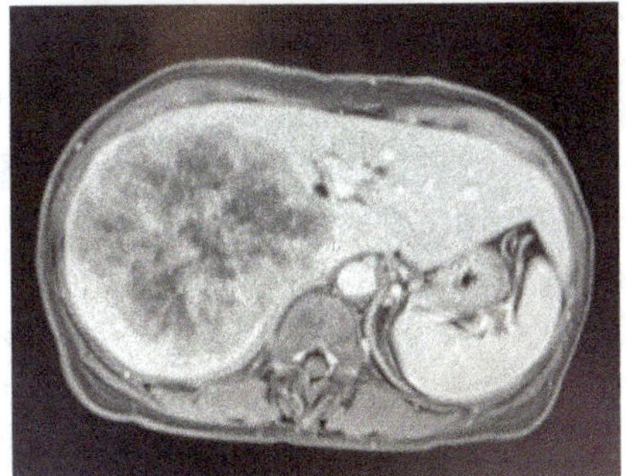

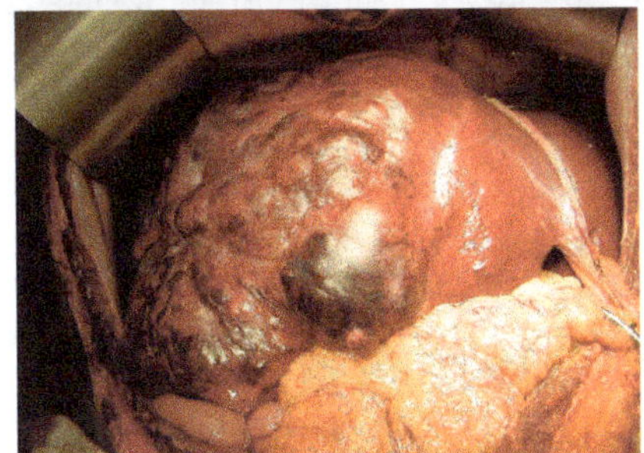

A5.15

1. The liver is cirrhotic. It is characterized by fibrosis of the liver. There is a lesion in the right lobe of the liver.

2. Palmar erythema.

3. Viral Hepatitis (B, C), autoimmune, alcoholic liver disease, non-alcoholic steatohepatitis (NASH).

4. Portal hypertension leading to ascites, oesophageal varices, splenomegaly with thrombocytopenia and hepatorenal syndrome.

5. The tumour in the right lobe of the liver is a hepatocellular carcinoma. Resection of the tumour was performed.

A5.16

1. A heterogenous hypodense large hepatic mass in the right lobe of the liver.

2. A large liver tumour has been resected. (Right hepatectomy)

3. Hepatocellular carcinoma (HCC).

4. In the background of hepatic cirrhosis, there is impairment of hepatic function. We have to determine the adequacy of hepatic functional reserve after partial liver resection and hepatic regenerative potential to mitigate the risk of post-operative liver failure.

5. Serum Alpha-fetoprotein or Des-Carboxyl prothrombin.

Q5.17

This is a 60-year-old male with hepatitis B.

1. What is seen in the CT scan?

2. What is the diagnosis?

3. What is the likely clinical presentation?

4. What procedure was attempted to manage the problem?

5. What is the next step if this procedure fails?

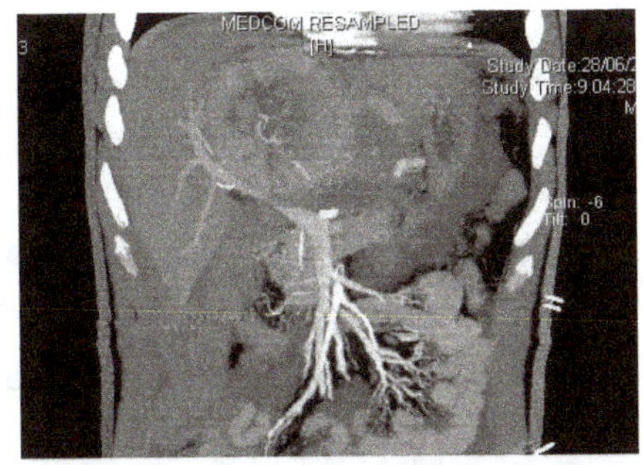

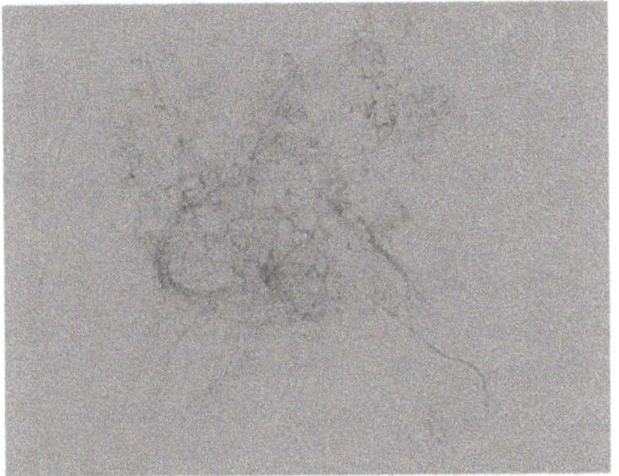

Q5.18

This is a 60-year-old male who had a colectomy for a colon cancer 5 years ago.

1. What is the likely diagnosis?

2. What tumour marker blood test would be likely to be elevated?

3. What surgery was performed?

4. What options are available if the patient is unfit for surgery?

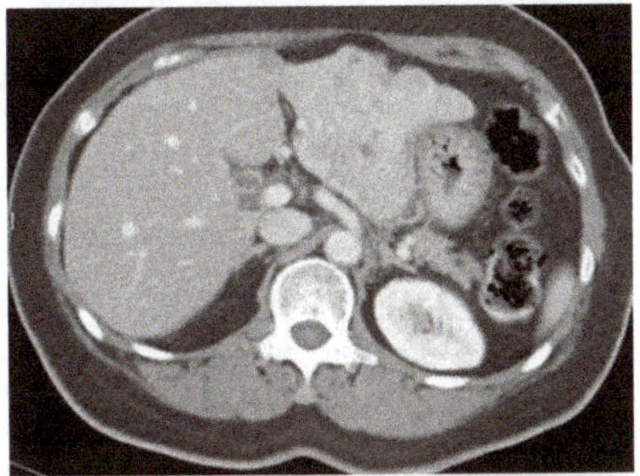

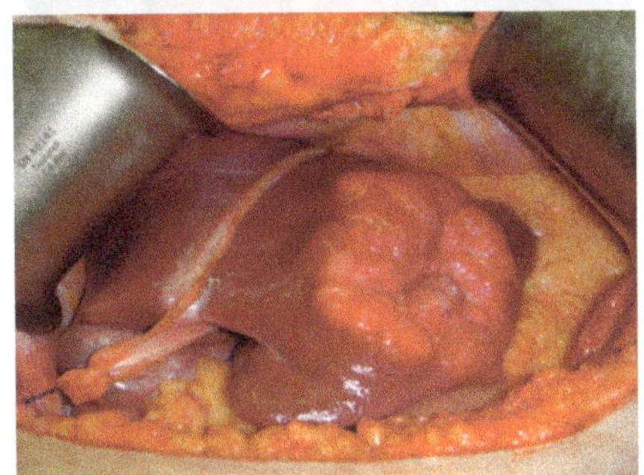

A5.17

1. There is a large tumour in the left lobe of the liver. There is blood in the peritoneal cavity (haemoperitoneum in upper abdomen).

2. Intraperitoneal bleeding from ruptured HCC.

3. Acute abdominal pain and distension with haemodynamic circulatory shock.

4. Transarterial embolization of the tumour to arrest the tumour haemorrhage.

5. Emergency open surgery either to resect the tumour or hepatic arterial ligation to arrest the bleeding.

A5.18

1. A colon metastasis to the left hemi-liver. The liver is non-cirrhotic. Nearly 20% to 25% of patients diagnosed with colorectal cancer will develop liver metastases.

2. Carcinoembryonic antigen (CEA).

3. Resection of the metastasis. It is indicated when there is no other extrahepatic metastasis.

4. Loco-regional therapy which include targeted tumour therapy (radiofrequency ablation), radiotherapy, trans-arterial chemoembolization, systemic chemotherapy or immunotherapy.

Q5.19

This is a 40-year-old male.

1. What is the abnormality seen in the CT scan?

2. What is the most likely diagnosis?

3. What is the likely clinical presentation?

4. What blood investigations can confirm the diagnosis?

5. Why did this patient complain of discomfort with right hip flexion?

6. What is the management?

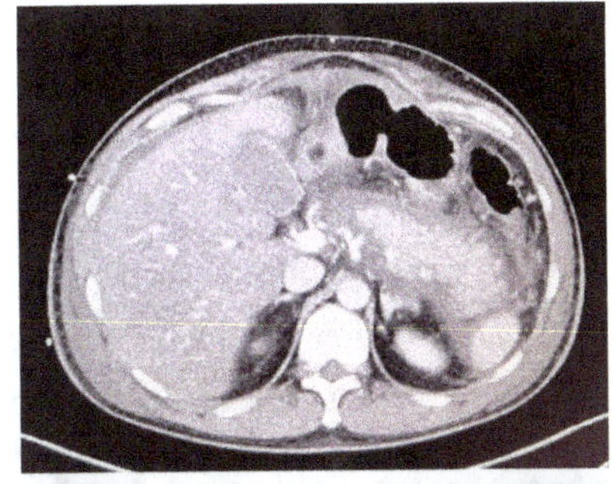

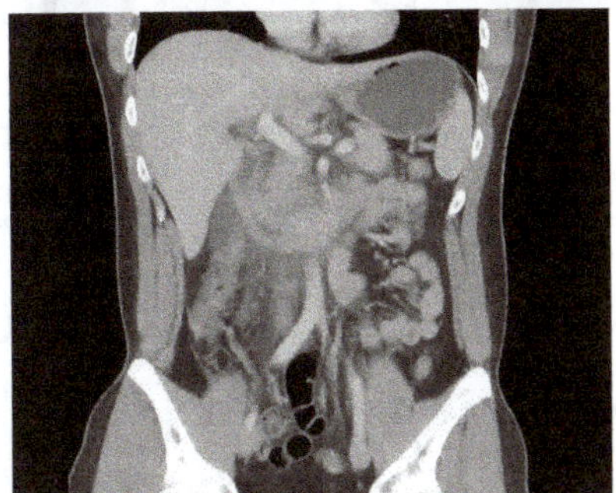

Q5.20

This is a 30-year-old female who has pancreatitis. She developed sepsis and emergency surgery was performed one week after the onset.

1. What is seen in the CT scan and what does it suggest?

2. What emergency surgery was performed and what was removed as seen in the kidney dish?

3. What are possible long-term morbidities to the pancreas if the patient survives?

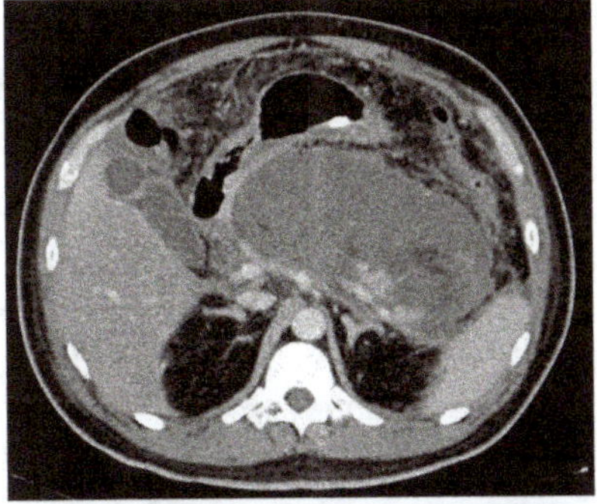

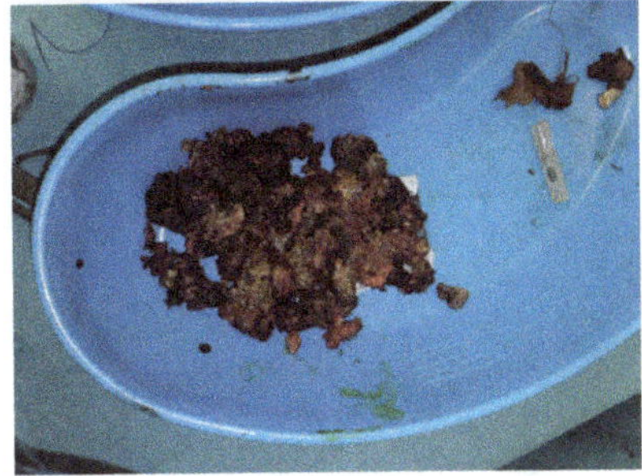

A5.19

1. The pancreas is homogenously enhancing and swollen with surrounding fat stranding. Peripancreatic oedema/fluid collection.

2. Acute oedematous pancreatitis.

3. Acute upper/central abdominal pain that radiates to the back.

4. Elevated serum lipase and amylase.

5. In the coronal view of the CT scan, there is fat stranding in the uncinate process of the pancreas. The inflammation extended retroperitoneally and inferiorly, causing irritation of the right psoas muscle.

6. Management is non-surgical but supportive. Early management is directed at timely adequate fluid resuscitation to address hypovolemia due to fluid sequestration during pancreatitis and associated systemic inflammation. Intensive care may be needed if other organs are affected.

A5.20

1. There is a collection in the pancreas with no contrast enhancement suggestive of a necrotic pancreas.

2. Emergency pancreatic necrosectomy was performed to remove infected necrotic tissues and drainage of infected fluid. Acute necrotising pancreatitis is an infrequent clinical entity, often accompanied by serious complications, with a mortality rate ranging from 15% to 30%.

3. If the patients survive the pancreatitis, they are at risk of exocrine and endocrine pancreatic insufficiency.

Q5.21

This is a 60-year-old male who had surgery.

1. What is seen in the x-ray?
2. What is the diagnosis?
3. What was his clinical presentation?
4. What surgery was performed?

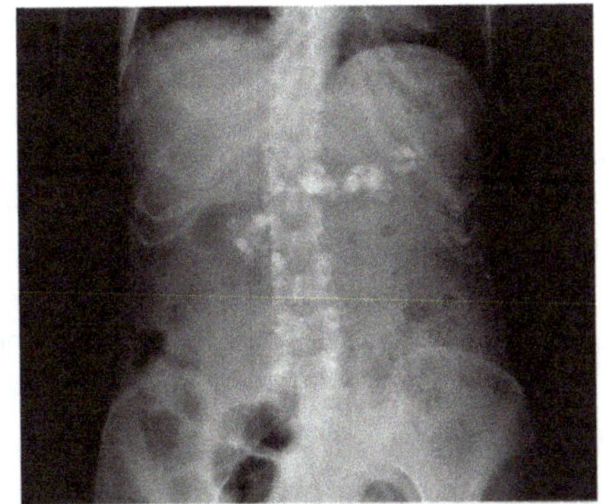

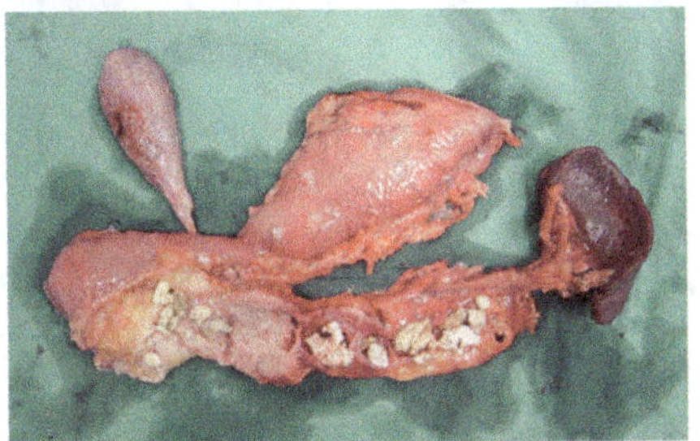

Q5.22

This is a 50-year-old male who recovered from pancreatitis 6 months ago.

1. What is the pathology seen in the CT scan?
2. What is the diagnosis?
3. What is the likely clinical presentation?
4. What is the management?
5. What procedure was performed as seen in the ultrasound?

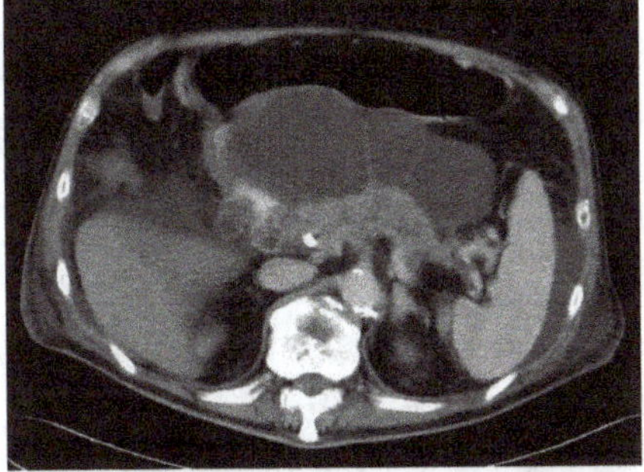

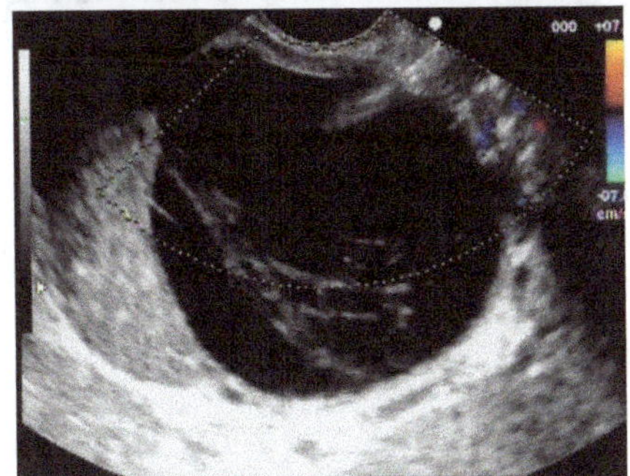

A5.21

1. There are multiple calculi seen in the pancreas.

2. Chronic pancreatitis with calculus formation.

3. Recurrent episodes of abdominal pain radiating to the back. The pain is caused by obstruction of pancreatic ducts and its branches by the calculi leading to ductal hypertension.
   He may have exocrine and endocrine impairment with pancreatic parenchymal damage.

4. Total pancreatectomy with removal of the gallbladder, distal stomach, duodenum and spleen.

A5.22

1. There is a homogenous hypodense lesion with internal septations anterior to the pancreas.

2. Pancreatic pseudocyst. It is fluid collection that is surrounded by a non-epithelialized wall made up of fibrous and granulation tissue.

3. Symptoms are often non-specific. A large pseudocyst may cause vague upper abdominal pain, dyspepsia symptoms or early satiety as it compresses the stomach.

4. If asymptomatic, the patient can be monitored with surveillance imaging.
   If symptomatic or the cyst is increasing in size, decompression of the cyst is recommended.

5. Endoscopic ultrasound (EUS) drainage of the cyst.

Q5.23

This is a 65-year-old female who had investigations for an elevated CA 19-9.

1. What is CA 19-9?

2. What does the PET MRI show?

3. What is the likely clinical presentation?

4. What procedure was performed with the ultrasound?

5. What is the differential diagnosis?

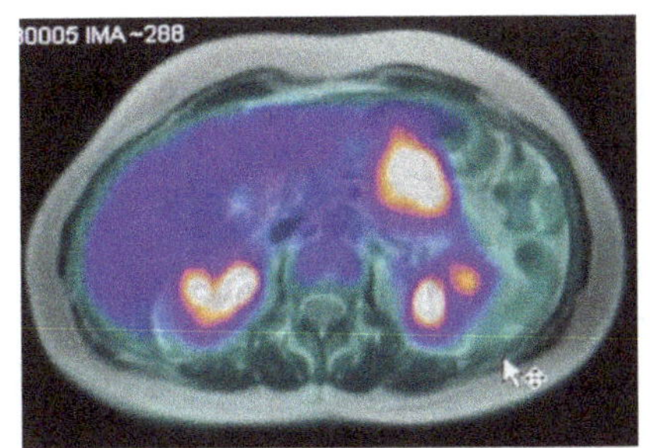

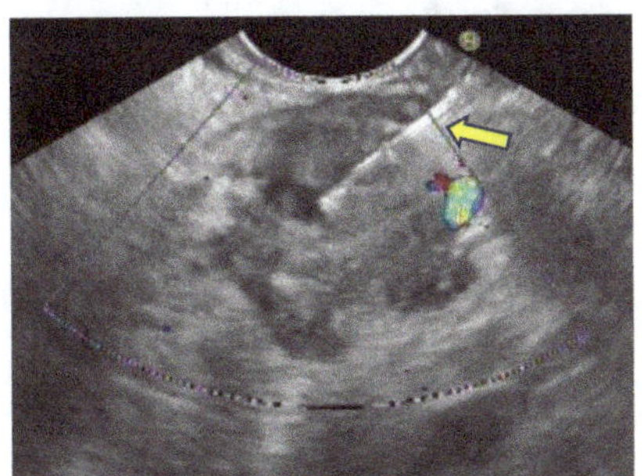

Q5.24

This is a 60-year-old female.

1. What is seen on the CT scan?

2. What is the likely clinical presentation?

3. What is the diagnosis?

4. What is the management?

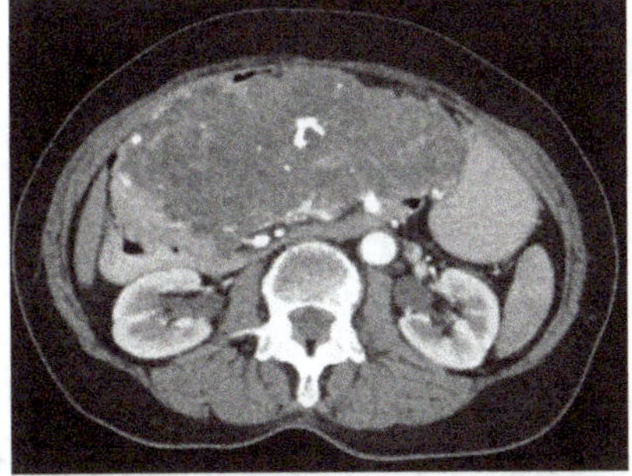

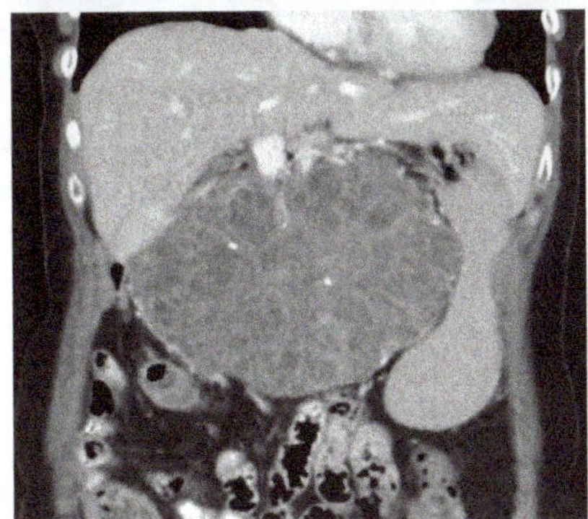

A5.23

1. Carbohydrate antigen (CA) 19-9 is a type of antigen released by pancreatic cancer cells.

2. There is a lesion in the distal pancreas that is FDG avid.

3. Patients are often asymptomatic.

4. Fine needle biopsy of the lesion was performed through the stomach via endoscopic ultrasound. (The needle is seen arrowed).

5. Pancreatic adenocarcinoma or invasive intraductal papillary mucinous neoplasm.

A5.24

1. There is a large complex cystic mass in the pancreas with multiple internal septations ("honeycomb like") and coarse calcifications. The normal pancreas parenchyma is almost completely replaced.

2. She would experience early satiety and upper abdominal discomfort. Clinical examination of the abdomen would reveal a palpable mass in the upper abdomen.

3. Serous cystic adenoma of the pancreas.

4. Surgical resection is considered if it is resectable.

6 Head and Neck

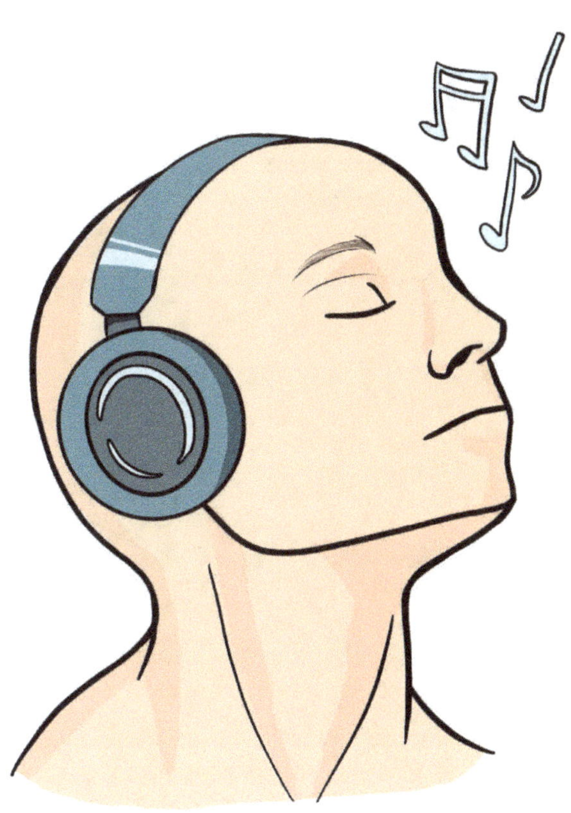

Q6.1

This 50-year-old female presented with a right neck lump. She experiences pain when eating.

1. What is the diagnosis?
2. What is the likely cause?
3. What physical examination can we perform to further evaluate the lump?
4. What is the management?

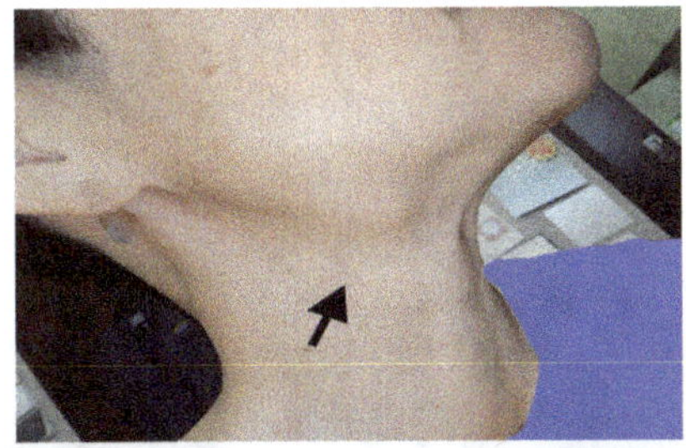

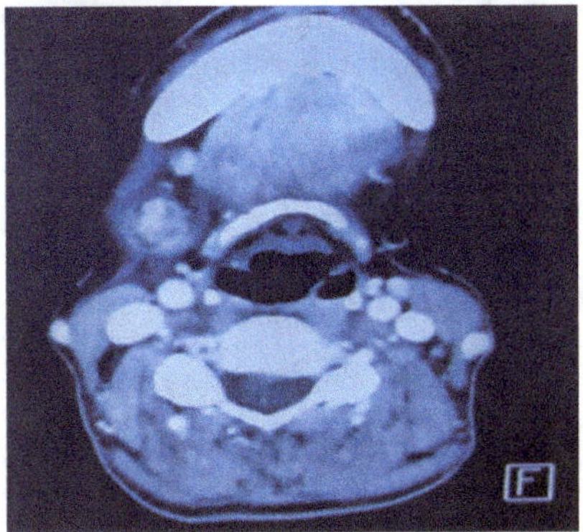

Q6.2

This is a 48-year-old man with a lump that fluctuates in size.

1. What is seen in the 2 pictures?
2. What is the most likely diagnosis?
3. What is the pathophysiology of this lesion?
4. What is the management?

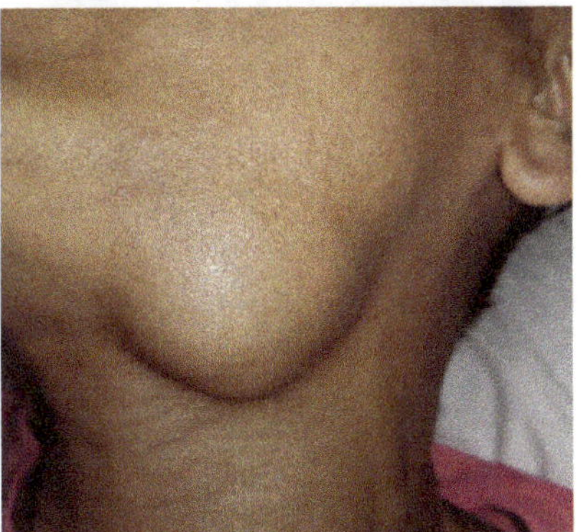

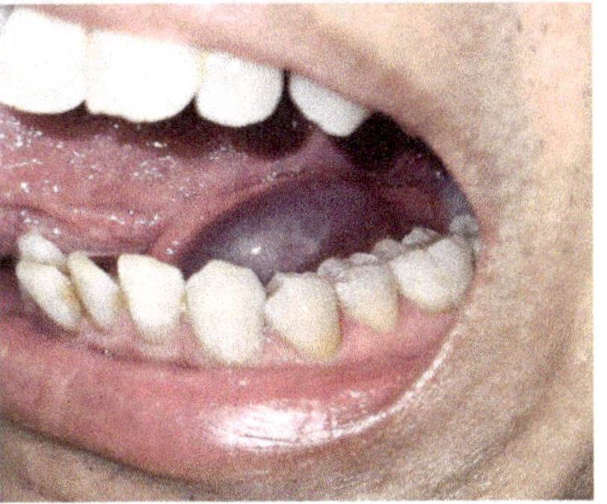

A6.1

1. An inflamed right submandibular gland (sialadenitis).

2. There is a blockage of the salivary duct (Wharton's duct) by a stone (sialolithiasis).

3. Bimanual examination (between the floor of the mouth and below the jaw) will confirm the size of the gland, elicit tenderness and possibly palpate a stone in the duct.

4. A single episode can be managed conservatively. Repeated episodes of inflammation may warrant surgical removal of the submandibular gland.

A6.2

1. There is a smooth round lesion arising from the lower border of his left jaw. Within the oral cavity, there is a bluish lesion arising from the left base of his tongue.

2. A mucocele or oral ranula.

3. Ranulas can form as a result of partial obstruction of a sublingual duct, leading to formation of an epithelial-lined retention cyst.

4. Mucoceles and ranulas may spontaneously resolve.
   Sclerotherapy: with OK-432 or bleomycin.
   Surgical: marsupialization (unroofing the cyst and tacking the edges of the cyst to adjacent tissue) or excision with its associated salivary gland.

Q6.3

This is a 70-year-old man.

1. Describe the pathology seen.
2. What is the most likely diagnosis?
3. What are other clinical symptoms?
4. What are the cell types?
5. What is the management?

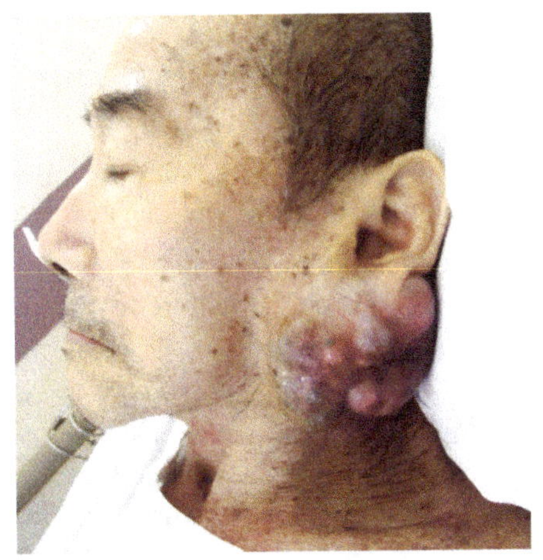

Q6.4

This is a 70-year-old man.

1. Describe the lesion seen.
2. What organ is it arising from?
3. What are possible pathologies?
4. What surgery was performed and what anatomical structure needs to be preserved?

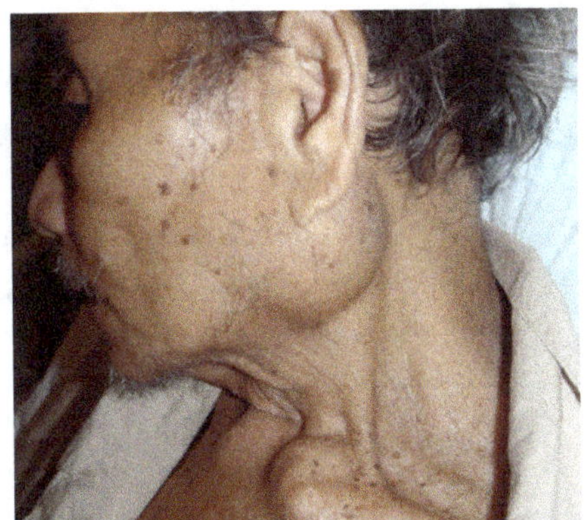

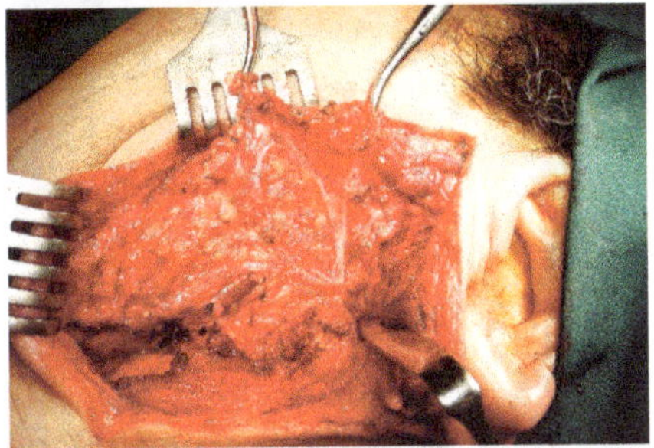

A6.3

1. There is a multilobulated mass inferior to his left ear lobe. There are overlying skin changes.

2. Parotid cancer.

3. The tumour grows rapidly. It may be painful with ipsilateral facial paralysis.

4. Mucoepidermoid, adenoid cystic carcinoma, acinic cell, adenocarcinoma, squamous cell, undifferentiated carcinoma and carcinoma ex-pleomorphic adenoma.

5. Complete surgical resection followed, by radiation therapy (when indicated). Conservative excisions are plagued by a high rate of local recurrence. The extent of resection is based on tumour histology, tumour size and location, invasion of local structures, and the status of regional nodal basins.

A6.4

1. There is a smooth mass arising at the angle of the mandible just under the left ear lobe.

2. The parotid gland.

3. Pleomorphic adenoma and Warthin's tumour.

4. Most tumours of the parotid (approximately 90%) originate in the superficial lobe. Superficial parotidectomy with preservation of the facial nerve was performed.

Q6.5

This is a 70-year-old man with a pulsatile lump in the right side of his neck.

1. What is the diagnosis?
2. What is the clinical presentation?
3. What is seen on the CT angiogram?
4. What further investigations can be performed?
5. What is the management?

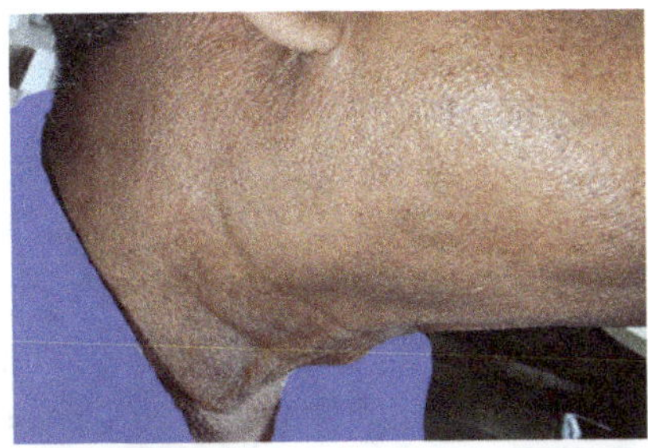

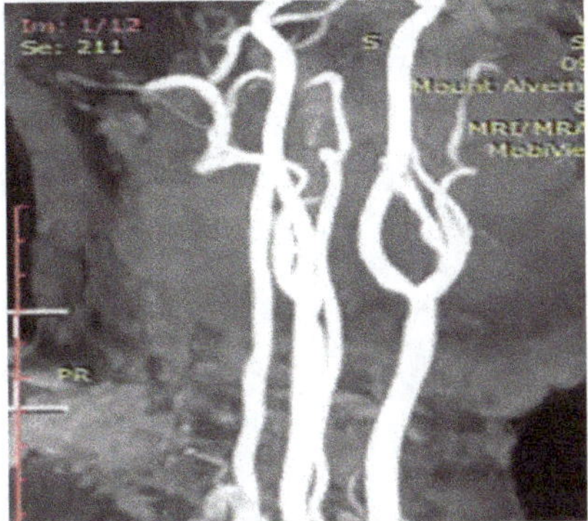

Q6.6

This is a 60-year-old man.

1. Describe what is seen in the neck.
2. What are differential diagnoses?
3. How can we confirm the diagnosis?

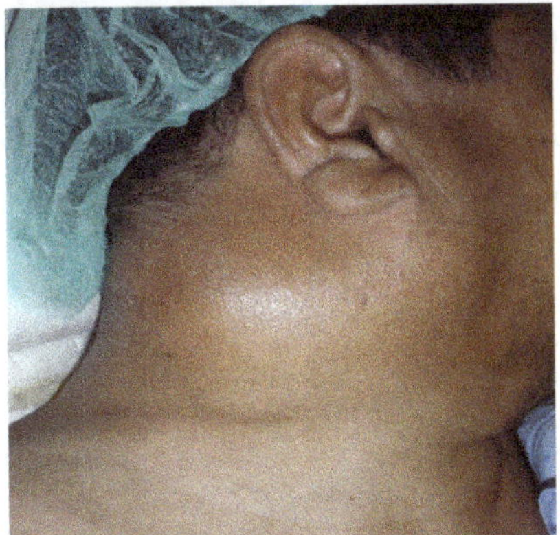

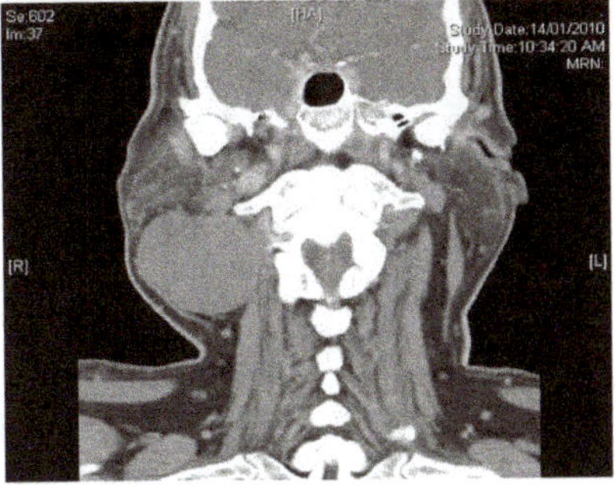

A6.5

1. Carotid body tumour (CBT).

2. It is commonly an asymptomatic palpable slow-growing mass in the anterior triangle of the neck. Characteristically, the tumour can be moved side to side but not up or down, due to its location within the carotid sheath.

3. There is splaying of the internal carotid and external carotid arteries.

4. Urinary catecholamines can be checked to exclude a functional CBT.

5. Surgery is usually the treatment modality of choice for younger, healthier patients with CBTs, and radiotherapy is reserved for elderly patients who are poor surgical candidates.

A6.6

1. There is a large mass arising in the upper neck lifting the earlobe.

2. Parotid tumour or cervical lymphadenopathy (primary or secondary).

3. Obtain histology with a biopsy. This patient had lymphoma.

Q6.7

This is a 60-year-old man.

1. What is the pathology seen?
2. What is the aetiology?
3. How are they classified?
4. What is the management?

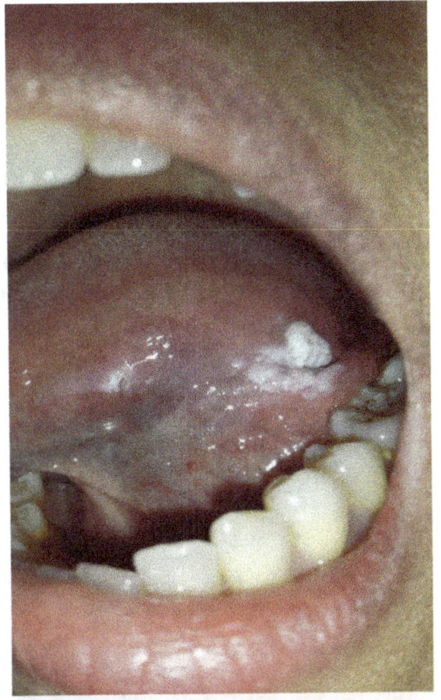

Q6.8

This is a 60-year-old man.

1. What is the diagnosis?
2. What are risk factors?
3. What is the likely cell type?
4. What is the clinical presentation?
5. What surgery was performed?

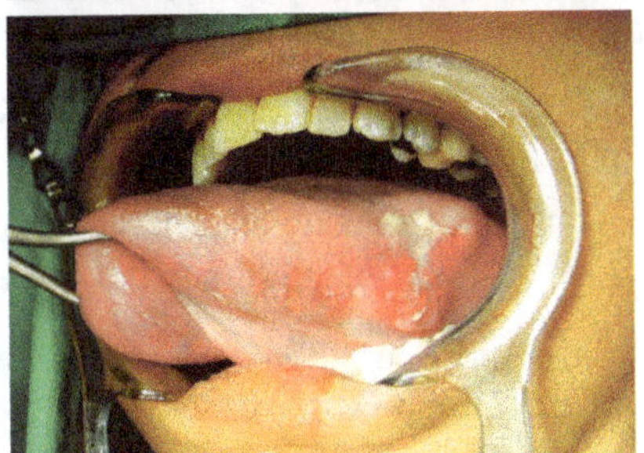

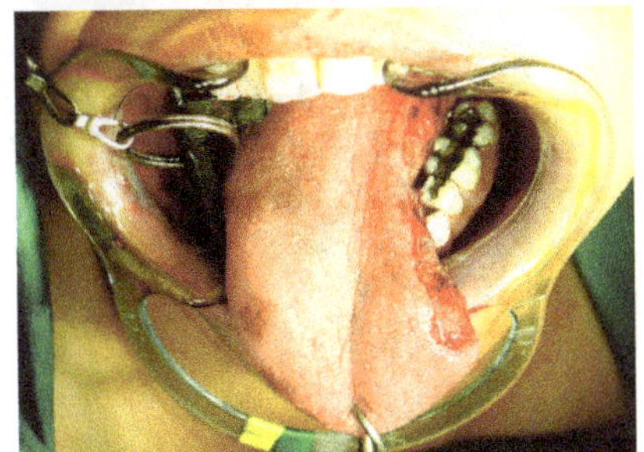

A6.7

1. Leukoplakia on the left side of the tongue.

2. The aetiology of most cases is unknown (idiopathic). Factors associated with it include tobacco use, alcohol consumption, chronic irritation, candidiasis, vitamin deficiency, endocrine disturbances, and possibly a viral infection.

3. Homogenous leukoplakia: most common, uniformly white plaques that are usually asymptomatic in nature. Low malignant potential.
    Non-homogenous leukoplakia: speckled or verrucous. Highest risk of malignant transformation.

4. Eliminate all contributing factors.
    Surgical excision or laser surgery of the lesions.
    Close surveillance and follow-up.

A6.8

1. Tongue cancer. There is an ulcerative mass on the lateral aspect of the tongue.

2. Smoking, drinking alcohol, and, human papilloma virus infection.

3. 90% of these neoplasms are squamous cell carcinomas.

4. The most common symptom is localized pain. They present with palpable neck lymphadenopathy.

5. Left Hemiglossectomy.
    Early-stage tongue carcinoma (T1 or T2) can be treated successfully with single-modality therapy, namely surgery or radiation.
    Patients with advanced disease (T3 or T4) have a poor response to single-modality treatment, hence surgery and postoperative chemoradiation would be recommended.

Q6.9

This is a 60-year-old man who presents with hoarseness of voice for 3 months.

1. What is seen in the CT scan?

2. What is the likely diagnosis?

3. How common is it?

4. What are other clinical presentations?

5. What is seen in the surgical picture?

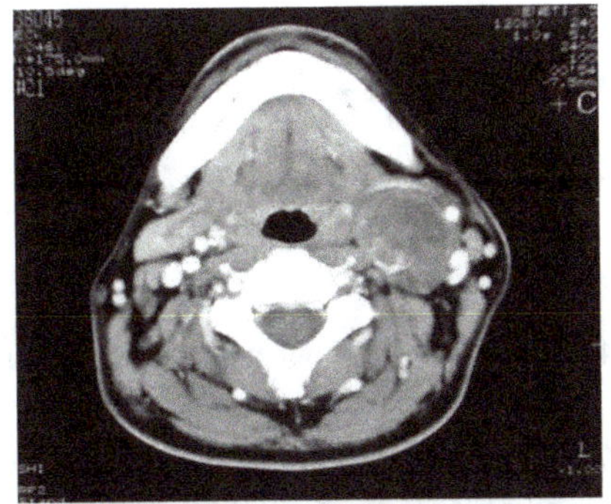

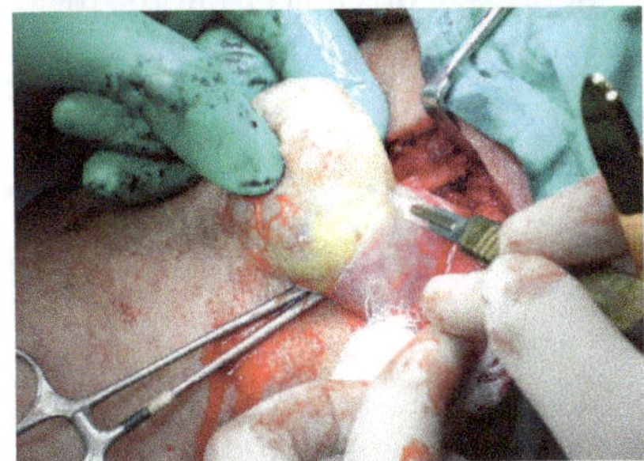

Q6.10

This is a 45-year-old man with a midline neck mass that moves with swallowing and moves up with tongue protrusion.

1. What is the diagnosis?

2. What is its aetiology?

3. What is its clinical presentation?

4. What surgery has been performed?

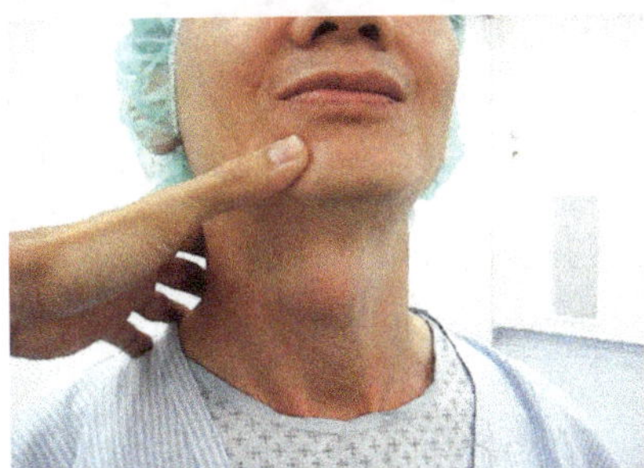

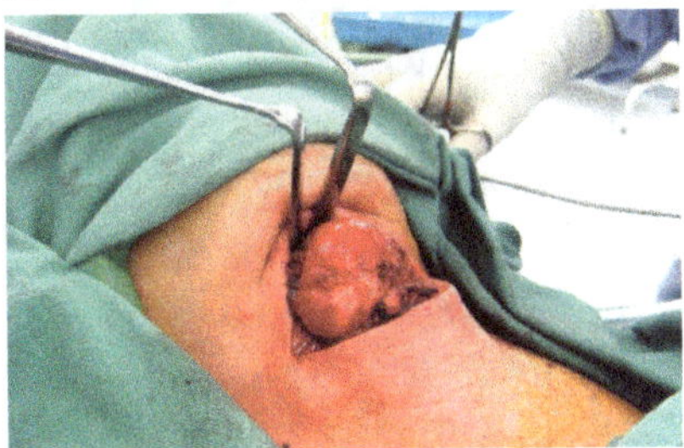

A6.9

1. There is a large well-circumscribed mass in the left side of the neck deep to the carotid vessels.

2. Nerve tumours arising from the vagus nerve, most probably a schwannoma. Hoarseness of voice would suggest recurrent laryngeal nerve involvement.

3. It is rare.

4. Patients may have paroxysmal cough during palpation of the mass due to vagal stimulation.

5. It is a benign tumour. Intracapsular enucleation of the tumour is the surgical approach of choice. Efforts to ensure nerve preservation during surgical excision are mandatory.

A6.10

1. Thyroglossal cyst.

2. A thyroglossal duct cyst is an embryologic remnant that forms due to the failure of closure of the thyroglossal duct extending from the foramen cecum in the tongue to the thyroid's location in the neck.

3. They are often asymptomatic. However, they can present as an abscess or intermittently draining sinus.

4. Thyroglossal duct cysts are surgically removed to prevent recurrent infections.
   The Sistrunk procedure is the resection of the cyst and its tract to the base of tongue. It includes removing the central third of the hyoid bone where the tract runs behind.

Q6.11

This is a 40-year-old lady who presented with a blocked right nostril.

1. What is seen at endoscopy of her right nostril?

2. What is seen on the right aspect of her neck?

3. What is the diagnosis and how can we confirm it?

4. What is the cancer cell type and who are at risk?

5. What are other possible clinical presentations of this disease?

6. What is the management?

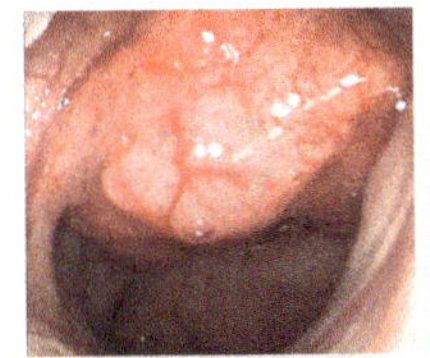
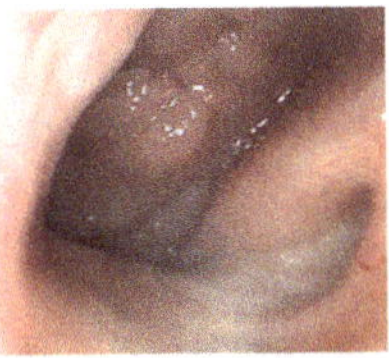
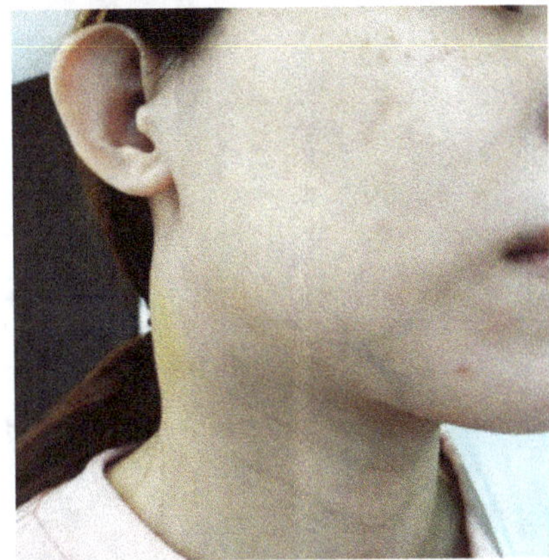

Q6.12

This is a 25-year-old female.

1. What is the abnormality seen?

2. What is seen in the CT scan?

3. What is the diagnosis?

4. What is the aetiology?

5. What is the clinical presentation?

6. What is the management?

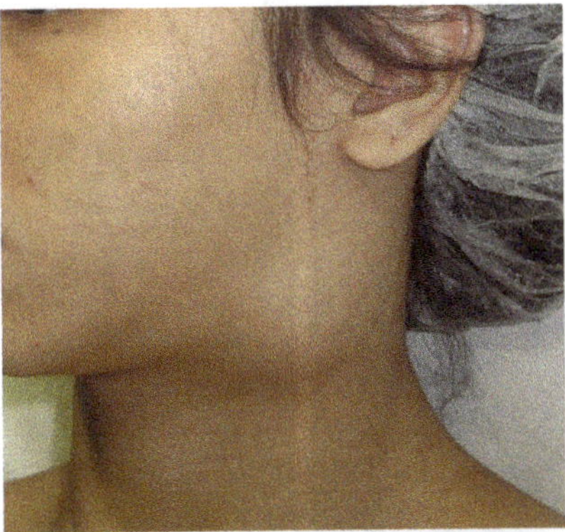
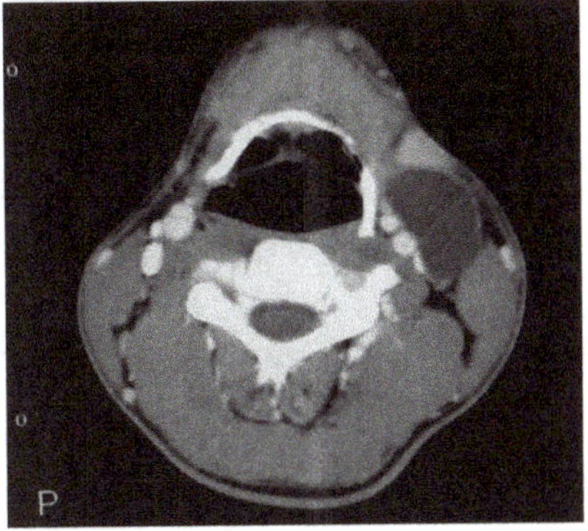

A6.11

1. There is a hyper-vascular tumour.

2. There is obliteration of the empty space between the angle of the mandible and upper sternocleidomastoid muscle, suggestive of enlarged level 2 cervical lymph nodes.

3. Nasopharyngeal carcinoma, which can be confirmed with a biopsy.

4. Squamous cell carcinoma. Chinese ethnicity and exposure to Epstein-Barr virus.

5. Most cases present at an advanced stage with palpable neck nodal metastasis. Associated symptoms such as hoarseness or voice changes, dysphagia or odynophagia, otalgia, nasal obstruction (unilateral versus bilateral), epistaxis, haemoptysis, hematemesis, diplopia, headache or facial pain, and persistent rhinorrhoea.

6. Nonsurgical treatment for nasopharyngeal carcinoma includes radiation therapy, chemotherapy, or a combination of modalities, depending on the stage of the tumour.

A6.12

1. There is a mass arising at the angle of his left jaw.

2. There is a cystic mass arising anterior to the sternocleidomastoid muscle superficial to the carotid vessels.

3. Branchial cleft cyst.

4. Branchial cleft anomalies form due to the incomplete involution of branchial cleft structures.

5. Branchial cleft cysts are often asymptomatic but can often become tender, enlarged, or inflamed with superinfection or abscess formation during episodes of upper respiratory tract infections. A fistula tract may develop.

6. The treatment of a branchial cleft cyst is excision due to the risk of infection and further enlargement.

Q6.13

This is a 70-year-old man.

1. What is seen in his oral cavity?
2. What is the diagnosis?
3. What are risk factors?
4. What is the clinical presentation?
5. What is the management?

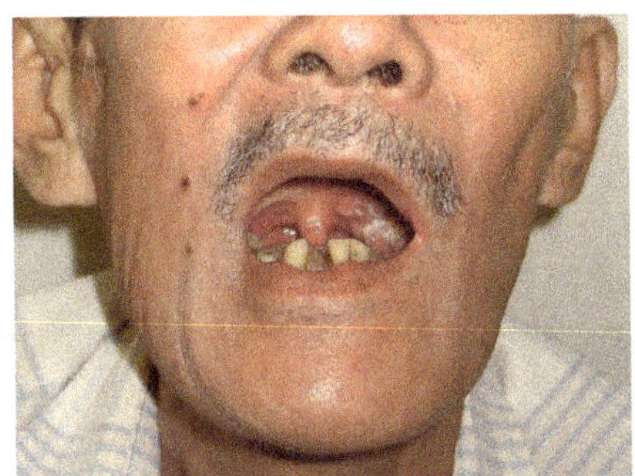

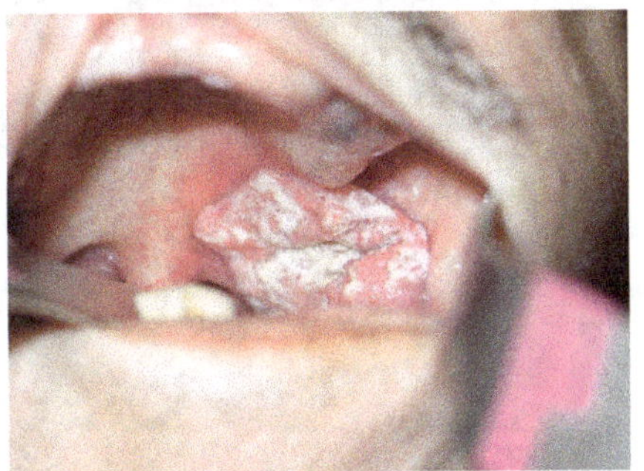

Q6.14

This is a 70-year-old man.

1. What surgery has been performed for this patient?
2. What is the purpose of the surgery?
3. What are variations of this surgery?
4. What are complications of this surgery?

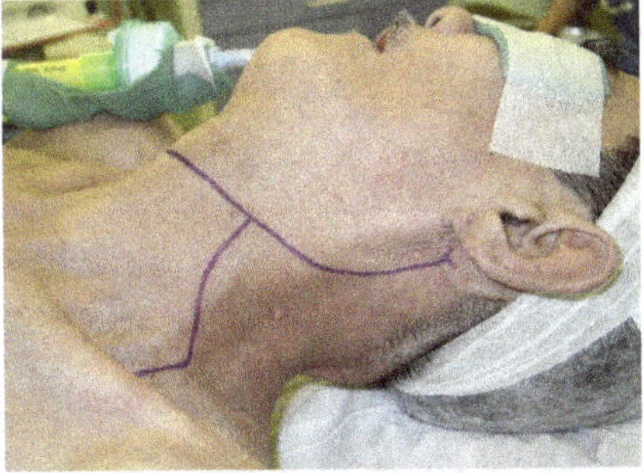

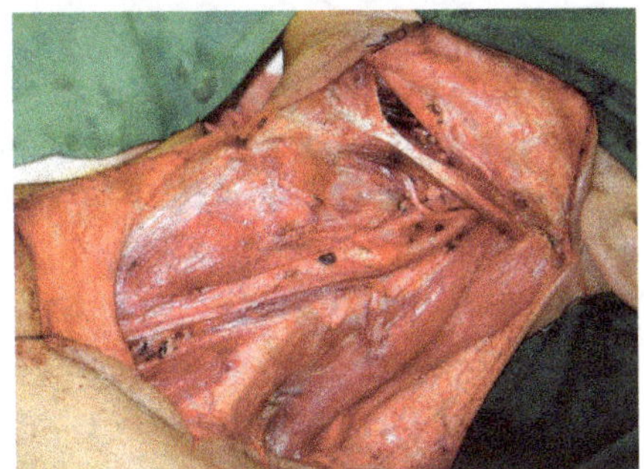

A6.13

1. There is a fungating tumour arising from the left tonsil.

2. Left tonsil cancer. It is the most common form of oropharyngeal malignancy.

3. Smoking and exposure to human papillomavirus (HPV). Its incidence is sharply rising due to the increasing prevalence of HPV.

4. Patients may be asymptomatic and referred as an incidental finding of asymmetrical tonsils.
   Others may complain of a sore throat, unilateral otalgia, or sensation of a mass in the throat, with trismus being a concerning sign of local invasion.

5. Early cancers are treated with single modality treatment — surgical excision or radiotherapy.
   Advanced cancers will need a combination of surgery and chemoradiotherapy.

A6.14

1. Radical neck dissection.

2. The procedure removes all lymph nodes in the lateral neck (levels I–V) the spinal accessory nerve (CN XI), internal jugular vein (IJV), sternocleidomastoid muscle (SCM).

3. Selective neck dissection is performed of the appropriate nodal basins based on the tumour's location.
   Modified radical neck dissection (MRND) are classified as type I, II, or III based on which structures (CN XI, IJV and SCM) are preserved.

4. Haemorrhage from major vessels, chyle fistula, pneumothorax, and damage to multiple nerves (particularly CN VII, CN X–XII, sympathetic chain, the brachial plexus, phrenic nerve, and lingual nerve).

Q6.15

This is a 50-year-old man.

1. Describe the lesion seen.
2. What is the diagnosis?
3. What is the clinical presentation?
4. What is the natural history of these lesions?
5. What is the management?

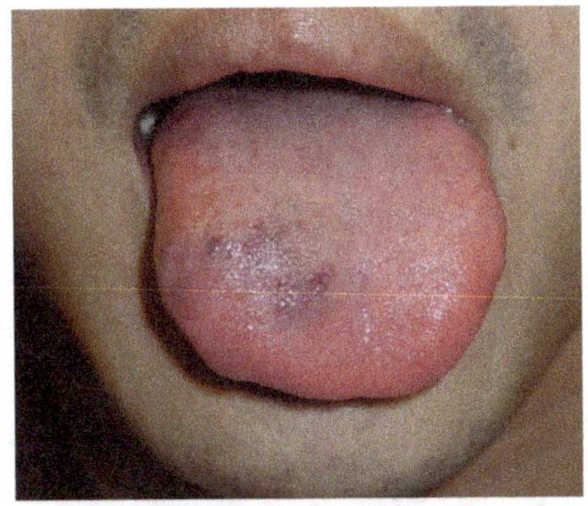

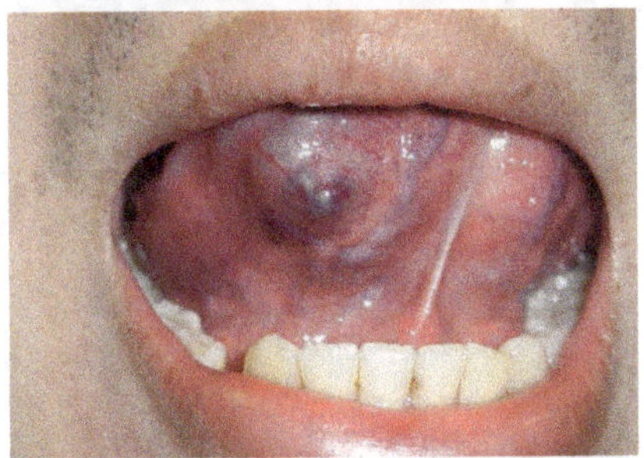

Q6.16

This is a 40-year-old male.

1. What is seen in the picture?
2. What is the diagnosis?
3. What is its aetiology?
4. What is the management?

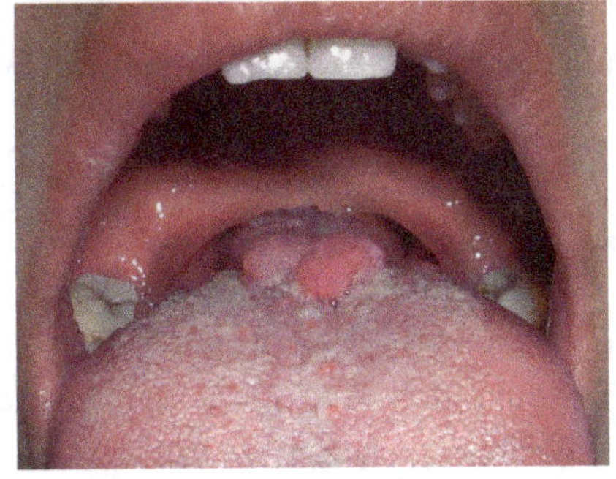

A6.15

1. There is a smooth purplish round lesion arising on the right side of the tongue's surface, which extends posteriorly. The mucosa of the tongue is preserved.

2. Haemangioma.

3. Smaller lesions are painless and asymptomatic.
   Larger lesions bleed easily with minimal trauma or cause speech impairment. The lesions are soft and compressible.

4. There is rapid growth in the early years, followed by a period of stabilization. In the later years, the lesions may enter a phase of spontaneous involution.

5. For lesions that persist into adulthood or are symptomatic, treatment is recommended.
   Medical: beta-blockers.
   Sclerotherapy: injection of a foreign agent into one of the major vessels of the lesion to cause endothelial damage and obliterate the lumen.
   Surgical resection of the lesion.

A6.16

1. There is a pinkish multilobulated lesion at the base of the tongue. There is no bleeding or ulceration.

2. It is a benign squamous cell papilloma.

3. It is a precancerous lesion of viral origin caused by the Human papilloma virus (HPV), types 6 and 11.

4. While most cases require no treatment, therapy options include cryotherapy, application of a topical salicylic acid compound, surgical excision and laser ablation.

Q6.17

This is a 70-year-old man.

1. What surgery was performed?
2. What would be his clinical presentation?
3. What is the "hole" in the neck?
4. How is he able to speak after the surgery?

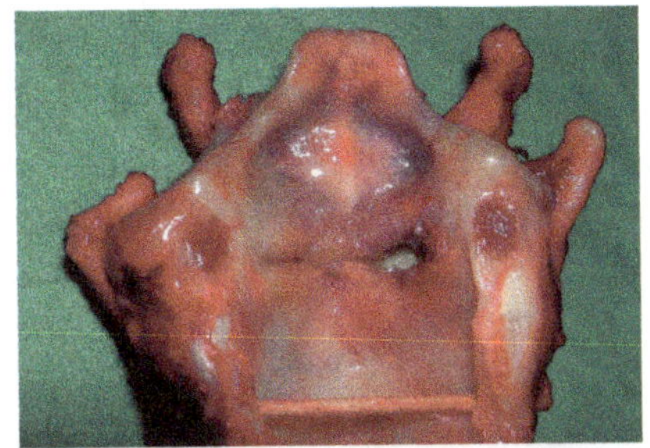

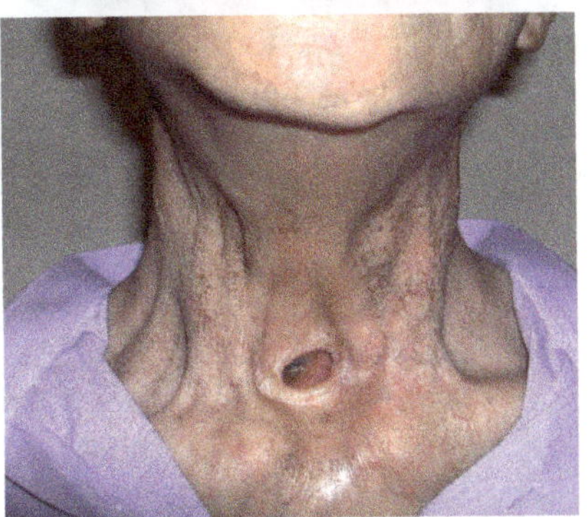

Q6.18

This is a 30-year-old female with a lingual thyroid.

1. Describe the abnormality seen.
2. How can we confirm the diagnosis?
3. What is its aetiology?
4. What is the clinical presentation?

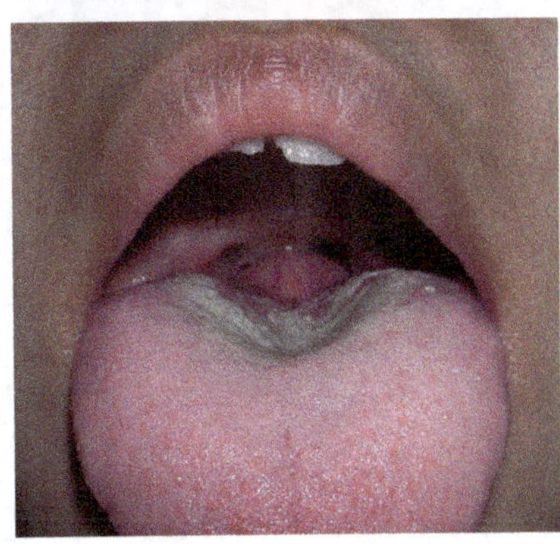

A6.17

1. A laryngectomy for a cancer of the larynx. It involves the removal of all supraglottic, glottic, and subglottic tissue from the tongue base to the superior trachea.

2. Hoarseness is the most common presenting symptom of glottic cancers due to vocal cord immobility or fixation. Pain with swallowing is the most common early symptom of supraglottic cancer.

3. A tracheostomy.

4. Tracheo-oesophageal puncture (TEP) with a voice prosthesis is the most common way to restore speech after a laryngectomy.

A6.18

1. There is a pinkish lesion at the base of the tongue.

2. Scintigraphy (radioactive iodine scan) will confirm the location of the functioning lingual thyroid and demonstrate the absence of the thyroid gland in the neck.

3. Normally the thyroid gland descends along a path from foramen cecum in the tongue to its final position in front of the trachea. The failure of migration of thyroid tissue along the path from ventral floor of the pharynx to its normal location, and sequestration within the tongue substance leads to the development of lingual thyroid.

4. Most lingual thyroids are small and asymptomatic. Large ones can cause dysphagia, dysphonia, cough, snoring, sensation of foreign body, sleep apnoea, bleeding and dyspnoea.
    Some may have hypothyroidism.

7 Endocrine

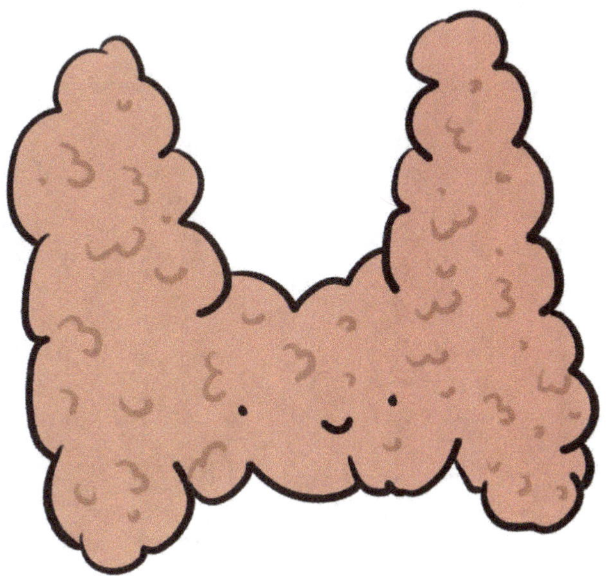

Q7.1

This is a 75-year-old female with a lump in the neck.

1. How can we ascertain whether the lump originates from the thyroid on clinical examination?

2. What could the contents of the lump be?

3. What investigation can we perform to determine whether it is benign or malignant?

4. What important structure (arrowed) is identified and preserved during surgery?

5. What morbidity would occur if the structure is damaged?

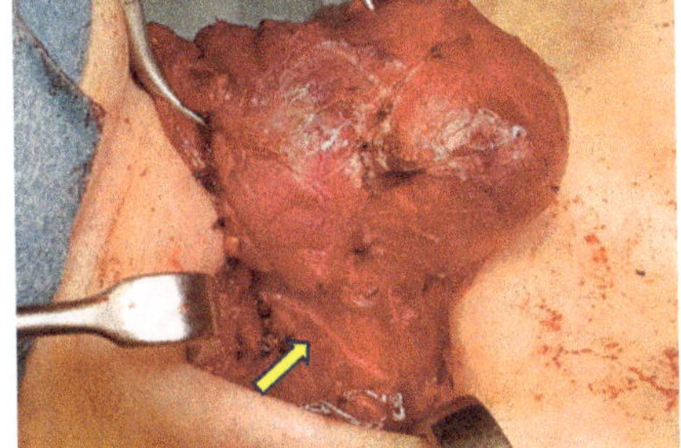

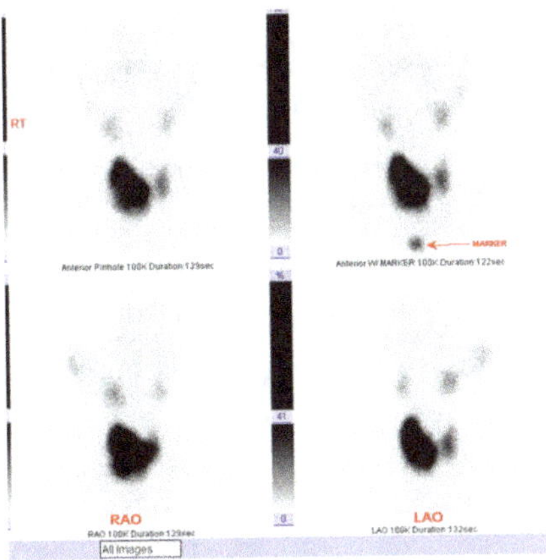

Q7.2

This is a 55-year-old female with a goitre.

1. What scan was performed?

2. What is the diagnosis?

3. What is the clinical presentation?

4. What is the management?

A7.1

1. The thyroid gland moves with swallowing. If the lump moves with swallowing, it is a lump originating from the thyroid gland.

2. It can be solid or cystic.

3. Needle biopsy to obtain cytology.

4. Recurrent laryngeal nerve.

5. Ipsilateral vocal cord paralysis.

A7.2

1. Nuclear scintigraphy was performed with radioactive iodine-123 or technetium-99m.

2. Solitary right toxic nodule of the thyroid gland. The left lobe has relative lower uptake.

3. She would present with an enlarged right thyroid nodule with signs and symptoms of hyperthyroidism.

4. Surgical removal of the right thyroid lobe would cure her hyperthyroidism.

Q7.3

This is a 70-year-old female.

1. What abnormality is seen in the picture?

2. What symptoms could she be experiencing?

3. What does the CT scan demonstrate?

4. What is a potential complication post-surgery?

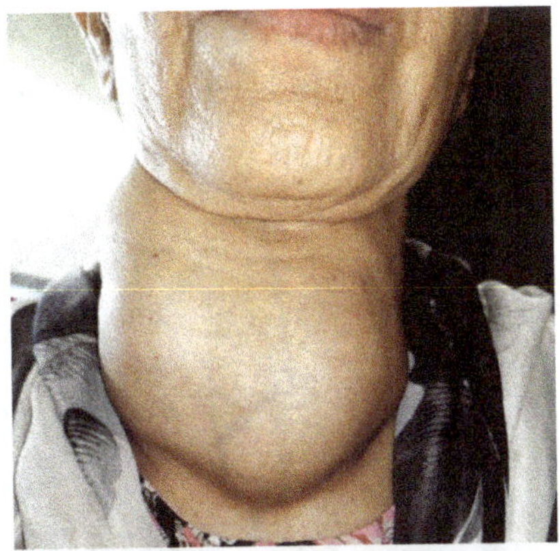

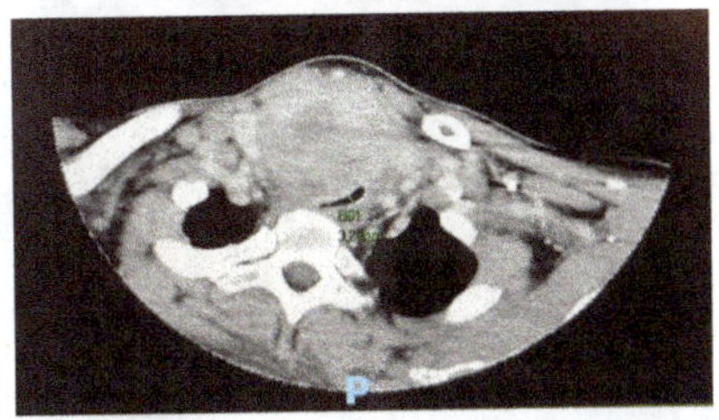

Q7.4

This is a 50-year-old female.

1. What is the abnormality on the CT scan?

2. What is the diagnosis based on the surgical specimen?

3. What is the likely clinical presentation?

4. What clinical manoeuvre is useful in diagnosis for this patient?

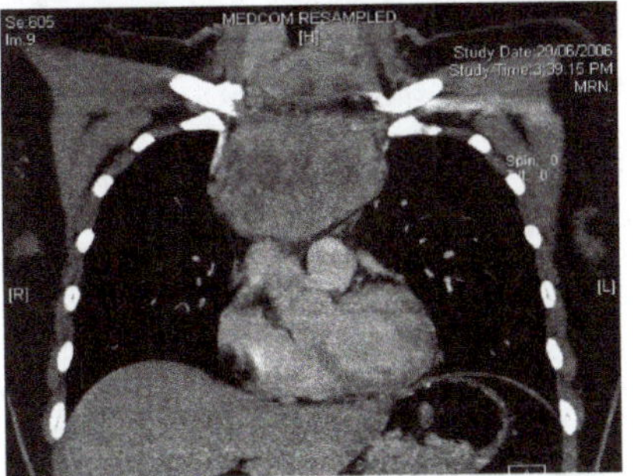

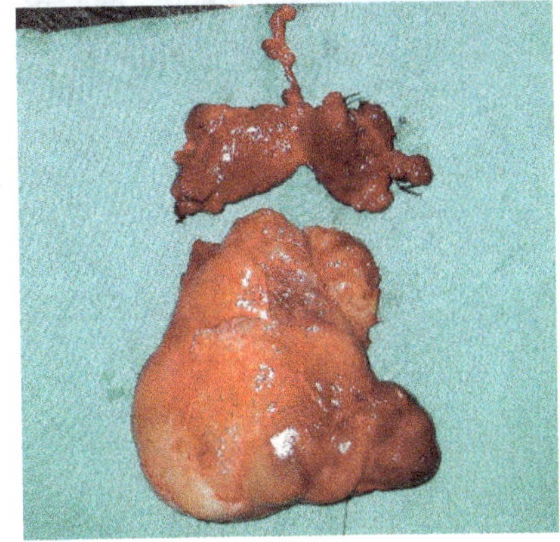

A7.3

1. There is a large multinodular thyroid gland.

2. Compression on the adjacent structures can cause dysphagia, dyspnoea and stridor.

3. A large goitre causing compression and severe narrowing of the trachea.

4. Tracheomalacia. The extrinsic compression by an enlarged thyroid gland over a prolonged period causes weakness of the tracheal wall due to softening of supporting tracheal cartilage, causing the trachea to collapse.

A7.4

1. There is a large mass in the superior mediastinum.

2. Retrosternal goitre. The larger retrosternal component corresponds to the findings on the CT scan.

3. Patients are often asymptomatic. The pathology is usually incidentally detected on radiological investigations. Large ones can cause dyspnoea, choking sensation, cough, and dysphagia. Progressive hoarseness, stridor, and superior vena cava syndrome are less common.

4. A Pemberton manoeuvre can indicate the presence of superior vena cava syndrome: The manoeuvre is performed by having the patient elevate both arms until they touch each side of their face. A positive Pemberton sign indicates compression at the thoracic outlet and is demonstrated by facial congestion, cyanosis, and/or respiratory compromise after 1 minute.

Q7.5

This is a 35-year-old female.

1. Describe what you see in the pictures.

2. What is the diagnosis?

3. What investigations can we use to confirm it?

4. What symptoms would she be experiencing?

5. What other eye problems could she have?

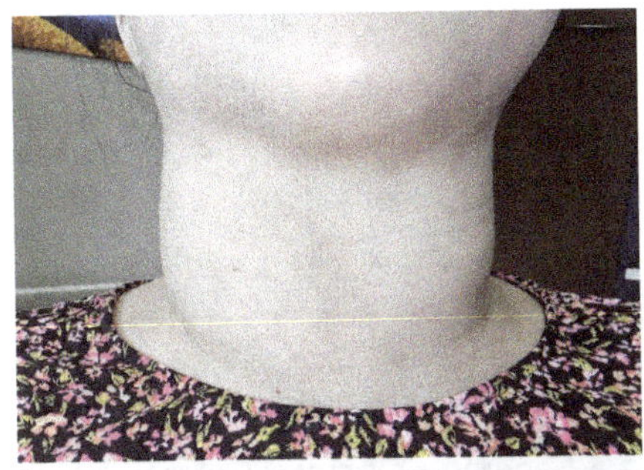

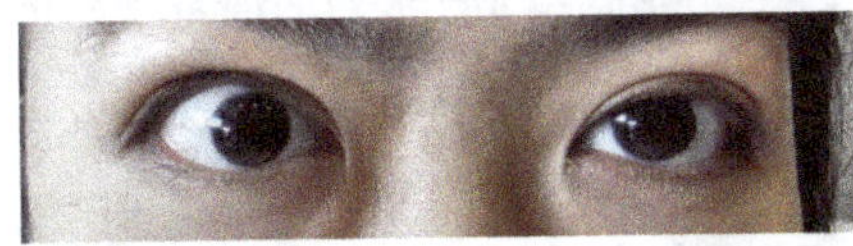

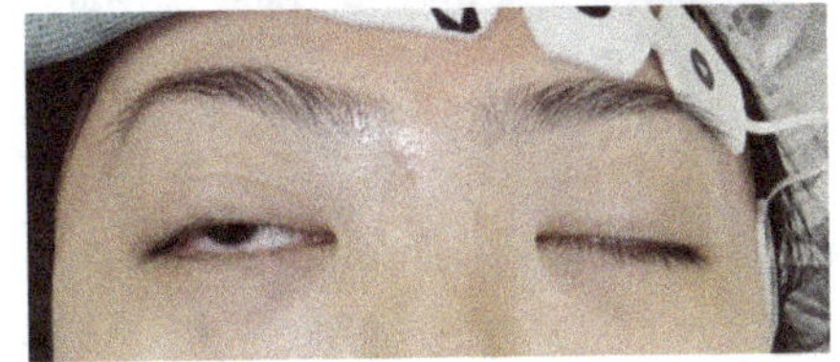

Q7.6

This 16-year-old girl had a total thyroidectomy 2 days ago. She presents with chest tightness and muscle discomfort.

1. What surgical complication has occurred and what clinical sign does she exhibit?

2. What is the pathophysiology?

3. How can we confirm the diagnosis?

4. How common is it?

5. What other clinical sign can we elicit?

6. How can we manage the problem?

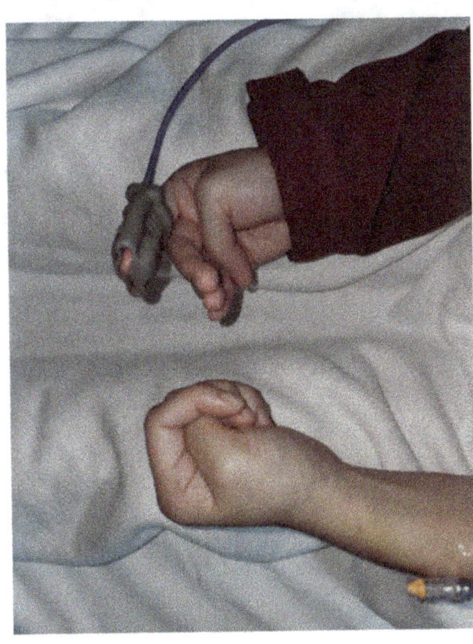

A7.5

1. She has a diffuse enlarged goitre. There is thyroid eye disease with proptosis affecting the right eye more than the left. She is unable to close her right eye fully (lagophthalmos) when she is asleep.

2. Graves' disease. It is an autoimmune disorder characterized by hyperthyroidism due to circulating autoantibodies.

3. Elevated thyroid function tests and assays for TSH-receptor antibodies are positive.

4. General — increased basal metabolic rate, weight loss despite increased appetite.
   Skin — increased sweating, fine hair, vitiligo, alopecia, pretibial myxoedema.
   Heart — tachycardia, irregular heart rate.
   Psychiatric — restlessness, anxiety, irritability, insomnia.
   Neurologic — hand tremor, hyperactive deep tendon reflexes.

5. In Graves', the periorbital tissues are attacked, causing inflammation and swelling.
   Decreased vision can occur when swollen tissues compress on the optic nerve. The extraocular muscles can be involved, leading to restriction of the normal eye movements, resulting in double vision.

A7.6

1. Trousseau's sign of latent tetany secondary to hypocalcaemia.

2. Inadvertent injury to the four parathyroid glands has occurred leading to hypoparathyroidism and hypocalcaemia.

3. Low serum parathyroid hormone and calcium levels.

4. It occurs in 1–5% of total thyroidectomies.

5. Chvostek's sign. The facial muscles twitch after the facial nerve is tapped lightly on the upper cheek.

6. Calcium replacement — intravenous and oral.

Q7.7

This is a 40-year-old female diagnosed with papillary thyroid cancer (PTC). There is no associated neck lymphadenopathy.

1. What abnormality is seen in the ultrasound of the thyroid gland?

2. How was the cancer confirmed?

3. What was performed for this patient as seen in the surgical picture?

4. What is the adjuvant management after surgery?

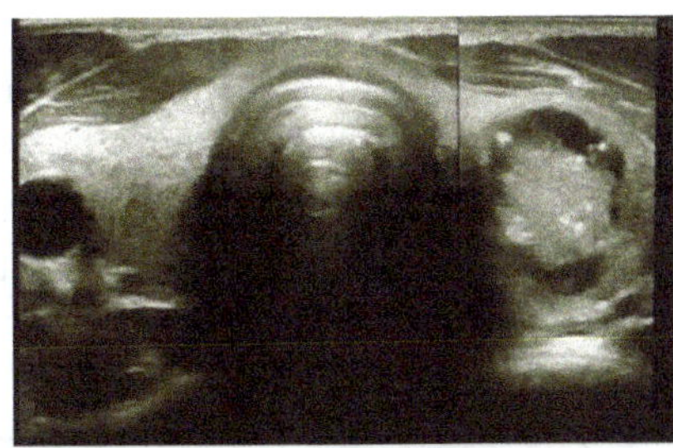

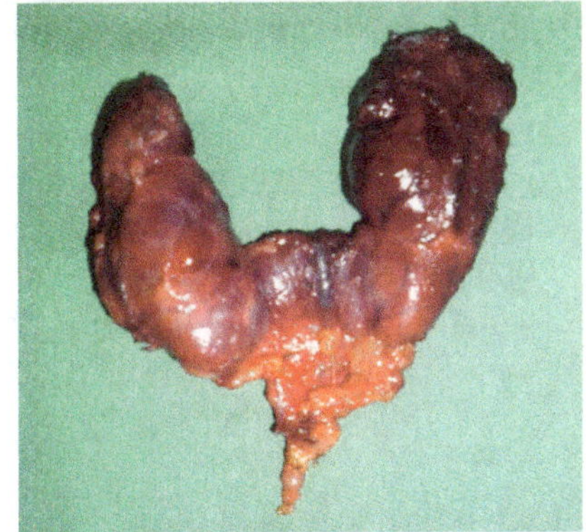

Q7.8

This is a 35-year-old female who had surgical removal of a right thyroid nodule.

1. What abnormality is seen on the pathology slides?

2. What is the diagnosis?

3. How does it commonly spread?

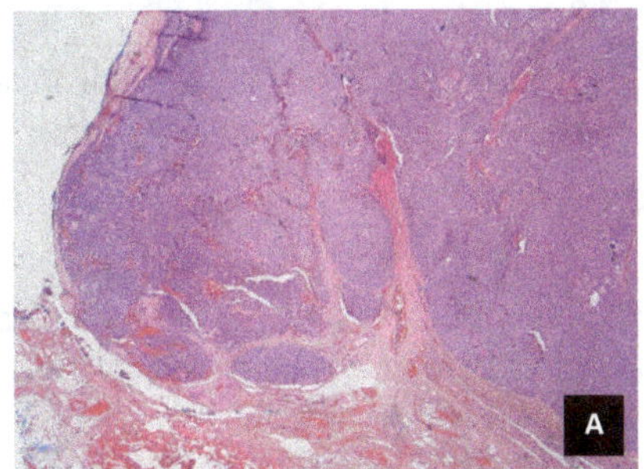

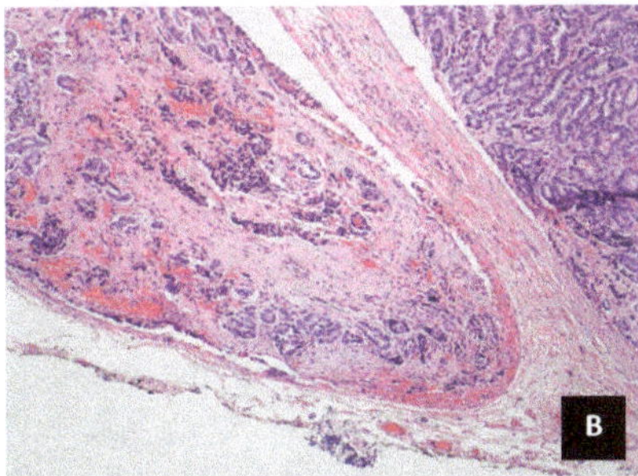

A7.7

1. There is a left thyroid nodule that is taller than it is wide. It has irregular borders with internal calcifications.

2. Fine needle aspiration cytology (FNAC) is the recommended method for diagnosing PTC with 95% sensitivity.
   Change in nuclear size and shape: nuclear enlargement, elongation and overlapping.
   Chromatin characteristics: chromatin clearing, margination and glassy nuclei.

3. Total thyroidectomy with left central level 6 lymph node dissection.

4. After thyroidectomy, radioiodine is used to ablate residual normal thyroid tissue. The patients will require lifelong thyroid hormone replacement, which will suppress TSH (TSH can promote the growth of remaining PTC cells). Patients will be monitored with serum thyroglobulin (TG). The TG would be undetectable after a total thyroidectomy. An elevated serum TG would suggest recurrence of the PTC.

A7.8

1. In picture A, there is capsular invasion of the thyroid nodule. In picture B, there is tumour vascular invasion.

2. Follicular thyroid cancer. It is not possible to diagnose it on cytology but by excision biopsy.

3. Because of its propensity for vascular invasion, it often spreads via the bloodstream to lungs and bones.

Q7.9

This patient just had a thyroidectomy.

1. What is seen in her neck?
2. What is seen in the drain?
3. What surgical complication has occurred?
4. What is the management?

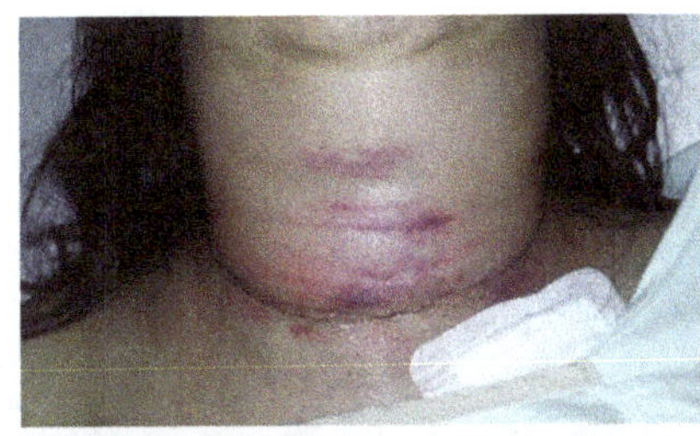

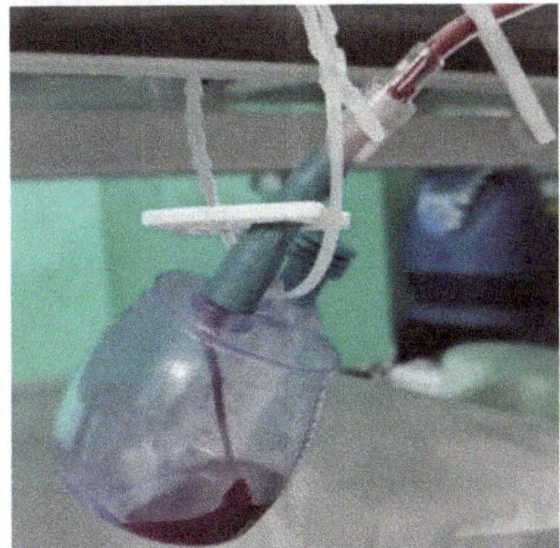

Q7.10

This is a 65-year-old male with a cancer in the left lobe of the thyroid gland.

1. What abnormality is seen in the trachea on the CT scan?
2. What is the likely diagnosis?
3. What is the patient likely to present with?
4. What further investigation can be performed?

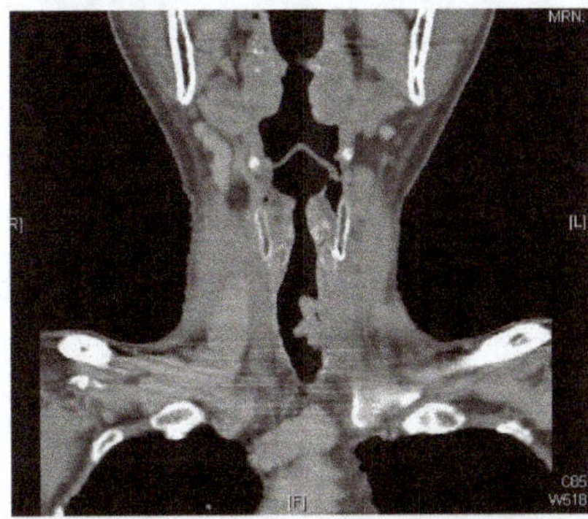

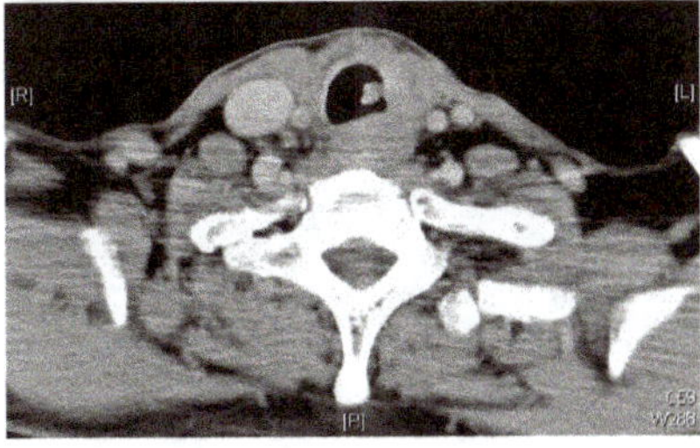

A7.9

1. The neck is swollen and there is evidence of superficial bruising.

2. There is fresh blood in the tube draining into the bottle, instead of haemoserous fluid.

3. Bleeding from the surgical bed resulting in a haematoma in the neck.

4. Emergency surgery to evacuate the blood as the haematoma will compress the trachea leading to airway compromise. The source of primary haemorrhage needs to be identified and secured.

A7.10

1. There is an intraluminal lesion arising from the left side of the trachea.

2. Left thyroid cancer with invasion into the trachea.

3. Haemoptysis and dyspnoea.

4. Bronchoscopy to confirm the tumour in the trachea.

Q7.11

This patient had surgery to remove a medullary thyroid cancer.

1. What is the originating cell type of this cancer?

2. What serum test is elevated?

3. What is its aetiology?

4. What surgeries were performed as seen in the pictures?

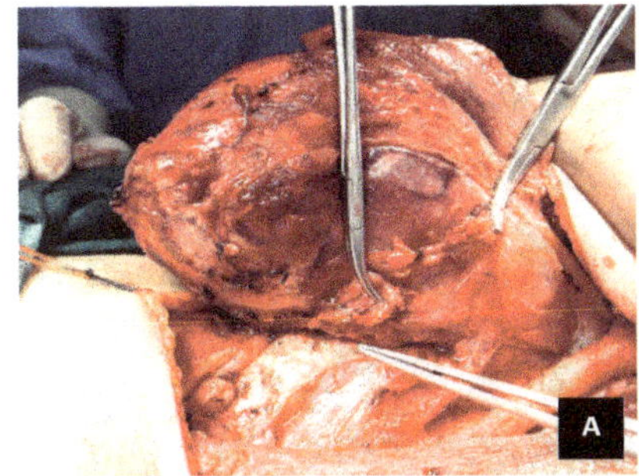

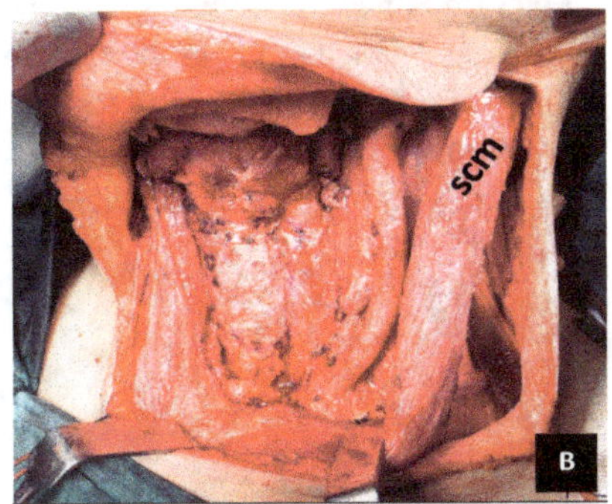

Q7.12

This is a 32-year-old male with MEN2a syndrome.

1. What pathology is seen in the PET scan of the neck?

2. What intra-abdominal tumour is shown in the picture?

3. What other pathology would this patient have?

4. What is the genomic anomaly?

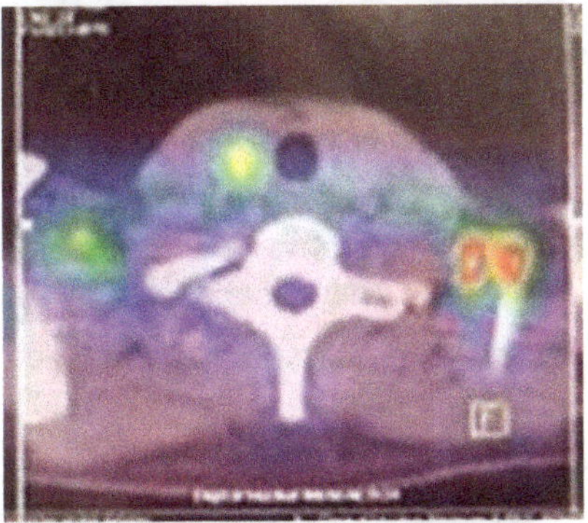

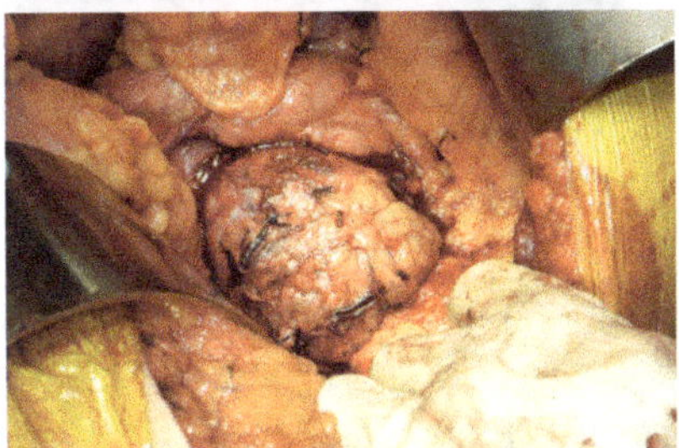

A7.11

1. Parafollicular cells, or C cells of the thyroid gland.

2. Elevated serum calcitonin level is an essential feature.

3. 75% of medullary thyroid cancers (MTC) are sporadic, and the remainder are familial as part of multiple endocrine neoplasia (MEN 2a, MEN 2b) and familial medullary thyroid cancer (FMTC). 50% of sporadic medullary thyroid cancers have acquired RET mutations.

4. Picture A: resection of the thyroid gland.
   Picture B: neck dissection of the cervical lymph nodes. The left sternocleidomastoid muscle (SCM, as seen in the picture) and carotid artery are visualised.
   MTCs do not respond to radioactive iodine (RAI) or conventional chemotherapy, hence an aggressive surgical approach is recommended.

A7.12

1. There are 3 nodules that are demonstrating avid uptake. It is a medullary thyroid cancer involving the right lobe with bilateral lymphadenopathy. Medullary thyroid cancer develops in all patients with MEN2a.

2. A phaeochromocytoma. They present in approximately half of MEN2a patients. They are bilateral in 60–80% of such cases.

3. Primary hyperparathyroidism. Four-gland parathyroid hyperplasia is present in nearly half of patients with MEN2a.

4. MEN 2a results from germline mutations in the RET proto-oncogene localized to 10q11.2 and is transmitted in an autosomal dominant fashion.

Q7.13

This is a 45-year-old male with end stage renal failure.

1. What is expected in the x-rays of these patients?

2. What is the diagnosis?

3. What is the pathophysiology?

4. What surgery was performed based on the surgical specimen?

5. What are indications for this surgery?

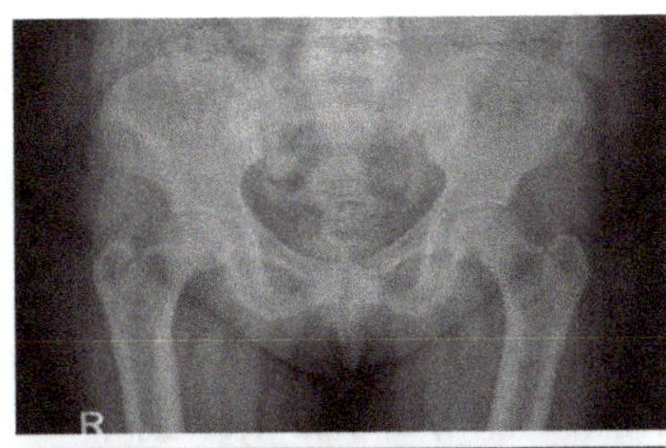
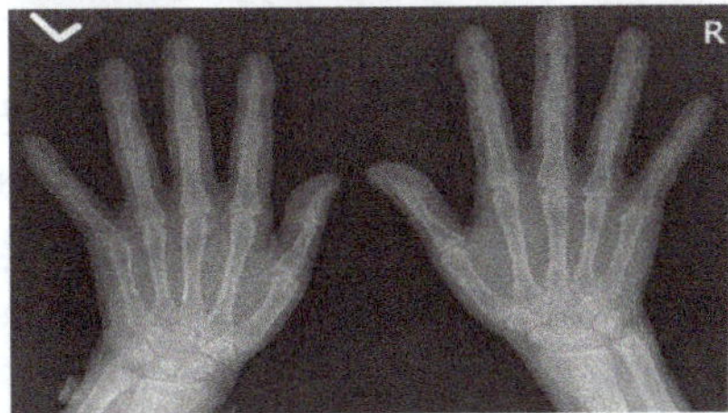
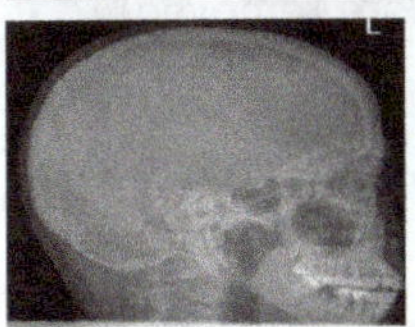
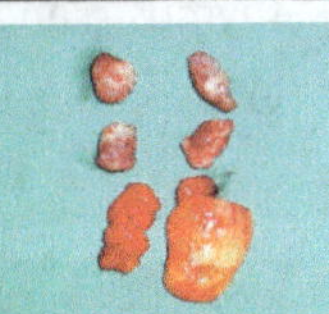

Q7.14

This is a 50-year-old female who presented with kidney stones.

1. What did the scan detect?

2. What is the diagnosis?

3. What other clinical symptoms could she be experiencing?

4. What biochemical test can confirm the diagnosis?

5. What surgery was performed?

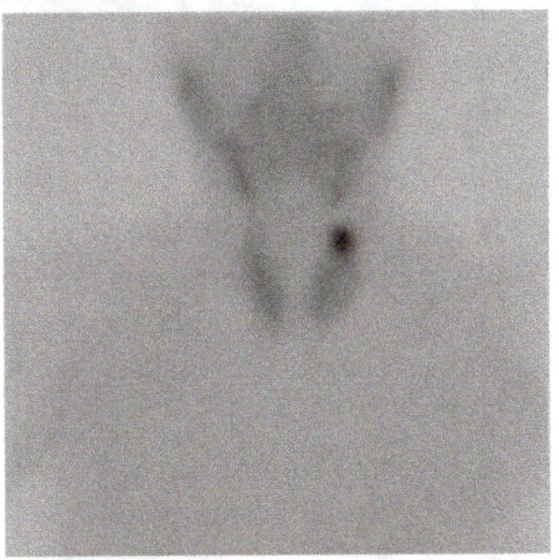
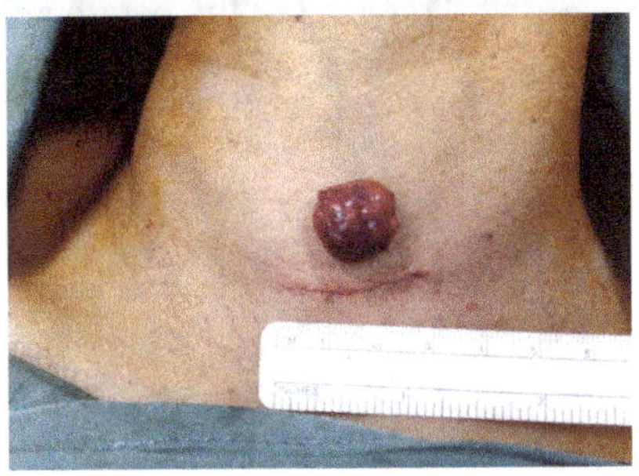

A7.13

1. These patients have renal osteodystrophy and are at risk of high bone turnover causing a spectrum of bone changes. Osteitis fibrosa cystica occurs in the long bones. There is increased subperiosteal bone resorption classically affecting the radial aspects of the proximal and middle phalanges of the 2nd and 3rd fingers. Lateral radiograph of the calvarium reveals punctate trabecular bone resorption that has a salt-and-pepper appearance.

2. Tertiary hyperparathyroidism.

3. There is autonomous release of parathyroid hormone (PTH) while in a hypercalcaemic state. During prolonged secondary hyperparathyroidism, increased blood phosphate levels drive hyperplasia of the parathyroid glands and this acts to reset calcium sensitivity at the calcium-sensing receptors leading to tertiary hyperparathyroidism.

4. Total parathyroidectomy (the 4 hyperplastic parathyroids and bilateral thymus glands are removed).

5. Osteopenia, bone pain, pathological fractures and calciphylaxis.

A7.14

1. There is a nodule demonstrating avid-uptake superior to the left lobe of the thyroid gland on the Sestamibi-scan.

2. Parathyroid adenoma causing primary hyperparathyroidism.

3. Renal: polyuria, hypercalciuria.
   Gastrointestinal: abdominal pain, peptic ulcer disease, acute pancreatitis.
   Neuromuscular: fatigue and muscle weakness.
   Psychological: depression, inability to concentrate, memory issues and confusion.

4. An elevated serum parathyroid hormone level and calcium level is diagnostic of primary hyperparathyroidism.

5. Surgical removal of the parathyroid adenoma.

Q7.15

This is a 69-year-old male who presented with acute confusion.

1. What is seen in the Tc-99m parathyroid SPECT-CT scan?

2. What is seen on the ultrasound scan?

3. What is the cause for the confusion?

4. What is the management?

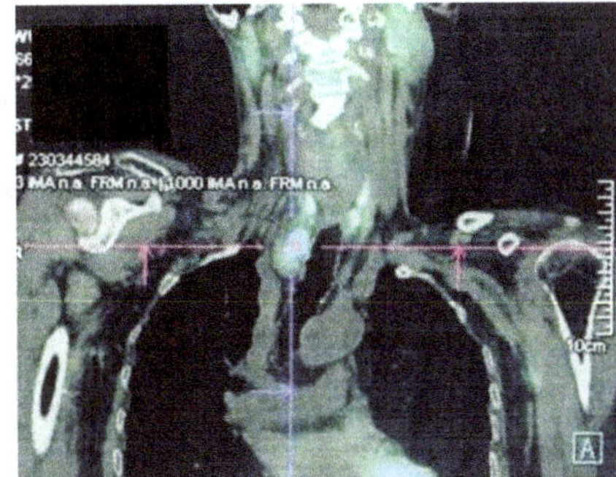

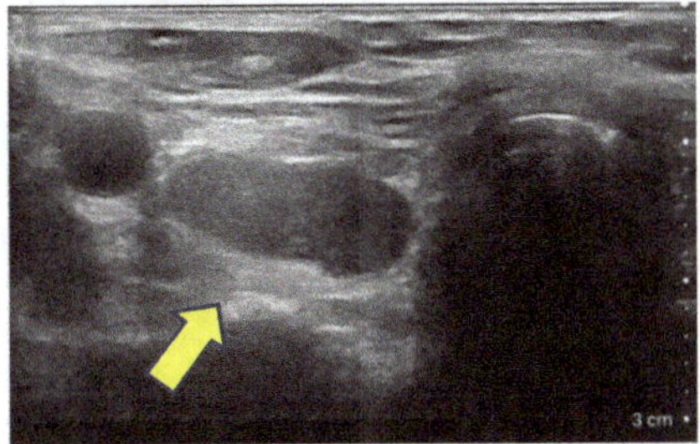

Q7.16

This is a 41-year-old female who presented with hypertension. An enlarged tumour was seen in her right adrenal gland on the CT scan.

1. What is the most likely diagnosis?

2. What is the likely clinical presentation?

3. What biochemical tests can be used to confirm the diagnosis?

4. What was the management for this patient?

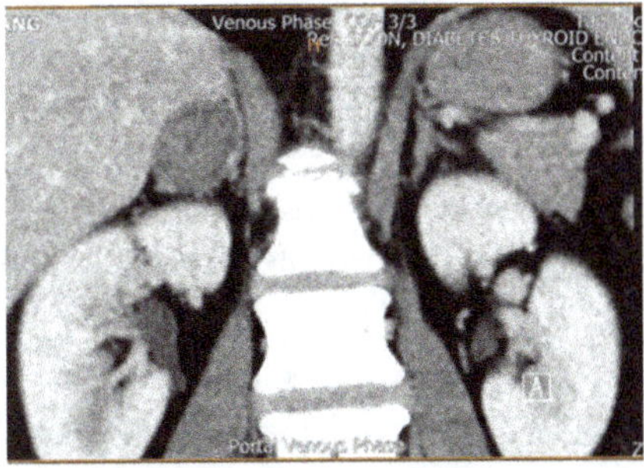

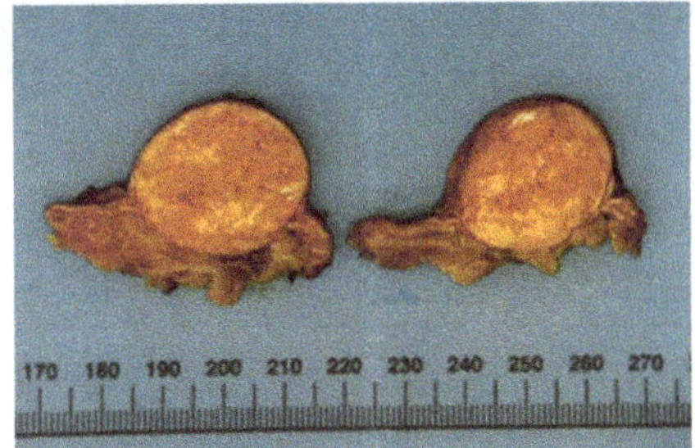

A7.15

1. There is a Sestamibi-avid nodule inferior to the right lower pole of the thyroid gland.

2. There is a smooth hypoechoic ovoid shaped lesion between the trachea and right carotid artery.

3. Hypercalcaemia due to a parathyroid adenoma. (His serum calcium was >3.75 mmol/L)

4. Intravenous fluids, bisphosphonates and removal of the parathyroid adenoma.

A7.16

1. Conn's syndrome — hyperaldosteronism. It is the most common cause for secondary hypertension.

2. Patients are often asymptomatic.
   Hypertension-related: headaches, facial flushing.
   Hypokalaemia-related: constipation, polyuria and polydipsia, weakness.

3. Elevated serum sodium and low potassium.
   A high aldosterone-to-renin ratio.

4. This lady had a single benign aldosterone secreting tumour, hence surgical removal (laparoscopic approach) was curative.

Q7.17

This is a 40-year-old male who had surgical removal of a tumour. Attached are his urine tests.

1. What is the diagnosis?
2. What are the genetics associated with this?
3. What are the likely presenting symptoms?
4. How can the patient be optimized prior to surgery?

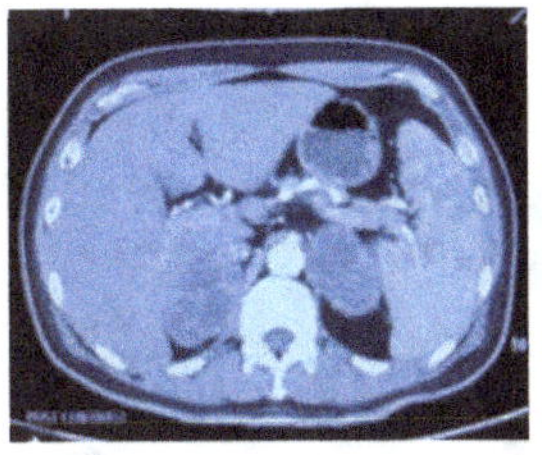

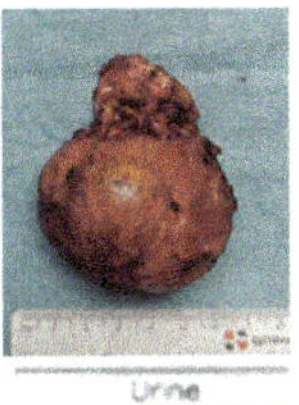

Metanephrine, Urine, 24HR (MAYO)

```
------------------REFERENCE VALUE------   Value
44-261 (Normotensive)                       321
<400 (Hypertensive)
```

Normetanephrine, Urine, 24HR (MAYO)

```
------------------REFERENCE VALUE------
111-419 (Normotensive)                     6503  (H)
<900 (Hypertensive)
```

Total Metanephrine, Urine, 24HR (MAYO

```
------------------REFERENCE VALUE------
200-614 (Normotensive)                     6824  (H)
<1300 (Hypertensive)
```

Q7.18

This is a 45-year-old male who presented with hyperandrogenism.

1. What is seen in the CT scan?
2. What is the likely diagnosis?
3. How common is it?
4. What are the possible clinical presentations?

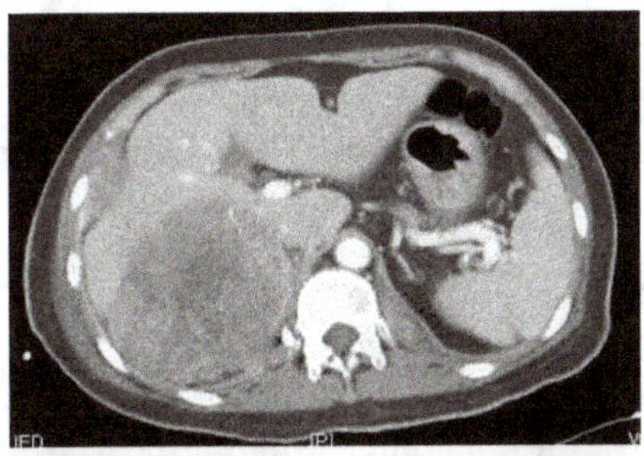

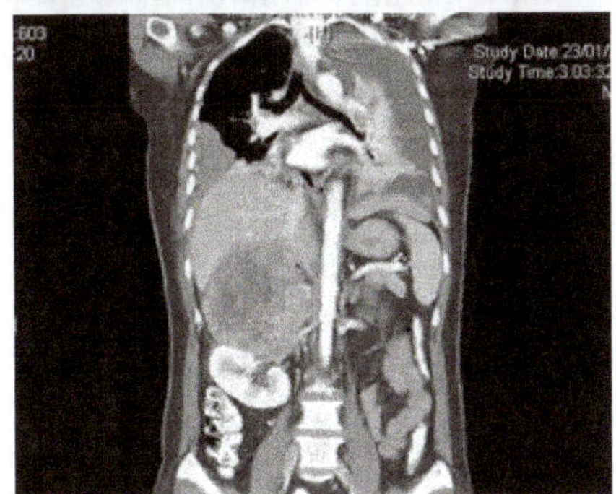

A7.17

1. A pheochromocytoma. The urine normetanephrines are very elevated. It is a catecholamine-secreting tumour derived from chromaffin cells. About 85% of pheochromocytomas are located within the adrenal glands.

2. Most are sporadic. About 30% of pheochromocytomas occur as part of hereditary syndromes such as Von Hippel-Lindau (VHL) syndrome, multiple endocrine neoplasia type 2 (MEN 2), and neurofibromatosis type 1 (NF1).

3. He may experience headaches, palpitations, diaphoresis and hypertension. Occasionally, they can be asymptomatic and detected incidentally.

4. Careful preoperative treatment with alpha and beta blockers is required to control blood pressure and prevent intraoperative hypertensive crises.
   - Start alpha blockade with phenoxybenzamine 7–10 days preoperatively.
   - Provide intravascular volume expansion.
   - Encourage high salt intake.
   - Initiate a beta blocker after adequate alpha blockade.

A7.18

1. There is a large tumour posterior and inferior to the liver, displacing the right kidney inferiorly. There is also pleural effusion.

2. Right adrenal carcinoma.

3. It is rare.

4. 50% of patients are asymptomatic. The other 50% are hormonally active. 30–40% of patients present with Cushing syndrome, while 20–30% present with virilization symptoms.
   A tumour of this size can present with right sided abdominal pain and a palpable abdominal mass.

Q7.19

This is a 54-year-old female who noticed she was frequently experiencing ecchymosis with minimal trauma.

1. What change is visible in the facial appearance?
2. What lesion is seen in the CT scan?
3. What is the likely diagnosis?
4. What are other possible clinical presentations?
5. What clinical test can we use to confirm the diagnosis?
6. What is the management?

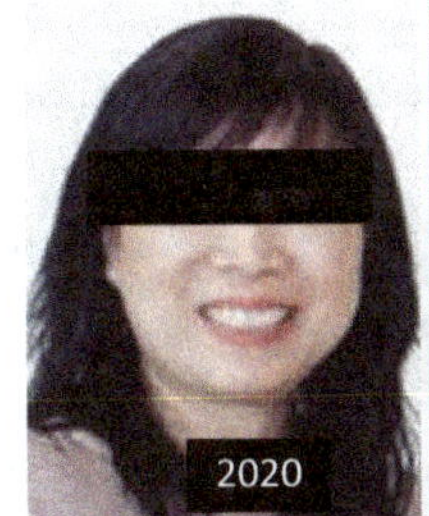
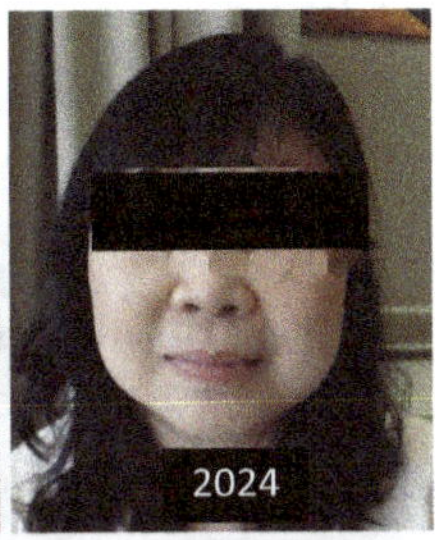

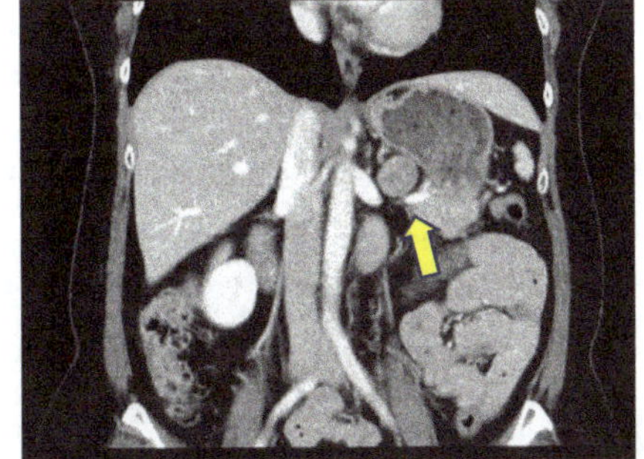

Q7.20

This is a 60-year-old male with a primary neuroendocrine tumour (NET).

1. What are NETs?
2. What scan was performed?
3. What does the scan show?
4. What is the likely clinical presentation?
5. How was the patient managed?

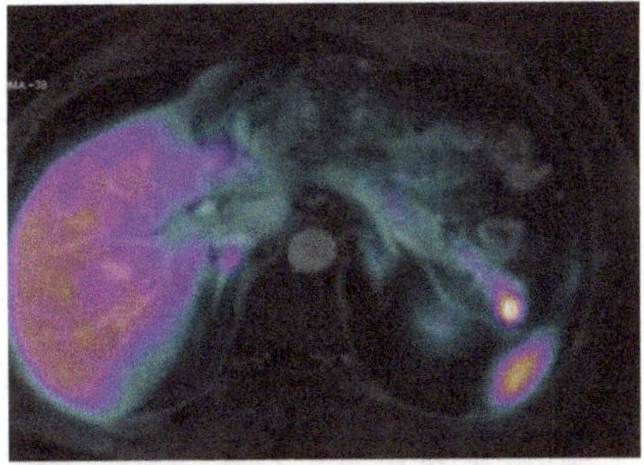

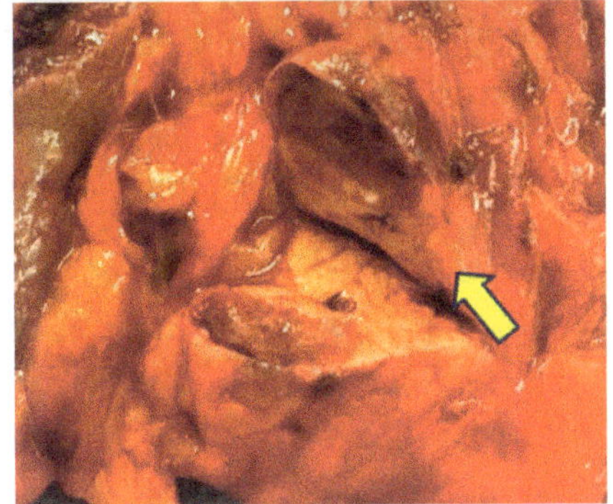

A7.19

1. She has developed a moon face. Fat deposits built up along the sides of her face making it look round and puffy.

2. There is an enlarged left adrenal tumour.

3. Cushing syndrome due to endogenous hypercortisolism secreted from the left adrenal tumour.

4. She may experience weight gain, fatigue, delayed wound healing, back and bone pain, depression or mood swings, loss of libido, irregular menstrual cycles and infertility.
   Physical examination may reveal "Buffalo torso," thin arms and legs, acne, abdominal wall striae, hirsutism, proximal muscle weakness of the shoulder and hip girdle muscles and paper-thin skin.

5. 24-hour urine free cortisol test.
   48-hour low-dose dexamethasone suppression test.

6. Surgical removal of the left adrenal tumour.

A7.20

1. NETs are a genetically diverse group of malignancies that sometimes produce peptides that cause characteristic hormonal syndromes.

2. Somatostatin Receptor Scintigraphy (SRS) is a type of radionuclide scan that uses a radioactive substance that can bind to a tumour's somatostatin receptors and illuminate them. The radioactive tracer used is Ga-68 dotatate.

3. There is uptake in the tumour at the tail of the pancreas.

4. The patient can be asymptomatic.
   Symptomatic patients may experience flushing, diarrhoea, constipation, palpitations, hypertension, shortness of breath and headaches.

5. Asymptomatic patients with small tumours can be managed conservatively with monitoring and surveillance.
   This patient was symptomatic and the tumour was resected with a distal pancreatectomy.

8 Thorax

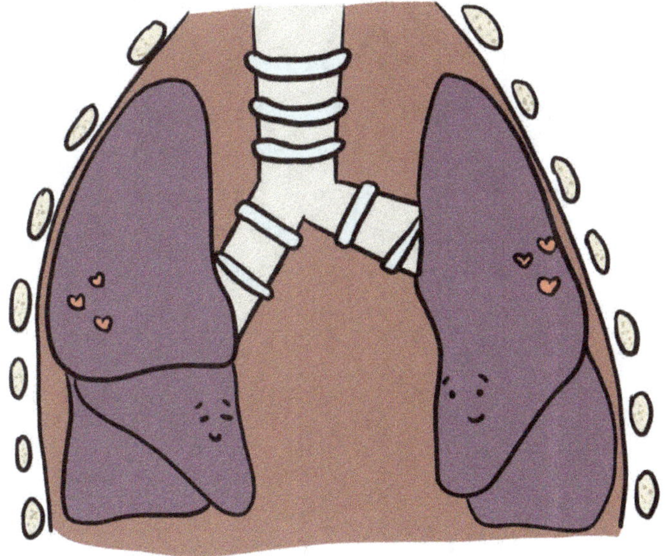

Q8.1

This is a 19-year-old female who had video-assisted thoracoscopic surgery.

1. What is this anatomical structure (arrowed)?

2. What surgery was performed?

3. What were her symptoms?

4. What non-surgical treatments are available?

5. What is a potential undesirable sequelae of this surgery?

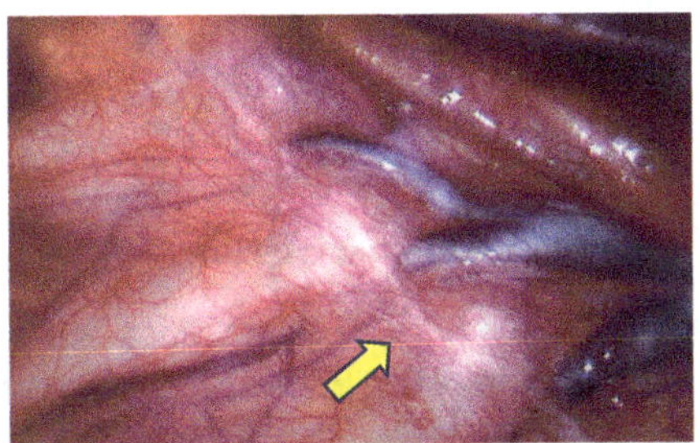

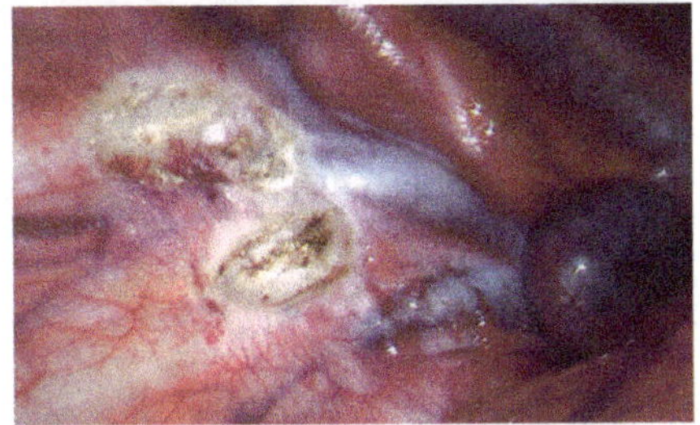

Q8.2

This is an x-ray of a 17-year-old female. She has no prior history of trauma.

1. What abnormality is seen in the chest x-ray?

2. What is her clinical presentation?

3. If left untreated, what is a feared sequelae?

4. What is the management?

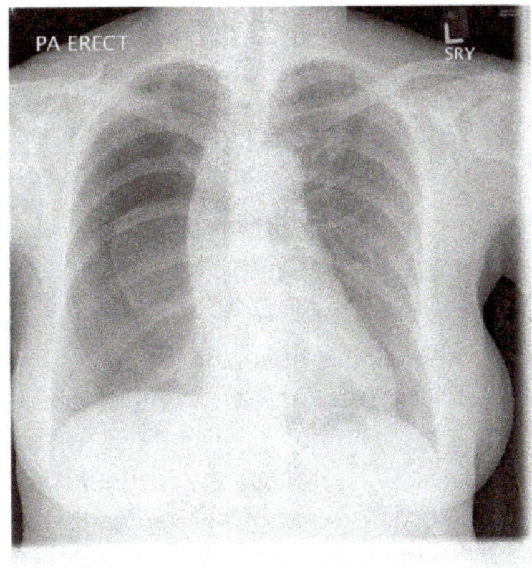

A8.1

1. Sympathetic chain.

2. Thoracic sympathectomy.

3. Palmar hyperhidrosis (sweaty palms).

4. Anticholinergic drugs
    Botulinium toxin injections
    Iontophoresis
    Sweat gland ablation by energy-based devices

5. Compensatory hyperhidrosis elsewhere in the body. It occurs in 20% of patients.

A8.2

1. A spontaneous right pneumothorax.

2. Symptoms include right chest discomfort/pain, tachycardia and dyspnoea. There will be decreased breath sounds on the right side.

3. A tension pneumothorax may develop.

4. The main goal for the treatment of spontaneous pneumothorax is to evacuate the gas from the pleural space and the prevention of recurrences. Clinically unstable patients with symptoms suggestive of tension pneumothorax are treated with emergent needle decompression.
    Large primary spontaneous pneumothorax can be managed with video-assisted thoracoscopy surgery (VATS) or thoracotomy to perform bullectomy, pleurectomy and mechanical pleurodesis.

Q8.3

This is a 55-year-old male.

1. What is seen in the chest x-ray?

2. What is the diagnosis as seen in the CT scan?

3. What is the clinical presentation?

4. What is the management?

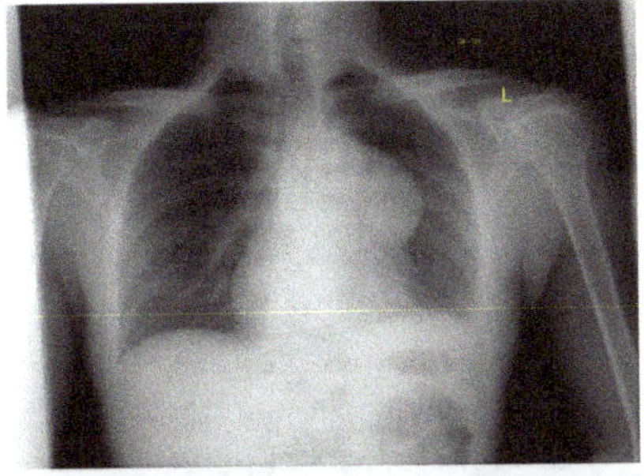

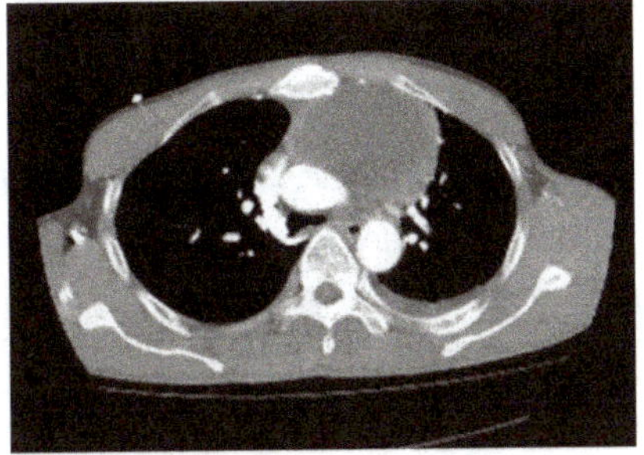

Q8.4

This is a 70-year-old male.

1. What is seen in the oesophagus during endoscopy?

2. What procedure has been performed as seen in the x-ray?

3. What is the diagnosis?

4. What are possible clinical presentations?

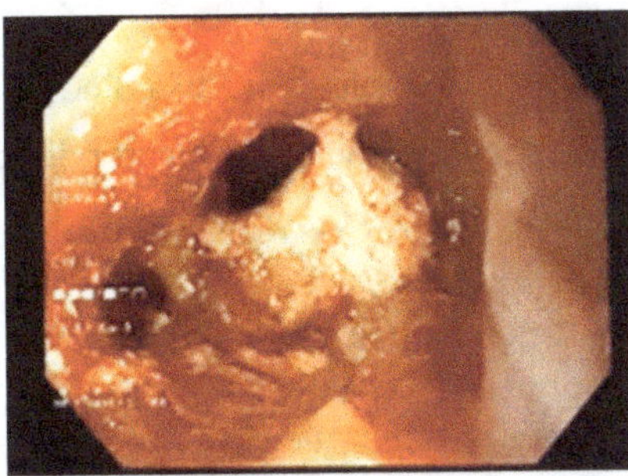

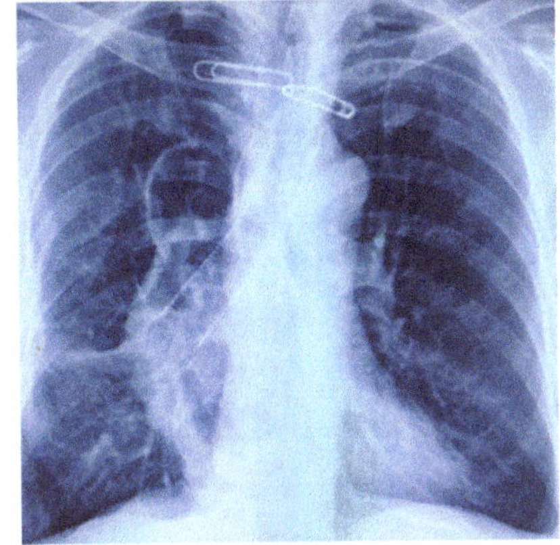

A8.3

1. The mediastinum is widened.

2. Thoracic aortic aneurysm.

3. Most patients are asymptomatic.
    Patients experience chest pain. If this pain radiates to the back, it may be a sign of dissection.
    Some patients can present with difficulty breathing due to airway compression. Hoarseness of voice can occur due to compression of the recurrent laryngeal nerve.

4. Small aneurysms can be managed conservatively with medication to lower the blood pressure.
    Symptomatic or large ones need intervention to prevent dissection or rupture.
    Open surgery involves replacing the diseased aorta with a prosthetic tube graft.
    Thoracic endovascular aortic repair (TEVAR) with branched or fenestrated grafts are other options.

A8.4

1. There is an ulcerative bleeding tumour in the oesophagus.

2. Stenting of the trachea and right bronchus.

3. Cancer of the oesophagus invading into the bronchus causing an oesophageal bronchial fistula.

4. Patients often present with paroxysmal coughing after ingestion of liquids. Others develop recurrent aspiration pneumonia, haemoptysis, or a productive cough with particles of food in the sputum.

Q8.5

This is a 40-year-old male who had previous surgical removal of a dermatofibrosarcoma protuberans (DFSP) 3 years ago.

1. What abnormality is seen in the chest x-ray?

2. What is the clinical presentation?

3. What is seen in the PET CT scan?

4. What is the likely cause for the effusion?

5. What is the management?

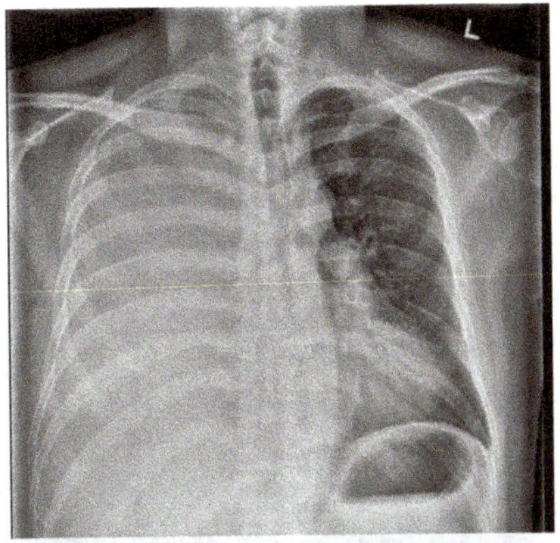

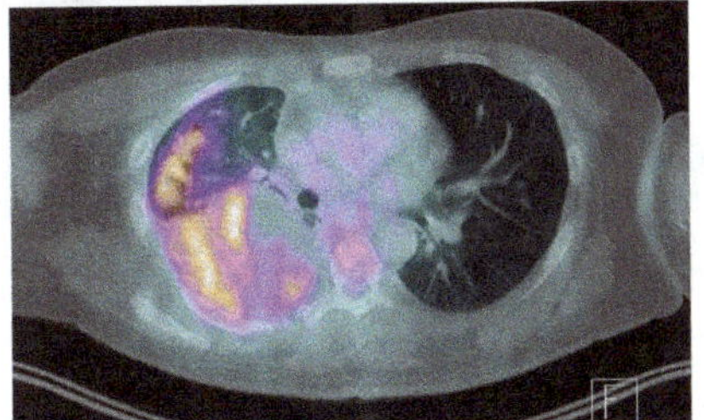

Q8.6

This is a 60-year-old male. He is asymptomatic. He was a motorcyclist involved in a road traffic accident 40 years ago.

1. What is seen on the x-rays?

2. What abnormal findings can be detected on physical examination?

3. What is the diagnosis?

4. How do you think the patient developed this problem?

5. What is the management?

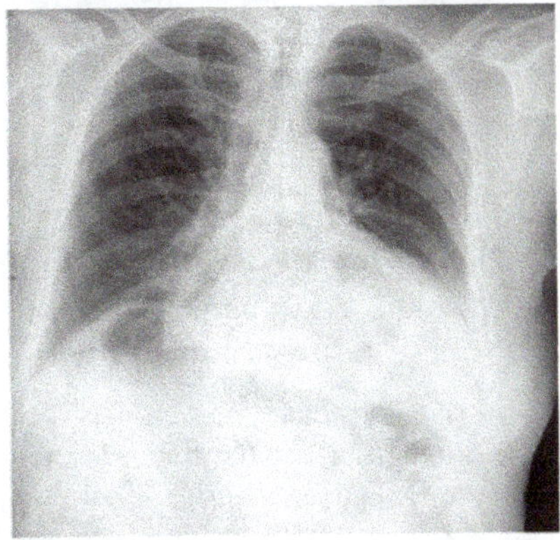

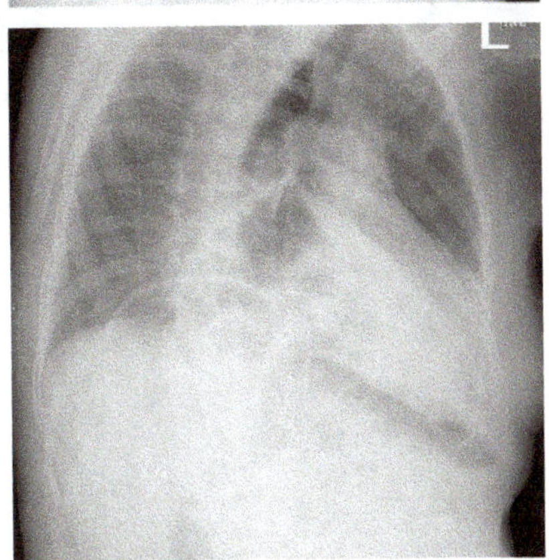

A8.5

1. There is a large pleural effusion in the entire right thorax with midline shift to the left.

2. The patient will be breathless. This will be associated with percussion dullness and decreased breath sounds over the right thorax.

3. There is a malignant tumour in the right thorax.

4. The effusion is caused by the metastatic DFSP.

5. The effusion needs to be drained for symptomatic relief. No more than 1,500 ml of fluid should be extracted in a single session, otherwise re-expansion pulmonary oedema can occur.
   Pleurodesis may be considered if frequent drainage in necessary.
   Biopsy of the tumour is necessary to confirm metastatic disease.

A8.6

1. There are radiolucent shadows in the mediastinum and lower thorax.

2. Bowel sounds with absent breath sounds on auscultation of the lower chest.

3. Diaphragmatic hernia.

4. The road traffic accident he suffered 40 years ago resulted in a small traumatic diaphragmatic hernia which was undetected then. All hernias increase in size as a result of increased intra-abdominal pressure over time.

5. Surgical repair of the hernia is recommended to prevent further enlargement of the hernia into the thoracic cavity which can cause ventilatory compromise. The bowel in the hernia can be twisted and strangulated.

Q8.7

This is a 55-year-old male who had surgery.

1. What is this organ in picture A?

2. What equipment is used to facilitate this surgery as seen in picture B?

3. What are other common surgeries necessitating this set-up?

4. What are some complications in using this device?

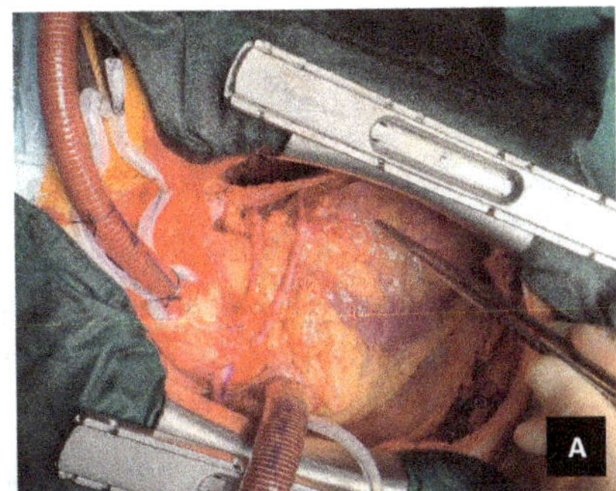

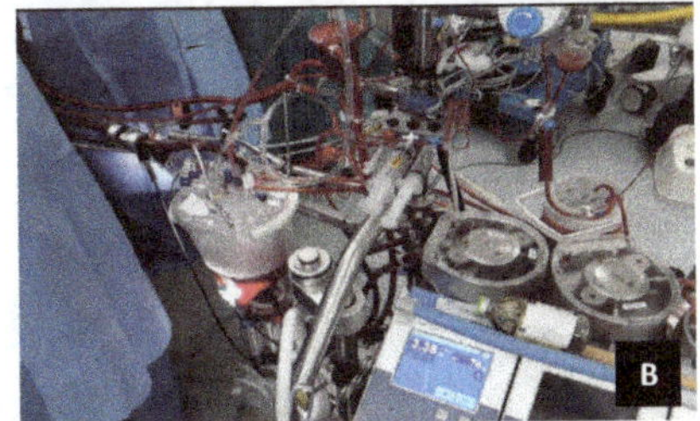

Q8.8

This is a 30-year-old male who sustained anterior chest trauma from a steering wheel injury.

1. What is the pathology detected on the CT scan?

2. What are some other injuries we need to exclude?

3. What is the management?

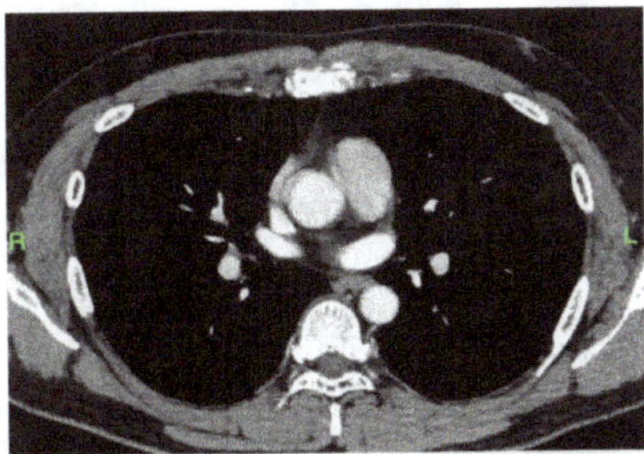

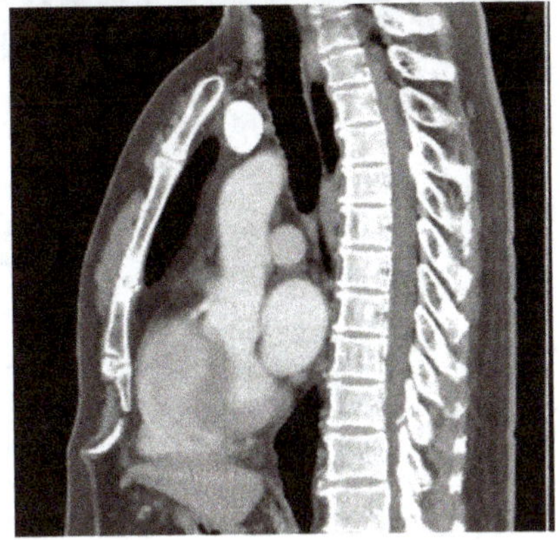

A8.7

1. Open heart surgery has been performed. The sternum has been separated and held in position by a retractor to access the heart. Arterial and venous cannulation is performed into the superior vena cava and ascending aorta respectively. Cardioplegic solution is used to protect the heart.

2. The cardiopulmonary bypass (CPB) circuit is a form of extracorporeal circulation to provide circulatory and respiratory support along with temperature management.

3. Coronary artery bypass surgery, cardiac valve repair or replacements, repair of large septal defects and repair of congenital heart defects.

4. The most common complication associated with CPB is a protamine reaction during anticoagulation reversal. Others include thrombosis, aortic dissection, gas embolism and dislodgement of the cannulas.

A8.8

1. There is a fracture between the middle and lower third of the sternum.

2. Sternal fracture is considered a marker for significant transmission of energy. During evaluation of these patients, carefully assess for cardiac, pulmonary, mediastinal, and thoracic spine injuries, as well as associated injuries unrelated to chest trauma.

3. Most sternal fractures heal without the need for surgery. Ensure adequate analgesia to alleviate the pain which can persist for 8 to 12 weeks. Pain on inspiration can result in atelectasis, pneumonia, and other pulmonary complications.

Q8.9

This is a 65-year-old male.

1. What abnormality is seen on the PET CT scan?

2. What is the diagnosis?

3. What are risk factors?

4. What is the clinical presentation?

5. Based on the surgical picture, what was performed?

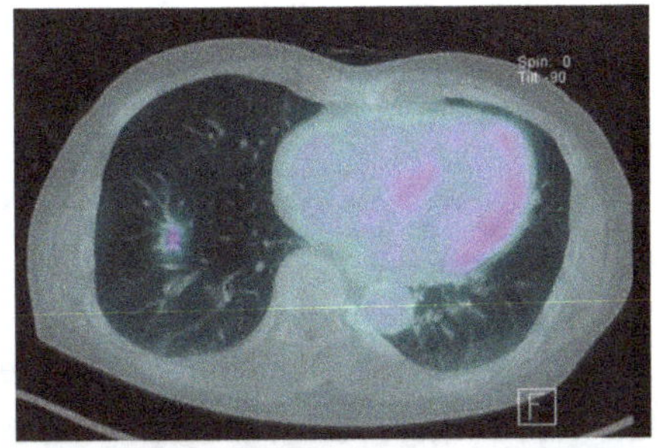

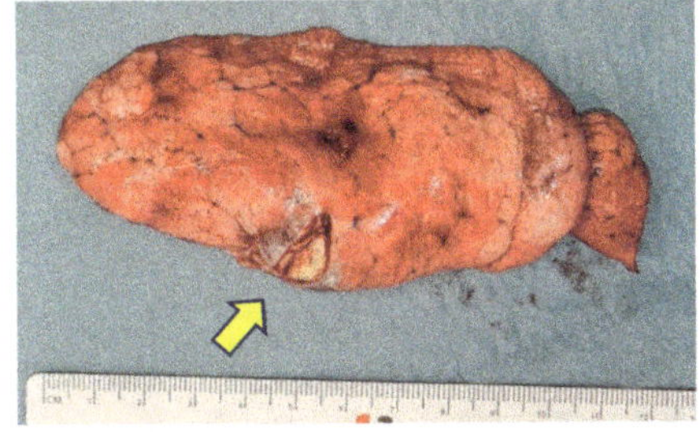

Q8.10

This is a 40-year-old male who presents with diplopia, ptosis and weakness.

1. What abnormality is seen on the CT scan?

2. What is the likely diagnosis?

3. How can we confirm the diagnosis?

4. What is the management?

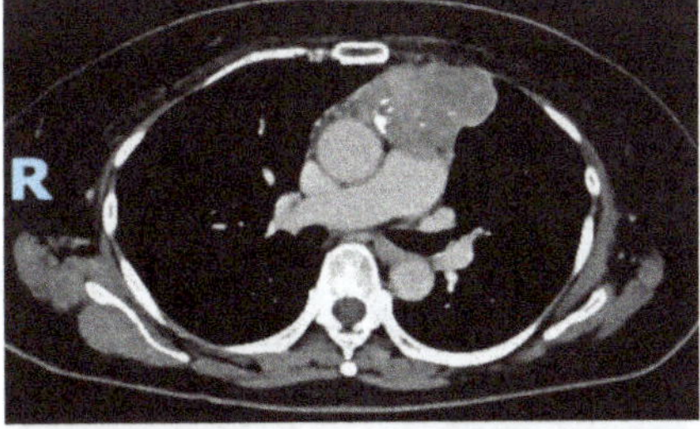

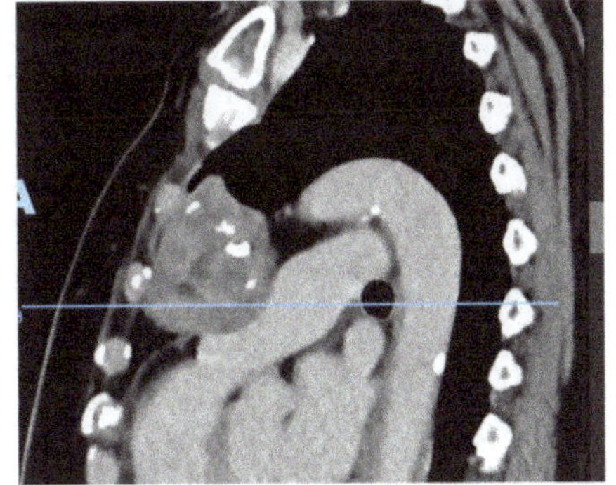

A8.9

1. There is a focal mass in the right lower lobe of the lung that is FDG-avid.

2. Lung or bronchogenic carcinoma. It is one of the commonest cancers.

3. Smoking and exposure to carcinogens (eg asbestos and radon).

4. Patients are often asymptomatic.
   Symptomatic patients can present with cough or haemoptysis.
   Chest pain or dyspnoea are less seen.

5. Wedge resection of the lung. The tumour is arrowed.

A8.10

1. There is a mass with internal calcification situated in the anterior mediastinum.

2. Myasthenia gravis with a thymoma.

3. The presence of anti-acetylcholine receptor antibodies.

4. Thymectomy. It can be performed trans-sternal or through a video-assisted thoracoscopic approach.

Q8.11

This is a 30-year-old male who had severe bouts of vomiting after an alcohol binge.

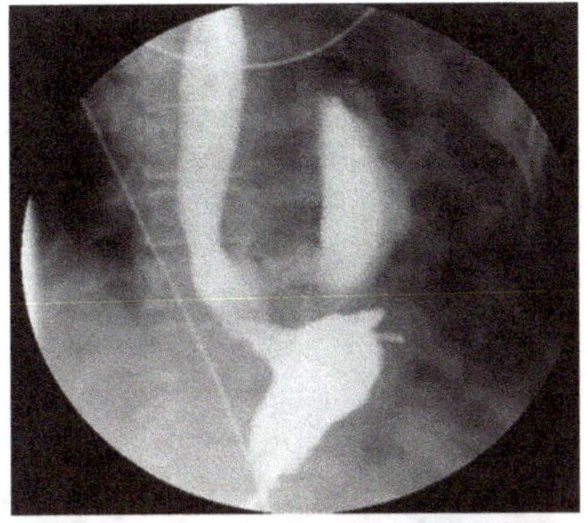

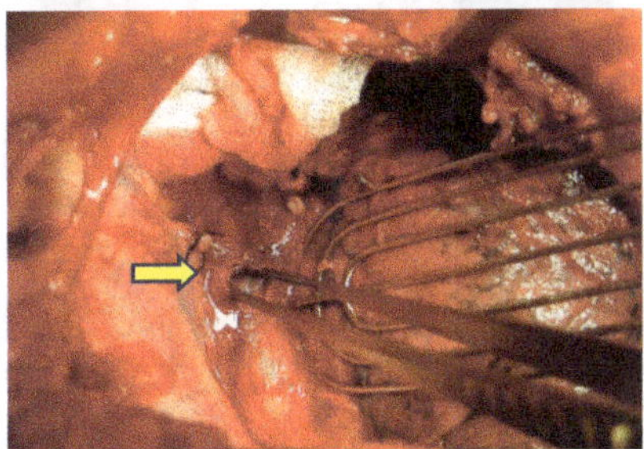

1. What is seen in the contrast study of the oesophagus?
2. What is the diagnosis?
3. What is the likely clinical presentation?
4. What is the management?

Q8.12

This is a 34-year-old male who experienced fever, night sweats and weight loss.

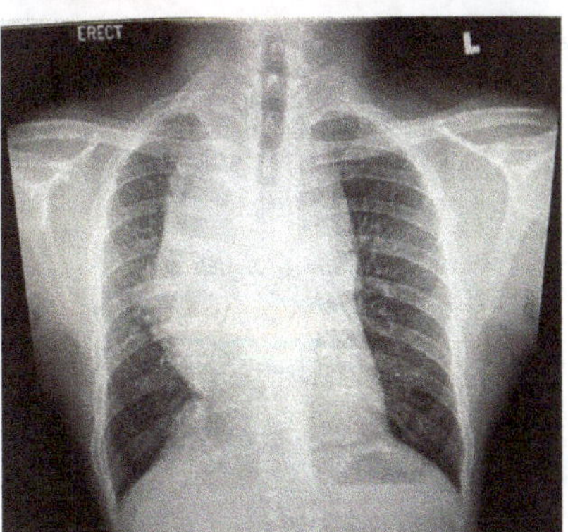

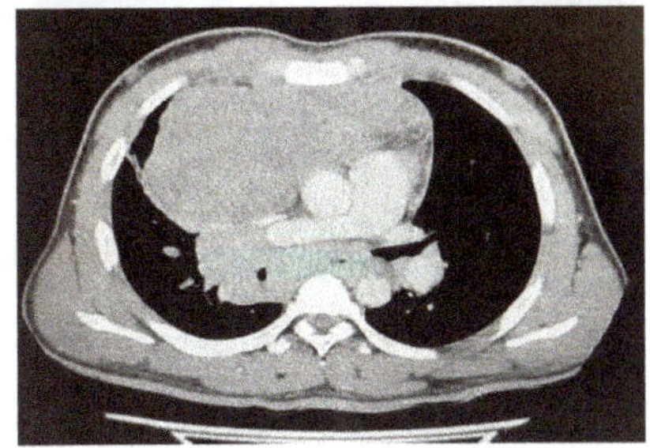

1. What abnormality is seen in the chest x-ray?
2. What abnormality is seen the CT scan?
3. What are other likely clinical presentation of this patient?
4. What is the likely diagnosis?
5. How can we confirm the diagnosis?

A8.11

1. Contrast has leaked out into the mediastinal space from the oesophagus.

2. Transmural oesophageal perforation. It is also known as Boerhaave syndrome.

3. The clinical presentation depends on the time elapsed since the injury and the extent of leakage. There must be a history of forceful vomiting. Symptoms are often non-specific. They may have chest or lower thoracic pain and subcutaneous emphysema. Sepsis can occur with mediastinitis.

4. Control the sepsis with antibiotics.
   Control the leak — based on size and location of the perforation.
   Surgical repair and stenting of the perforation or oesophageal resection or diversion are options.

A8.12

1. There is a widened upper mediastinum.

2. There is a large solid mass in the upper mediastinum between the sternum and great vessels.

3. He will present with compressive symptoms as a result of the large mass. These include cough, dyspnoea, hoarseness and dysphagia.

4. Mediastinal lymphoma.

5. A tissue biopsy is done to obtain histology. This can be achieved through percutaneous needle biopsy, mediastinoscopy, thoracoscopy or open surgical biopsy.

9
Vascular

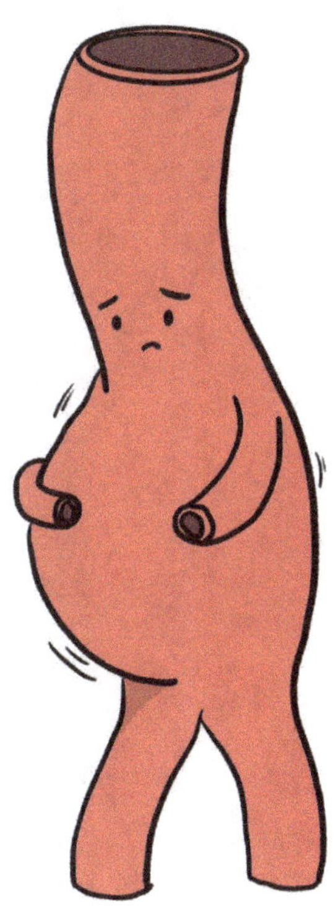

Q9.1

This is a 65-year-old female.

1. What clinical test has been performed?

2. What information does this test provide?

3. What pathology does this patient have?

4. What are her other possible clinical signs and symptoms?

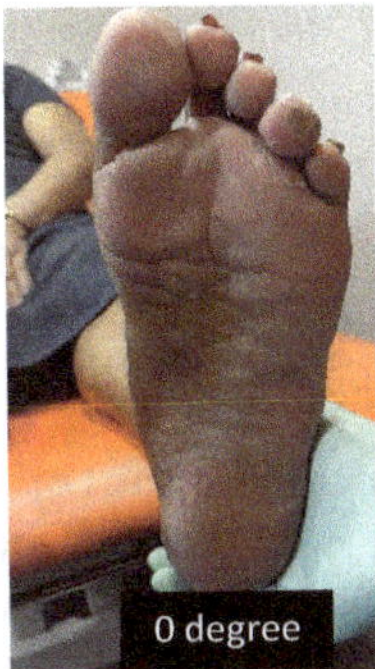
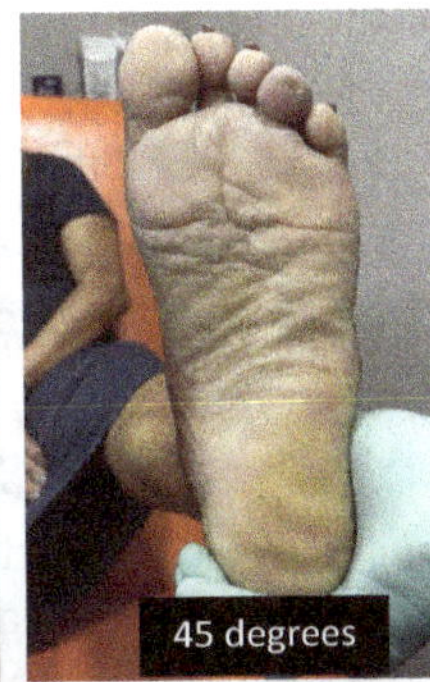

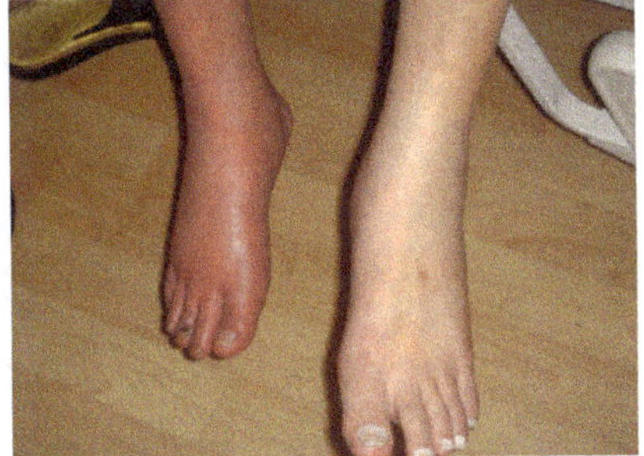

Q9.2

This is a 60-year-old diabetic male.

1. What is seen on his left foot?

2. What other signs on his left foot are likely to be present on clinical examination?

3. What is the diagnosis?

4. What investigations would you do?

5. What is the management?

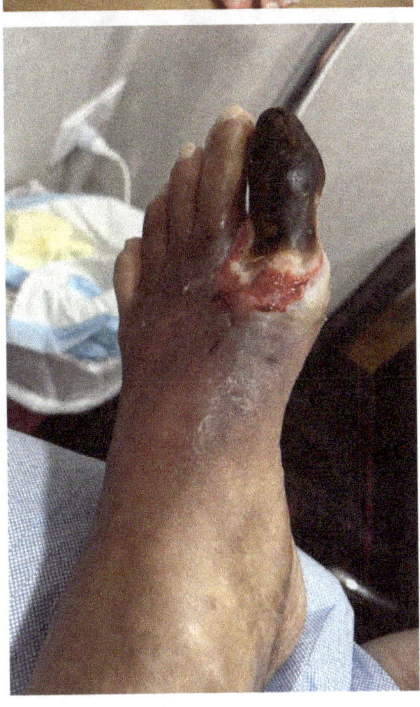

A9.1

1. Buerger's test. At 0 degrees, the foot is normal colour. When elevated to 45 degrees, the foot is pale. Reactive hyperaemia occurs on leg dependency.

2. The Buerger's angle, is the angle at which the foot becomes pale, corresponding to the severity of arterial insufficiency.

3. Peripheral artery disease.

4. She may experience intermittent claudication brought on by walking and relieved with rest. Her calf and foot may be painful when her leg is elevated. Physical examination may reveal loss of distal pulses, slow capillary refill, pallor and loss of hair.

A9.2

1. The left big toe is gangrenous. There are surrounding skin changes in the forefoot.

2. The left foot may be cooler in temperature and the pulses are absent.

3. Critical limb ischemia (CLI). He would have intermittent claudication with exertion that progressed to chronic rest pain. If a concurrent neuropathy is present (commonly seen in diabetics), there may not be a consistent history of pain, and tissue loss may be the first presentation of ischemia.

4. Foot x-rays, Ankle brachial pressure index (ABPI), Arterial duplex ultrasound, CT angiogram of the lower limb.

5. The foot will require revascularisation (either angioplasty or bypass) to prevent further gangrene.
   If there is wet gangrene of the big toe, the sepsis needs to be treated with antibiotics and amputation.

Q9.3

This is a 65-year-old diabetic male who presented with fever and a gangrenous toe.

1. How is gangrene classified?
2. What type of gangrene is this?
3. What is the pathogenesis?
4. What surgery was performed?

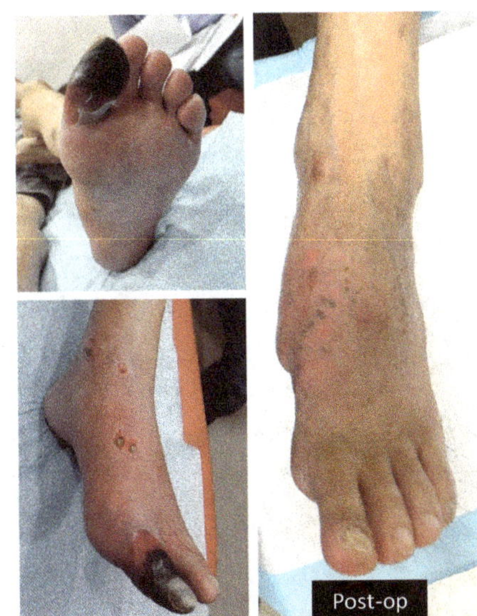

Q9.4

This is a 70-year-old male.

1. What is seen in picture A?
2. No surgery was performed. What is seen in picture B?
3. How can we further manage the patient?

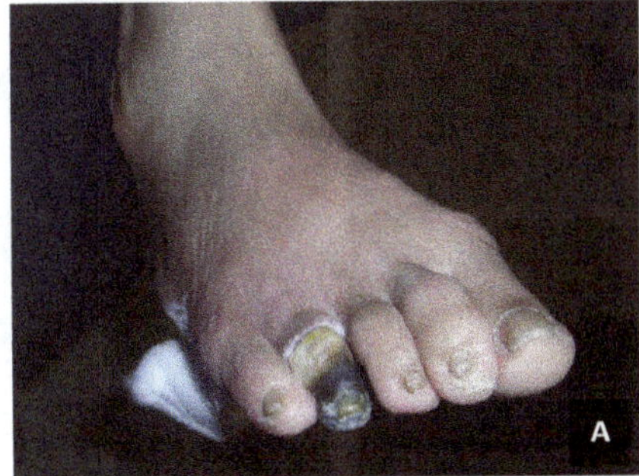

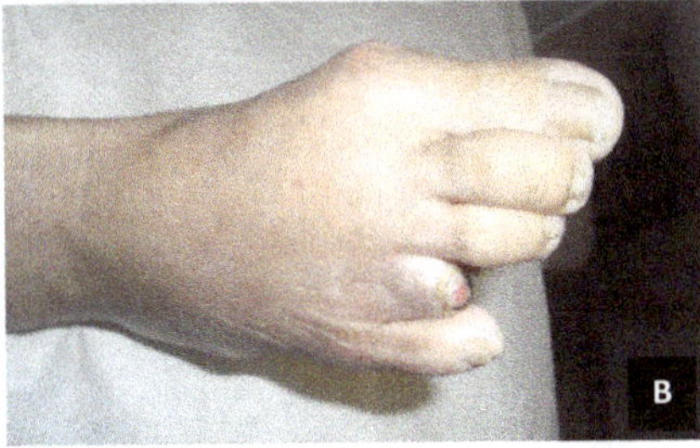

A9.3

1. The three main types of gangrene are:
   Dry: dehydrated ischemic tissue.
   Wet: ischaemic tissue complicated by secondary infection, which is associated with oedema and erythema but no crepitus.
   Gas: necrotizing infection with oedema, crepitus, and subcutaneous gas on x-ray.

2. Wet gangrene. He is septic with a fever.

3. Poorly controlled diabetic patients have peripheral arterial disease and are susceptible to these infections due to poor wound healing.

4. Ray amputation of the big toe to control sepsis.

A9.4

1. There is dry gangrene of the right 4th toe.

2. Autoamputation of the gangrenous toe has occurred.

3. Gangrene is an indication of critical ischaemia. The patient needs to have further investigation of the lower limb arterial system to identify any areas of stenosis to prevent further tissue loss.

Q9.5

This is a 60-year-old male who has right big toe wet gangrene.

1. What is seen in the angiogram?
2. What surgery was performed?
3. What is the success rate of this surgery?

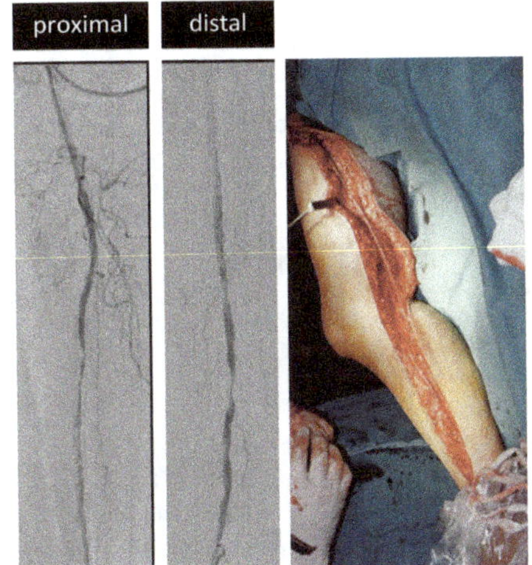

Q9.6

This is a 60-year-old male. An angiogram was performed on his right lower limb.

1. What does the pre-procedure angiogram show?
2. What is the likely clinical presentation?
3. What procedure was performed on him?
4. What does the post-procedure angiogram show?

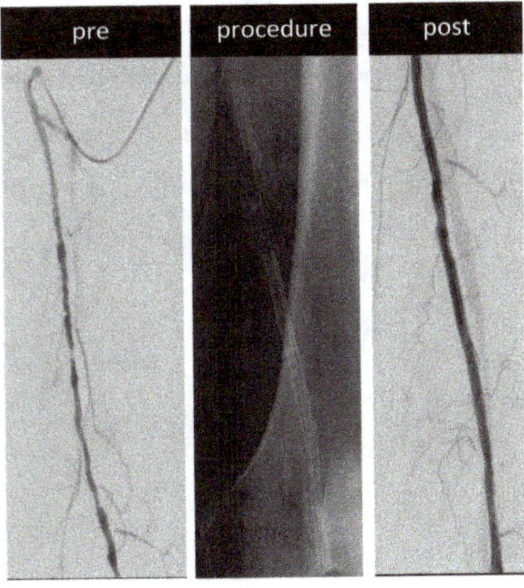

A9.5

1. It shows multiple stenoses of the superficial femoral artery.

2. Femoral popliteal bypass grafting, most often using an autologous great saphenous vein.

3. Up to 80% in 5 years.

A9.6

1. There are multiple stenoses of the superficial femoral artery.

2. Intermittent claudication progressing to rest pain.

3. Percutaneous transluminal angioplasty of the narrowed areas.

4. The check angiogram shows good patent flow through the artery after the procedure.

Q9.7

This is a 60-year-old male who presented with progressive worsening claudication pain of his right leg. Surgery was performed on his groin artery.

1. What diagnostic tests would have been performed before surgery?

2. Which artery in the groin is this?

3. What pathology is seen and removed from the artery?

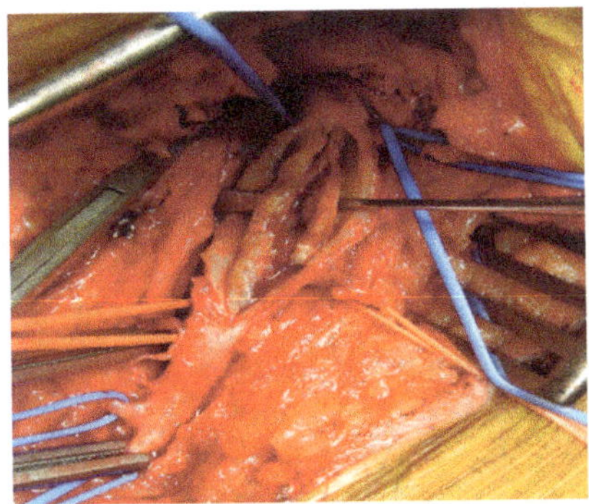

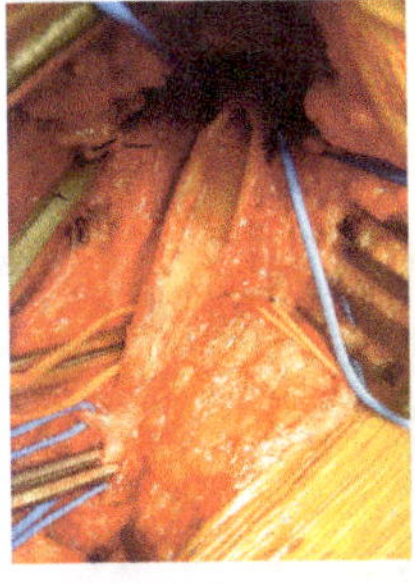

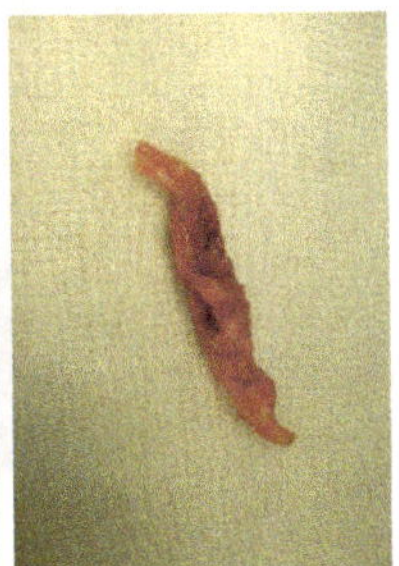

Q9.8

This patient had emergency surgery of the calf after a femoral endarterectomy.

1. What emergency surgery was performed for this patient?

2. What was the indication for this surgery?

3. What is the likely clinical presentation of the patient prior to surgery?

4. What other organs can be affected?

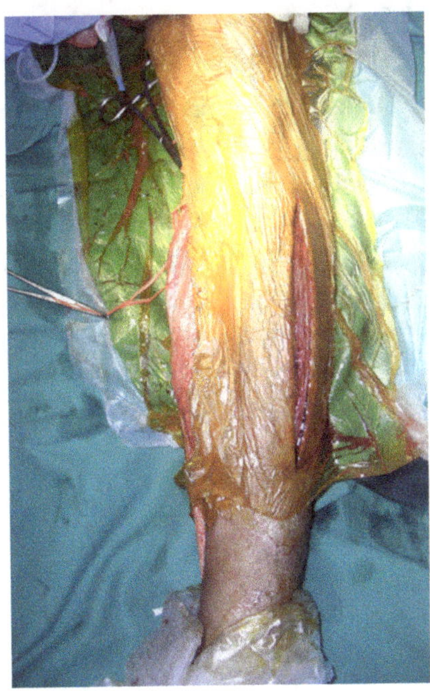

A9.7

1. ABPI, Duplex ultrasound scan and CT angiogram of the lower limb arteries.

2. Common femoral artery.

3. Atheromatous plaque in seen in the common femoral artery. Endarterectomy was performed.

A9.8

1. Fasciotomy of the calf.

2. Acute compartment syndrome due to reperfusion syndrome.

3. The patient would experience severe pain and parasthesia, especially with passive stretching of the calf muscles. The classical findings are swelling, discoloration, and loss of pulses in the extremity.

4. Other organs usually involved in vascular reperfusion injury are heart, lung, liver, skeletal muscles, gut, and kidneys, but it can also induce systemic inflammation, eventually leading to multi-organ failure.

Q9.9

This is a 75-year-old male.

1. What abnormality is seen in the ultrasound report of the left carotid artery?

2. What is the likely clinical presentation?

3. What surgery was performed?

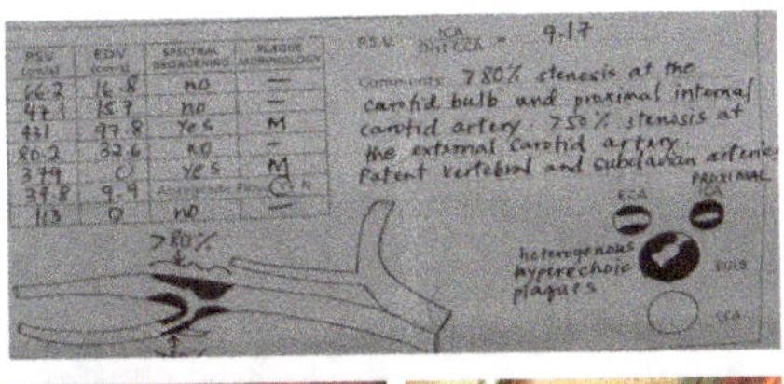

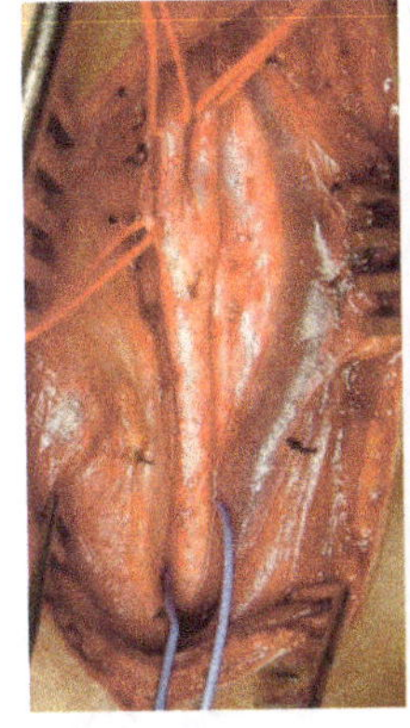

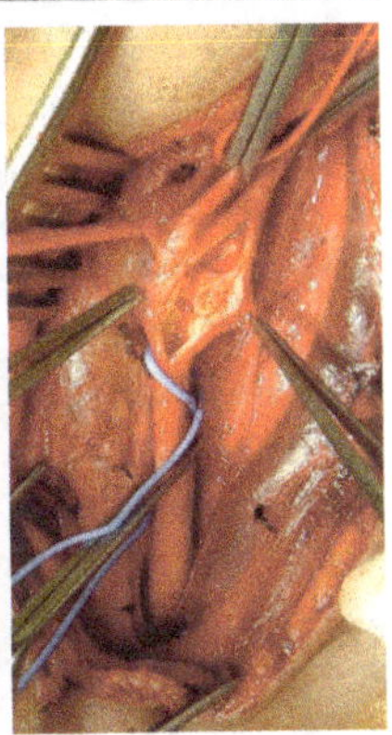

Q9.10

This is a 50-year-old male.

1. What is abnormality is seen in the CT scan?

2. What is the clinical presentation?

3. What is the pathogenesis of this condition?

4. What is the management?

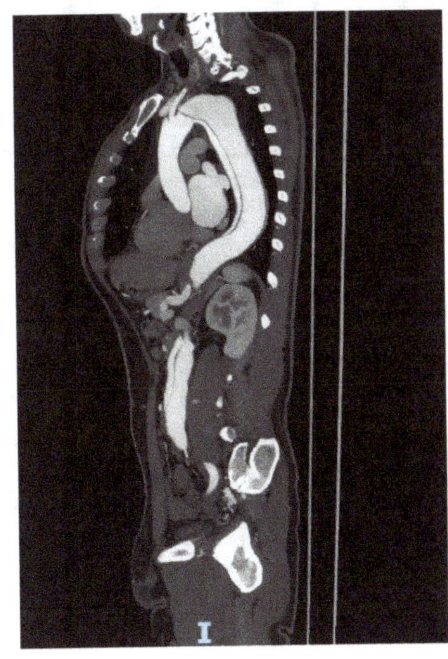

A9.9

1. There is a significant stenosis of the left internal carotid artery.

2. Patients may be asymptomatic. Others may present with neurologic symptoms — slurred speech, cranial nerve deficits, limb weakness, or visual disturbances. Amaurosis fugax is a common symptom of ipsilateral carotid stenosis. A carotid bruit may be present on clinical examination.

3. Carotid endarterectomy. It is recommended for patients with severe stenosis of 70% to 99%.

A9.10

1. Aortic dissection. A double lumen is seen in the thoracic aorta extending down to the abdominal region.

2. The patient will present with tearing chest pain that radiates to the back. Neurological deficits occur in 20% of patients. Hypertension and syncope are common. Some patients may have a difference of more than 20mmHg in blood pressure (BP) between the arms.

3. The aortic wall consists of three layers: the intima, media, and adventitia. Constant exposure to high pulsatile pressure and shear stress leads to a weakening of the aortic wall resulting in an intimal tear. Following this rent, blood flows into the intima-media space, creating a false lumen.

4. Adequate analgesia will decrease the sympathetic output. Optimisation of BP reduces aortic wall tension and limits extent of dissection. Surgical intervention with a synthetic vascular graft or endovascular stent-grafting.

Q9.11

This is a 75-year-old male.

1. What is the diagnosis?
2. What is the likely clinical presentation?
3. What surgery was performed?
4. What are complications of this surgery?

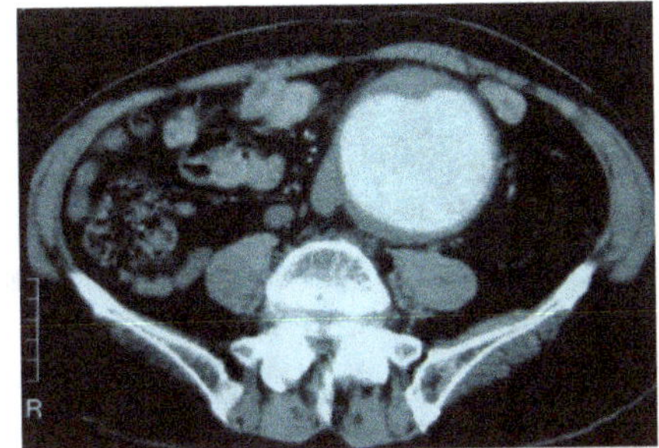

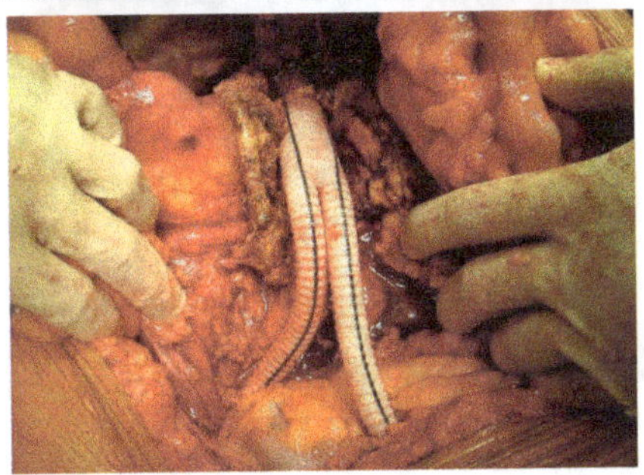

Q9.12

This is a 65-year-old male.

1. What is the diagnosis?
2. What are risk factors to developing this?
3. What is the natural history if left alone?
4. What are indications for intervention?
5. What treatment was performed?
6. What are complications of this procedure?

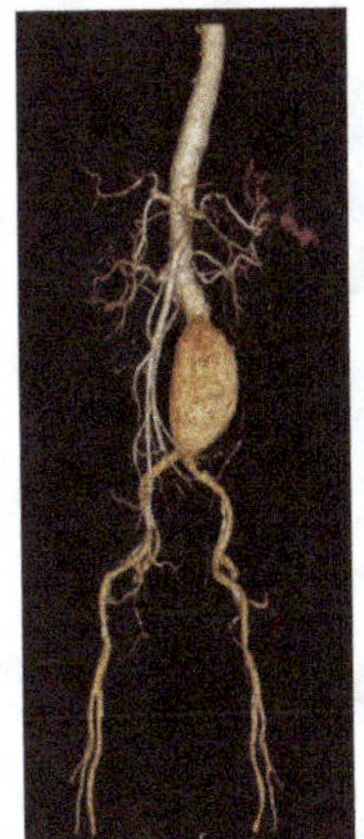

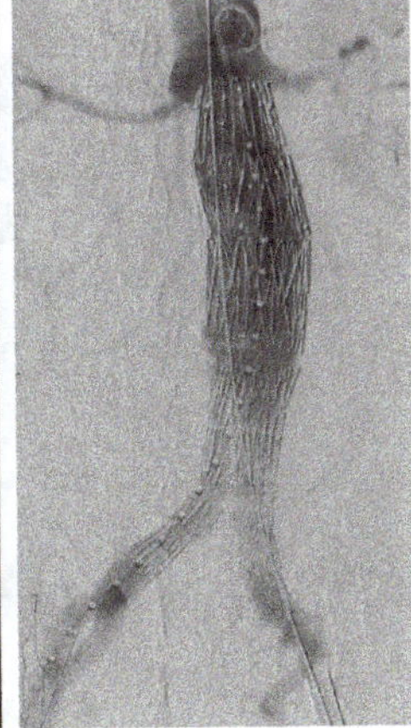

A9.11

1. There is a large abdominal aortic aneurysm.

2. They are often asymptomatic unless they leak or rupture. A large pulsatile central mass can be detected on abdominal examination.

3. Open surgical repair was performed with excision of the dilated aorta wall and placement of a sutured woven graft.

4. Complications are associated with cross-clamping of the aorta and blood loss during surgery.
   They include pulmonary, cardiac, renal, ischaemic colitis and wound infection.

A9.12

1. Abdominal aortic aneurysm (AAA) — fusiform shaped.

2. Risk factors include atherosclerosis (most common), smoking, advanced age, male gender, family history of AAA, hypertension, hypercholesterolemia, and prior history of aortic dissection.

3. They will slowly enlarge with corresponding increased risk of rupture.

4. The treatment of unruptured AAAs is recommended when the aneurysm diameter reaches 5.5 cm, shows a rapid enlargement of greater than 0.5 cm over 6 months, or if it becomes symptomatic.

5. Endovascular stenting of the aneurysm.

6. Graft migration and endo-leaks.

Q9.13

This is a 35-year-old female.

1. What is the abnormality seen in the splenic artery?

2. What is the clinical presentation?

3. What is the clinical management?

4. What was performed on this patient as seen in the specimen?

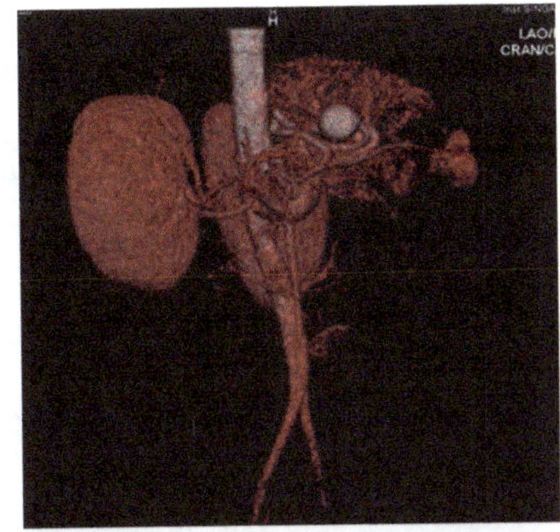

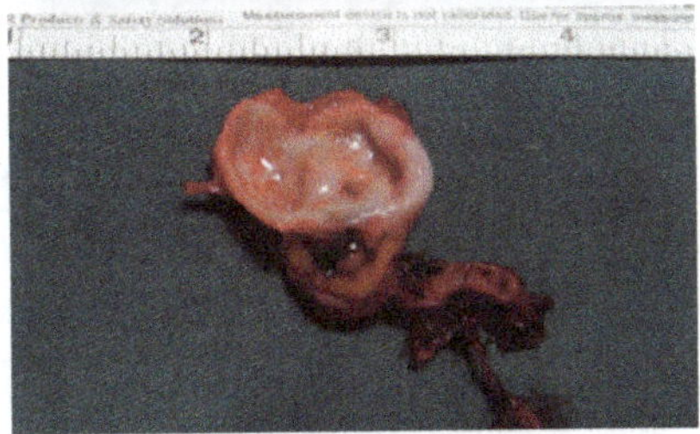

Q9.14

This is a 43-year-old male.

1. What is seen in the clinical picture?

2. What symptoms could he have?

3. What scan was done and what does it show?

4. What are the treatment options?

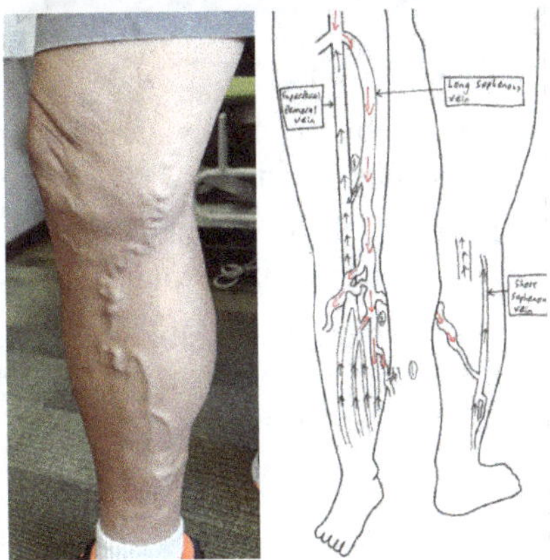

A9.13

1. There is an aneurysm arising at the distal aspect of the artery. (its size is the same as the diameter of the aorta).

2. It is mostly asymptomatic and are undetected. This aneurysm was an incidental finding on a CT scan.

3. Due to the increased risk of aneurysmal rupture, intervention rather than watchful waiting is advised.

4. The aneurysm was distal along the splenic artery adjacent to the hilum of the spleen. An en-bloc splenectomy with resection of the aneurysm was performed. The specimen picture shows the aneurysm sac.

A9.14

1. Varicose veins.

2. He may be asymptomatic, or experience a dull ache in the lower limb with prolonged standing.

3. Duplex ultrasound scan. It can be used to map all varicose veins, tributaries and incompetent perforating veins and rule out deep vein thrombosis.

4. Conservative management with elevation and compression stockings. More severe ones can be managed with stripping of the veins, sclerotherapy or endovenous thermal ablation.

Q9.15

This is a 65-year-old female. She has normal pulses on examination.

1. What is the pathological condition seen in picture A?
2. What is its pathogenesis?
3. What classification is used to stage the lesion?
4. What is the management?
5. What treatment was provided as seen in the picture?

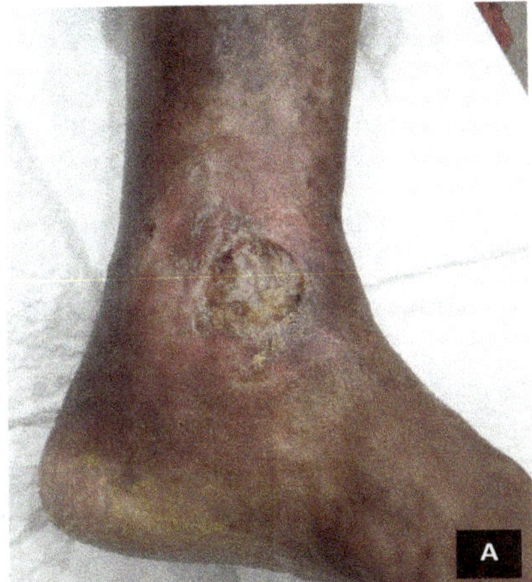

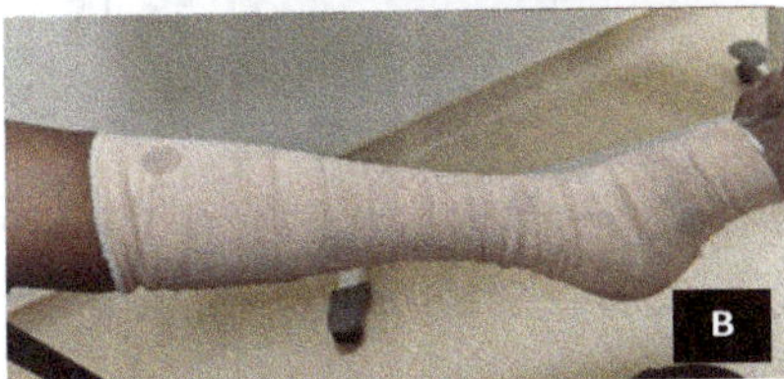

Q9.16

This is a 70-year-old diabetic male with a large foot wound.

1. How was the wound treated as seen in picture A?
2. What type of wounds are suitable for this form of treatment?
3. How often must the wound dressing be changed?
4. What are the principal actions of this treatment?
5. What is seen in picture B?

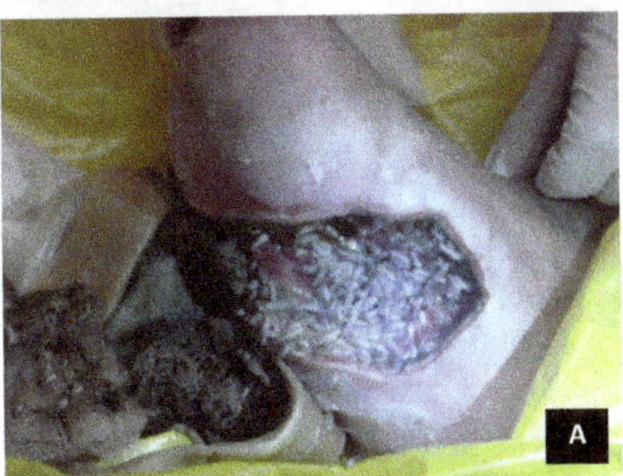

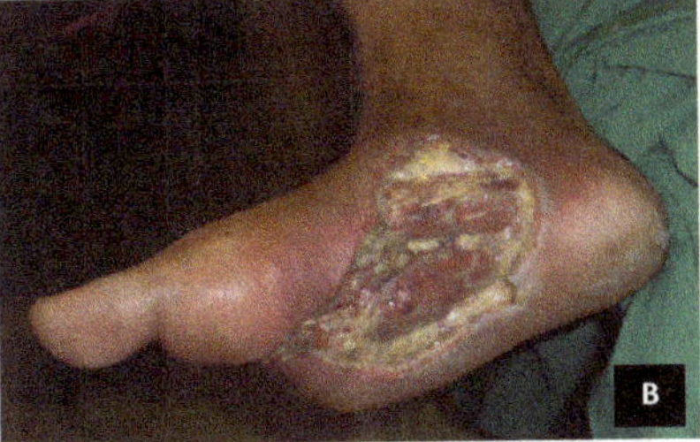

A9.15

1. A chronic venous ulcer. It is most commonly on the medial aspect of the lower limb. Description should include the ulcer area, depth, edges, wound base, signs of infection, and peripheral skin changes.

2. Two main factors are chronic venous insufficiency (CVI) and venous hypertension. The increased intraluminal pressure causes protein extravasation and fibrin cuff formation, which impedes the diffusion of oxygen and growth factors.

3. CEAP classification (clinical, etiological, anatomical and pathophysiological).

4. Two strategies: compression therapy and direct wound/ulcer management.

5. Compression therapy. It is the most practical and effective intervention for the treatment of venous ulcers. This involves the usage of various types of bandages, which can be elastic, inelastic, single- or multi-layered.

A9.16

1. Maggot debridement therapy. Sterile larvae of the Lucilia Sericata species of the green bottle fly.

2. A moist, exudating wound with sufficient oxygen supply is a prerequisite.

3. It takes 10–14 days for a newly hatched maggot to complete a lifecycle and turn into a fly. Dressings should be changed every 3–4 days, removing fully grown larvae before they are ready to pupate.

4. The larvae ingest necrotic tissue and digest bacteria.
   Bacterial growth is inhibited by the release of ammonia into the wound bed, which increases the wound pH.

5. The slough at the base of the wound has been debrided by the maggots.

Q9.17

This 60-year-old male had pelvic surgery 2 weeks ago.

1. What is the abnormality seen in the picture?
2. What is the likely diagnosis?
3. What would be found on clinical examination?
4. What are the risk factors?
5. How can we confirm the diagnosis?
6. What is the management?

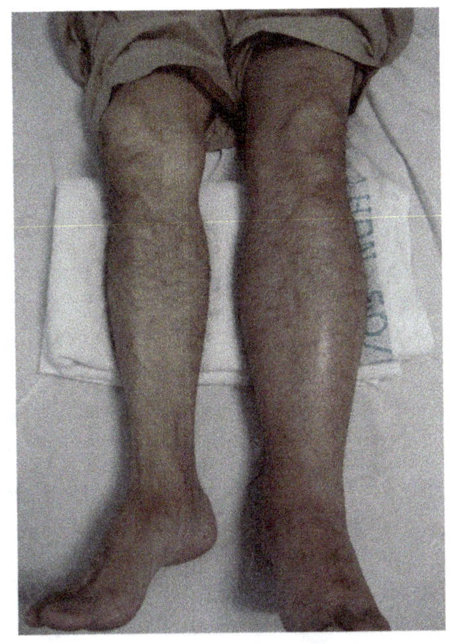

Q9.18

This is a 60-year-old male with a deep vein thrombosis (DVT).

1. What was inserted into the patient?
2. What was the indication?
3. Where is it normally sited?
4. What are complications of this procedure?
5. When should it be removed as seen in picture A?

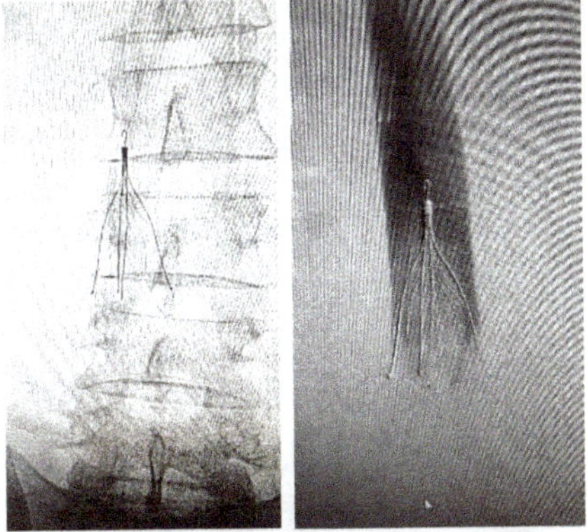

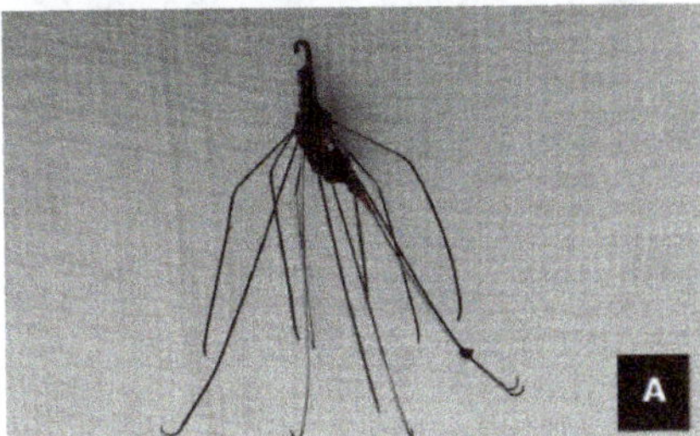

A9.17

1. His left lower limb is swollen and red as compared to the right.
2. Deep vein thrombosis.
3. The left lower limb will be warm and painful on passive dorsiflexion of the foot (Homan's sign).
4. Reduced blood flow: immobility, long surgery
   Increased venous pressure: hips in a flexed position
   Mechanical injury to the vein: previous DVT
   Increased viscosity: dehydration
   Increased risk of coagulation
5. Investigations include serum D-dimers, coagulation profile and an ultrasound of the lower limb veins.
6. The aim is to prevent pulmonary embolism and minimize the risk of developing post-thrombotic syndrome.
   The cornerstone of treatment is anticoagulation.

A9.18

1. An inferior vena cava (IVC) filter was inserted under imaging guidance via femoral vein or jugular vein access.
2. Patients with a DVT where anticoagulation was contra-indicated or failed. A pulmonary embolism needs to be avoided.
3. It is located just inferior to the inflow of the renal veins to lower the risk of thrombus occluding the renal veins.
4. Filter migration or fracture.
5. Removal should ideally take place once anti-coagulation is not required. IVC filters should be removed to decrease the risk of IVC thrombus formation. There is a clot seen at the apex of this filter.

Q9.19

This is a 19-year-old male.

1. Describe the abnormality seen on his face?

2. What does the MRI show?

3. What is the likely diagnosis?

4. How has the lesion been managed?

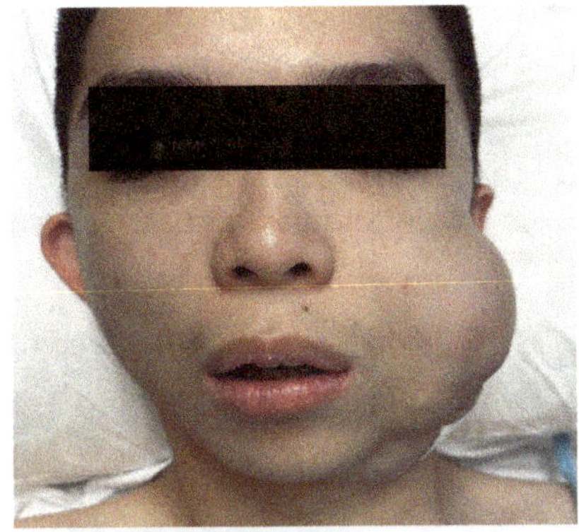

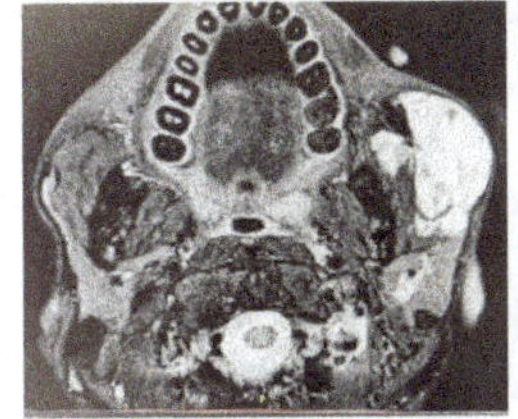

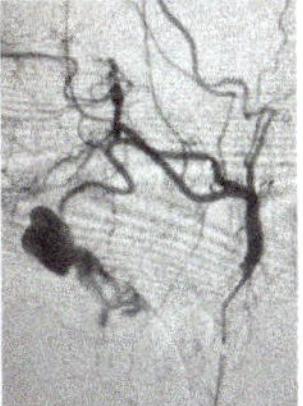

Q9.20

This is a 45-year-old male.

1. In picture A, what is seen in the right lower limb with him standing?

2. What characteristic of this lesion is demonstrated with the patient lying supine in picture B?

3. What is the likely diagnosis?

4. What is the management?

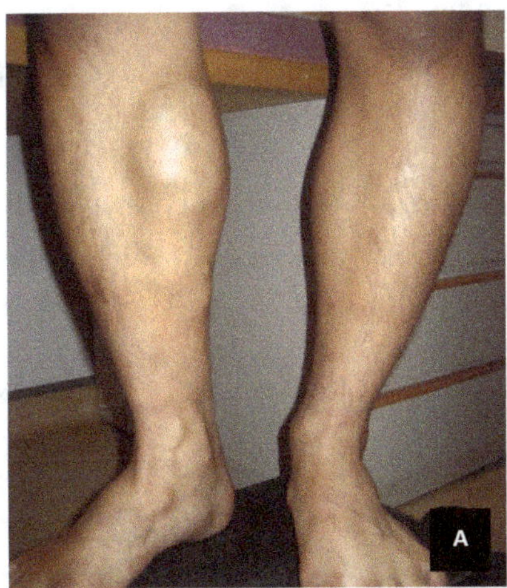

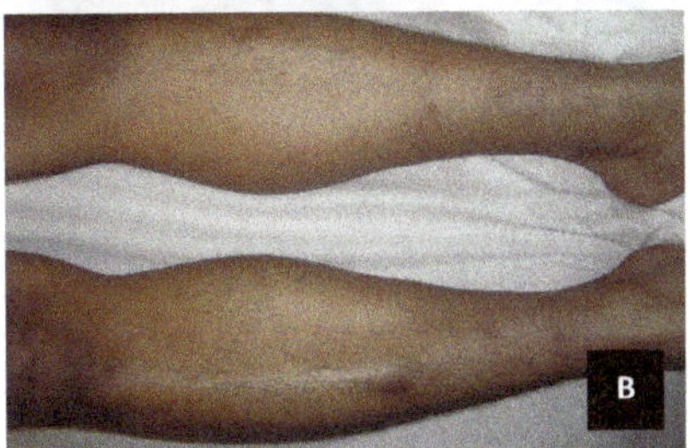

A9.19

1. There is a smooth swelling arising from the left side of the face. There are no overlying skin changes.

2. The is a smooth vascular lesion seen in the T2-weighted images. The lesion is adjacent to the left parotid gland.

3. Vascular anomaly.

4. Angio-embolization of the feeding vessel to the vascular lesion.

A9.20

1. There is an ovoid shaped lesion in the medial aspect of his inner right calf. There are no overlying skin changes. The veins around the right ankle are dilated.

2. The lesion has decompressed entirely, suggesting that it is venous in origin.

3. Vascular anomaly with large feeding veins.

4. It can be managed conservatively if the patient is asymptomatic, and if the lesion is not growing in size.
   Options for intervention include excision of the lesion.

Q9.21

This is a 55-year-old male.

1. What kind of vascular access is shown in the picture?

2. What is the indication for this?

3. What are other possible veins used for access with this catheter?

4. What are potential complications associated with prolonged use?

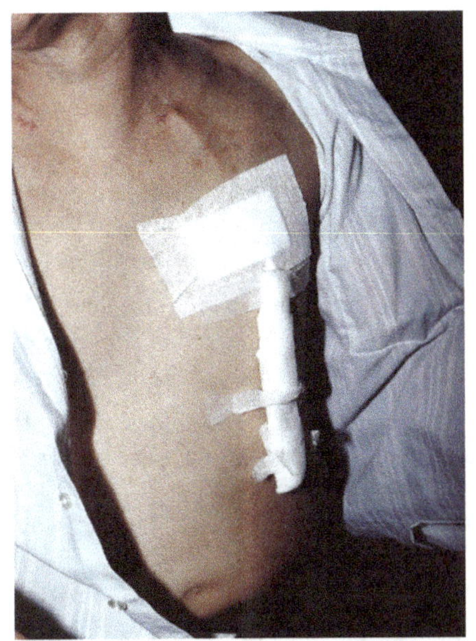

Q9.22

This is a 50-year-old male.

1. What is the diagnosis on the CT scan?

2. What is seen in the forearm?

3. What is the indication for this surgery?

4. What can be detected on palpation?

5. What are complications of this surgery?

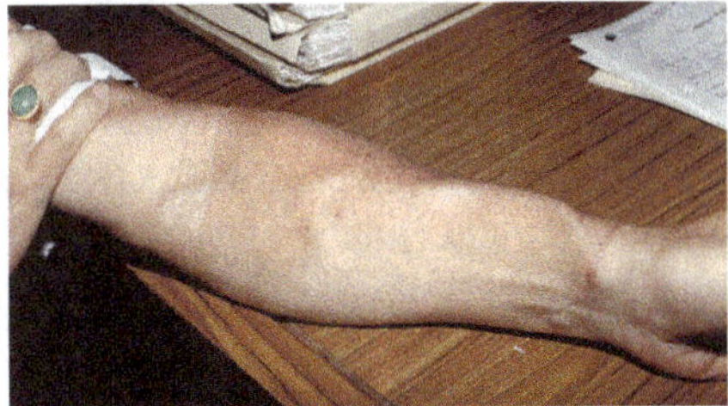

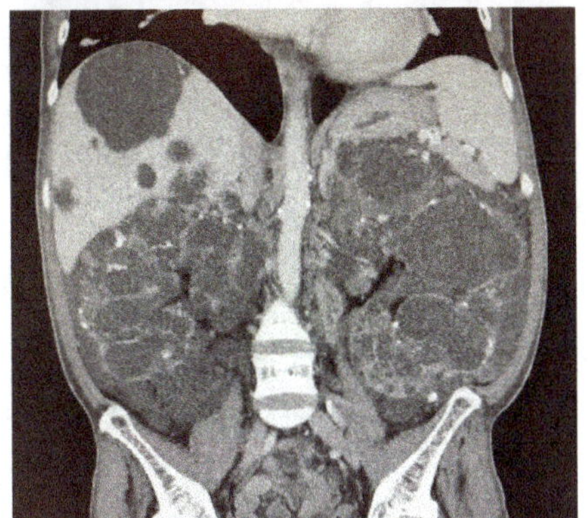

A9.21

1. This is a permcath. It is a double lumen tunnelled catheter used as an alternative access, in patients requiring haemodialysis. The 2 ports are for arterial and venous access.

2. This is an option in patients with no other alternatives for vascular access, patients with failed AVFs, or who are unable to create one, or for bridging during maturation of an AVF.

3. The right internal jugular vein (IJV) is the most popular as it has the most straightforward route into the superior vena cava. Alternatives are the external jugular, subclavian or femoral veins.

4. The catheter can be blocked by intraluminal clots, kink or get infected (being a foreign body). The vein can thrombose or be damaged by the catheter.

A9.22

1. Polycystic kidney disease leading to end-stage renal failure.

2. An arteriovenous fistula (AVF) was surgically created between the radial artery and cephalic vein.

3. It is created for vascular access for haemodialysis.

4. The matured fistula will be dilated with a distinct palpable thrill.

5. Mechanical failure due to anastomotic stenosis or thrombosis.
   Arterial steal syndrome occurs when arterial blood is redirected away from the hand.
   Pseudoaneurysm can develop from repeated cannulations.

10 Urology

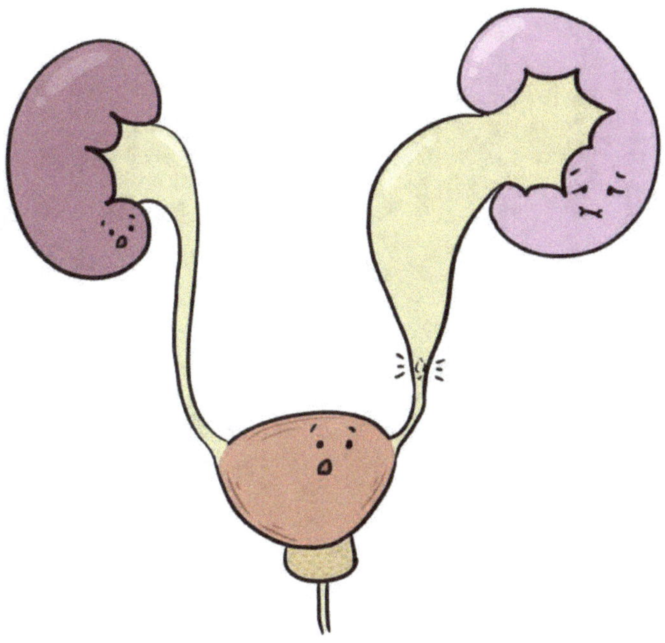

Q10.1

This is a 50-year-old male.

1. What is seen in the AXR and CT scan?

2. What is the pathogenesis?

3. What is the clinical presentation?

4. What is the management?

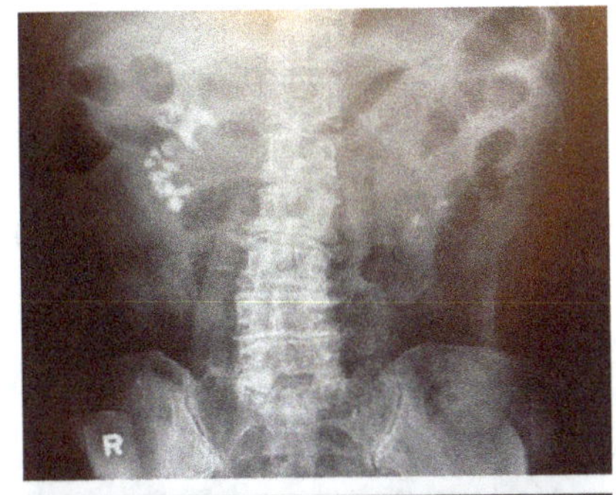

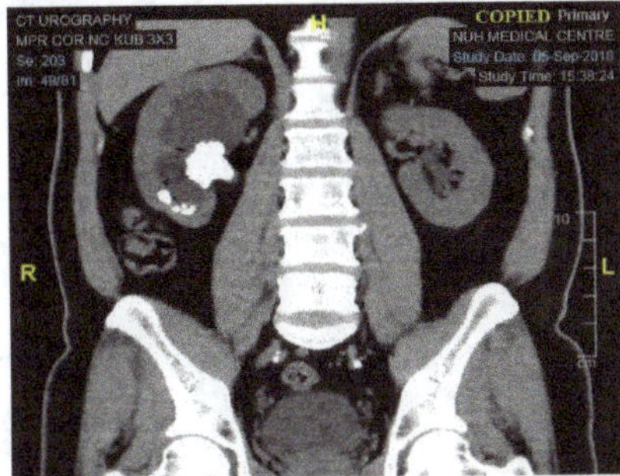

Q10.2

Ureteroscopy was performed on these 2 different patients.

1. What pathology is seen in both pictures?

2. Which locations are the pathologies likely to be lodged along the ureter?

3. What procedure is being performed to dislodge the pathology in the ureter as seen in picture B?

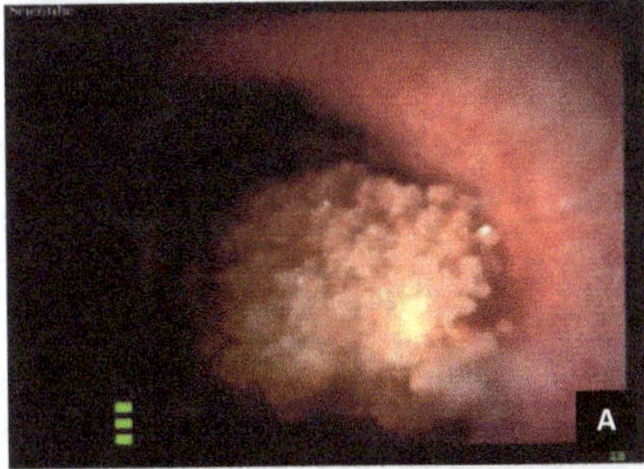

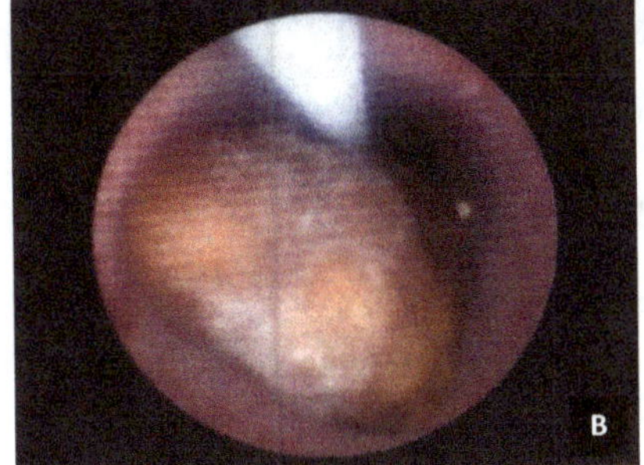

A10.1

1. Radio-opaque calculi in the right kidney.

2. Development of the stones is related to decreased urine production and increased excretion of stone-forming compounds such as calcium, oxalate, uric acid, cystine, xanthine, and phosphate. Calcium oxalate stones are the most common type.

3. Patients can be asymptomatic or may experience right flank pain (renal colic) and haematuria.

4. Small stones can be managed conservatively.
    Medium stones can be managed with extracorporeal shockwave lithotripsy (ESWL).
    This patient's stones are large and managed with percutaneous nephrolithotomy surgery (PCNL).

A10.2

1. Ureteric stones.

2. There are 3 sites of anatomical narrowing along the course of the ureter.
    *   The ureteropelvic junction (UPJ)
    *   The crossing of the ureter over the iliac vessels
    *   The intramural ureter at the ureterovesical junction (UVJ)

3. Intracorporeal (endoscopic) lithotripsy with laser, ultrasound or ballistic energy source.

Q10.3

This is a 50-year-old male.

1. What is seen in the KUB?

2. What is the likely clinical presentation?

3. How was the patient managed as seen from the surgical scar?

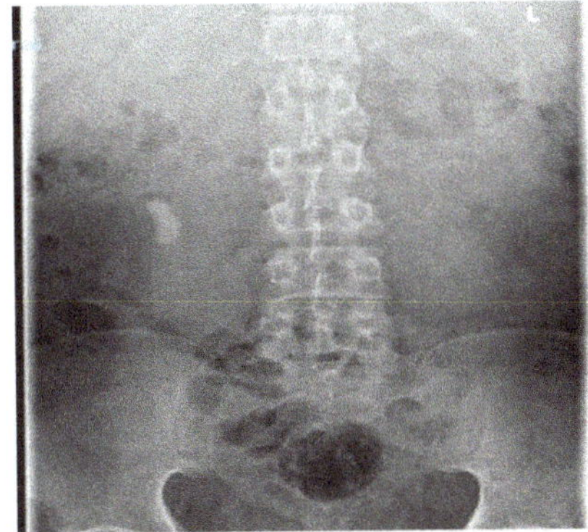

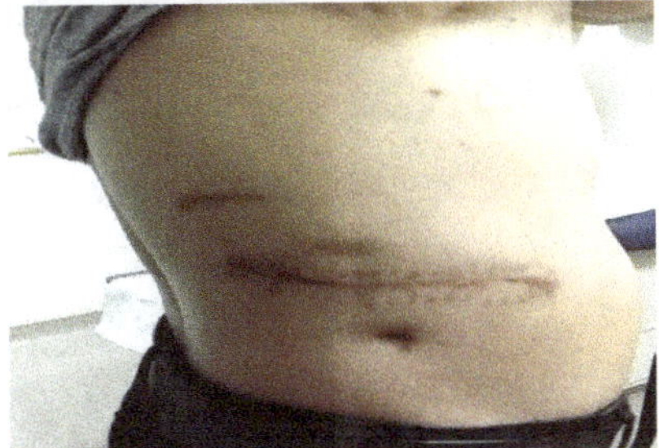

Q10.4

This is a 60-year-old male.

1. What is the pathology seen in the CT scan?

2. What are possible aetiologies?

3. What complications can develop if the pathology is not addressed promptly?

4. What procedure has been performed for the patient?

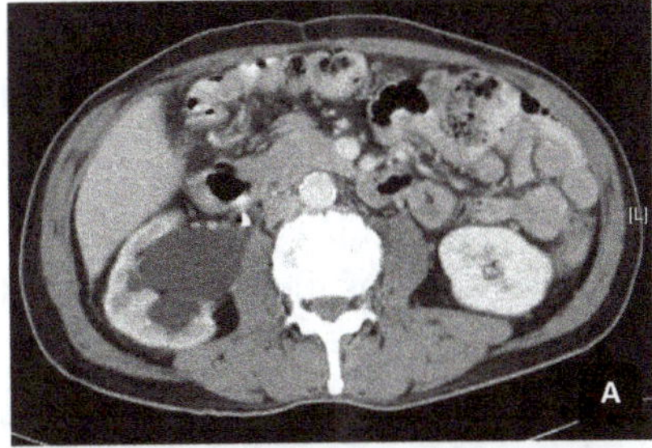

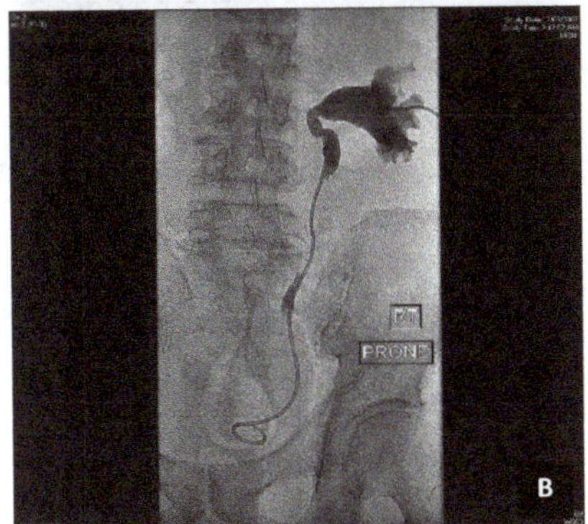

A10.3

1. There is a large radio-opaque stone in the upper right ureter.

2. The patient may experience episodes of sudden severe colicky flank pain that may become constant as time progresses.

3. The large stone failed other less invasive modalities of treatment and he needed an open ureterolithotomy via an incision along the 12th rib.

A10.4

1. There is hydronephrosis of the right kidney due to ureteric obstruction.

2. Intrinsic obstruction: renal stones, malignancy and ureteral strictures.
   Extrinsic compression: malignancy, trauma and retroperitoneal fibrosis.

3. Prolonged obstruction of outward flow of urine can lead to loss of kidney function.

4. Percutaneous dilation and stenting through the point of obstruction. A J-stent is seen in the bladder.

Q10.5

This is a 61-year-old female.

1. What pathology is seen in the CT scan?
2. What is the diagnosis?
3. What is the clinical presentation?
4. How was this patient managed as seen in picture B?

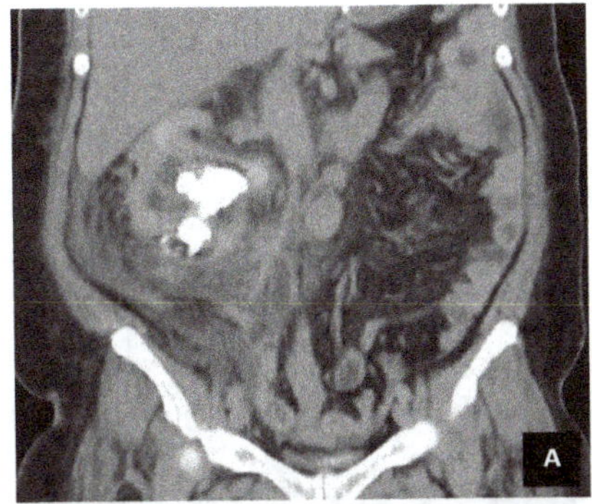

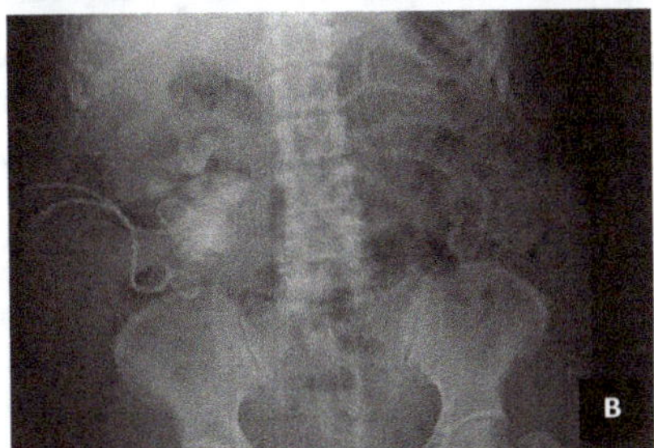

Q10.6

This is a 60-year-old male.

1. What is the abnormality seen in the x-ray?
2. What is seen in the CT scan?
3. What are likely findings on clinical examination?
4. What is the management?

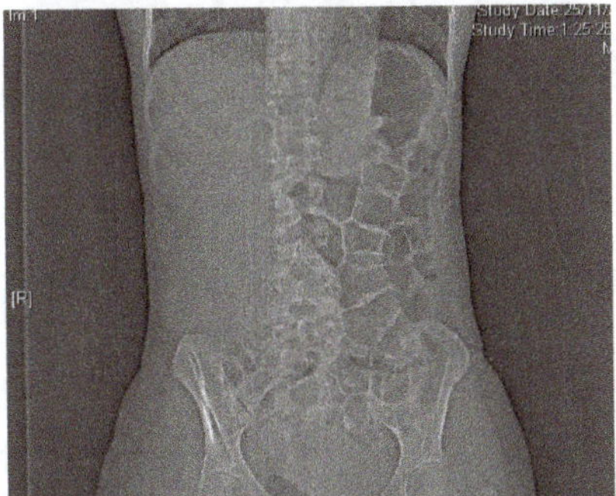

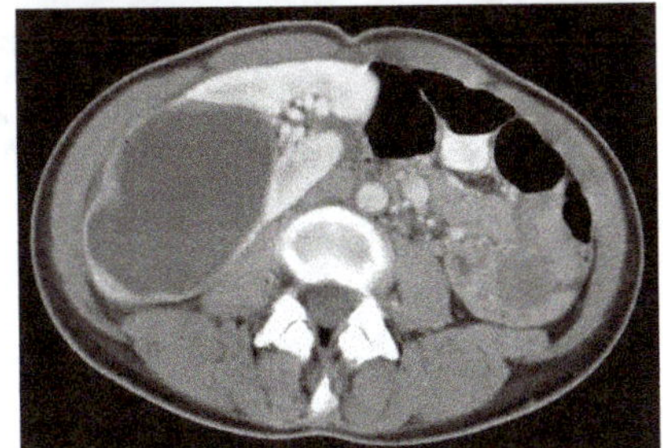

A10.5

1. There is a staghorn stone in the right kidney. The right kidney has surrounding fat stranding.

2. Pyelonephritis or pyonephrosis.

3. Fever with right sided abdominal or back pain. The right abdomen may be tender with a positive right renal punch.

4. The systemic sepsis was treated with intravenous antibiotics. Percutaneous nephrostomy with percutaneous drainage of pus. The stones will need to be removed.

A10.6

1. There is paucity of bowel shadows on the right side of the abdomen.

2. There is a large simple cyst in the right kidney. It has displaced all the intraperitoneal bowel to the left.

3. There will be a large ballotable and palpable mass on the right side of the abdomen.

4. Small cysts are asymptomatic and can be managed conservatively.
   This cyst is large and symptomatic. It can be managed with cyst aspiration and sclerotherapy (ethanol) or surgical resection.

Q10.7

This is a 70-year-old male with urinary symptoms.

1. What apparatus is seen in the picture?

2. What information does it provide?

3. What is the principle behind measuring urinary flow rate?

4. Based on the graph, what is the likely diagnosis?

5. What are the treatment options for this patient?

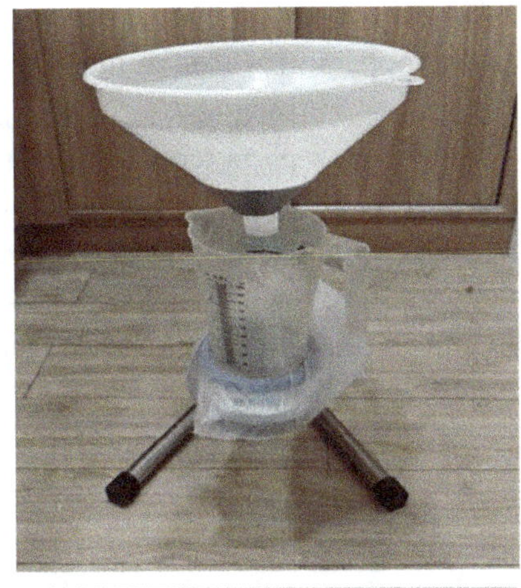

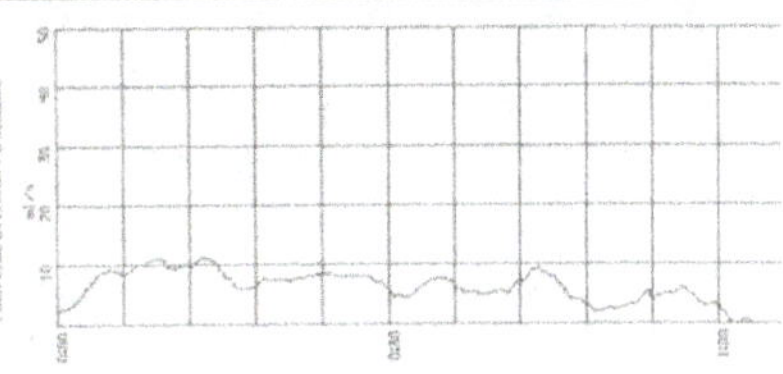

Q10.8

This is a 70-year-old male who had a surgical procedure for urinary symptoms.

1. What procedure was performed?

2. What symptoms might the patient present with?

3. What are indications for this surgery?

4. What are complications associated with this surgery?

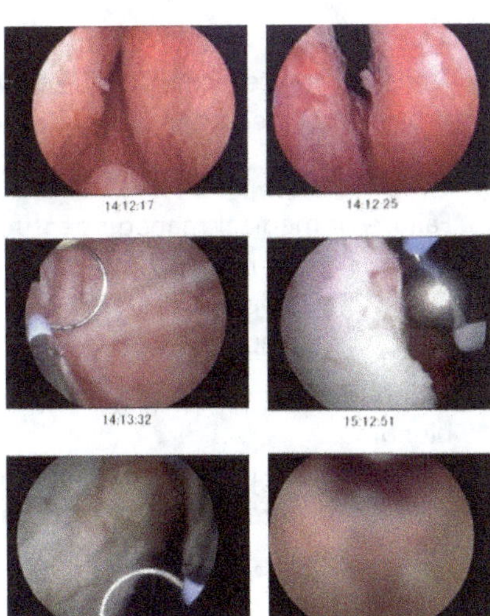

A10.7

1. This apparatus is used to measure urinary flow.

2. The urine flow pattern as well as flow rate (ml/s). This test is performed in the patient's preferred voiding position.

3. Urine flow curve plots the of velocity of voided urine against time. Uroflowmetry evaluates the interaction of the urinary bladder expelling strength (voiding pressure) and bladder outlet resistance.

4. Benign prostate hypertrophy (BPH). This is a typical uroflow pattern as there is a prolonged voiding pattern and low flow rate.

5. Medical therapy: alpha blockers, 5 alpha-reductase inhibitors.
   Surgical treatment: laser prostatectomy, water vapour therapy.

A10.8

1. Transurethral resection of the prostate (TURP). It is a procedure where the prostate is resected via an endoscopic approach.

2. Nocturia, poor stream, hesitancy, or prolonged micturition.

3. Failure of medical management for lower urinary tract symptoms (LUTS) or bladder outlet obstruction (BOO).
   Obstructive nephropathy.
   Two or more episodes of urinary retention.

4. Intraoperative: prostate perforation, ureteral orifice injury and excessive bleeding.
   Postoperative: Transurethral resection syndrome (TUR syndrome), retrograde ejaculation, infection (prostatitis) and urethral strictures.

Q10.9

This is a 60-year-old male.

1. What is seen in the right kidney on the CT scan?

2. What is the most likely diagnosis?

3. What is his likely clinical presentation?

4. What are the options for management?

5. What surgery was performed as seen in the intra-op photo?

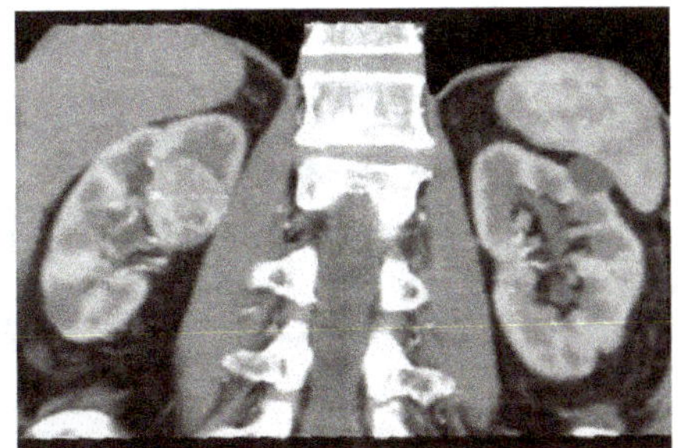

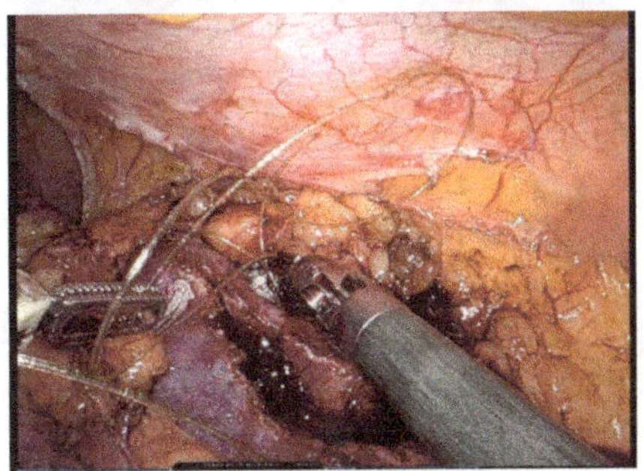

Q10.10

This tumour was removed from a 67-year-old male who presented with loin pain and gross haematuria.

1. What is the pathological specimen?

2. What is the aetiology?

3. What is the most common cell type?

4. What are risk factors associated with this?

5. Based on the pathological specimen, what vessel has the tumour invaded into?

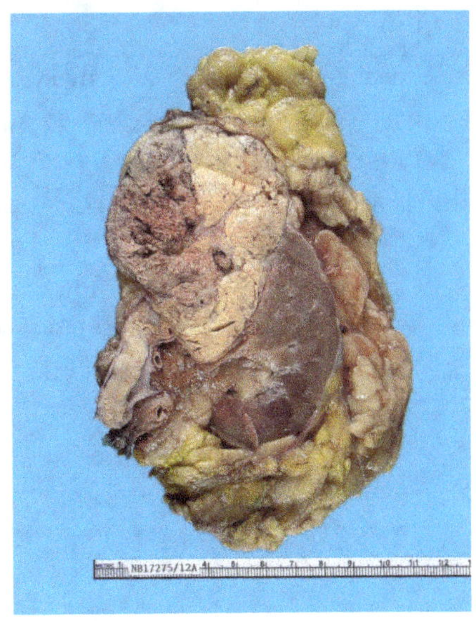

A10.9

1. There is a heterogenous lesion in the upper pole of the right kidney.

2. Right renal cell carcinoma (RCC).

3. 25% of patients are asymptomatic and the cancer is detected incidentally on imaging.
    Symptomatic patients may experience haematuria and abdominal or back pain.
    The classic triad of haematuria, mass and flank pain only occurs in 15% of patients.
    Paraneoplastic syndromes can occur causing hypercalcemia and erythrocytosis.

4. Surgical resection remains the only known curative treatment for localized RCC.
    Radiofrequency ablation can be considered as an alternative for small lesions in patients who are not candidates for surgery.

5. Partial nephrectomy. The photo shows repair of the kidney after resection of the tumour.

A10.10

1. Renal cell carcinoma (RCC) involving the upper pole of the kidney.

2. RCC mainly occurs sporadically but there are rare familial forms such as those associated with von Hippel-Lindau disease.

3. Clear cell (75%), papillary (10–15%) and chromophobe (5%) make up the others.

4. Cigarette smoking doubles the risk.
    Occupational exposure to certain chemicals — trichloroethylene, benzene.

5. There is extension of tumour into the renal vein.

Q10.11

This is a 76-year-old male who had a flexible cystoscopy performed.

1. What is the most likely diagnosis as seen in picture A?

2. What is the likely clinical presentation?

3. What are the risk factors for this pathology?

4. What was performed as seen in picture B?

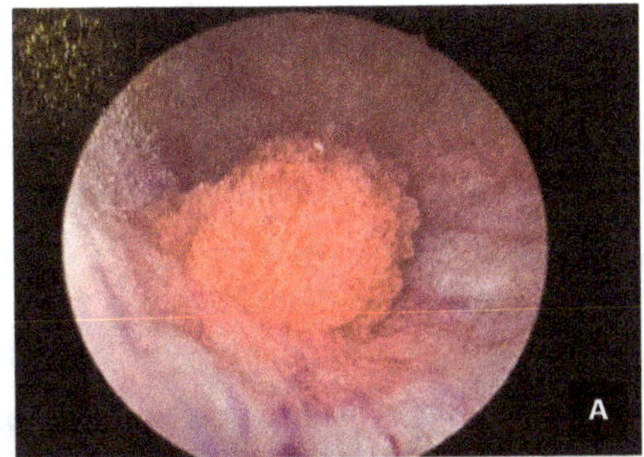

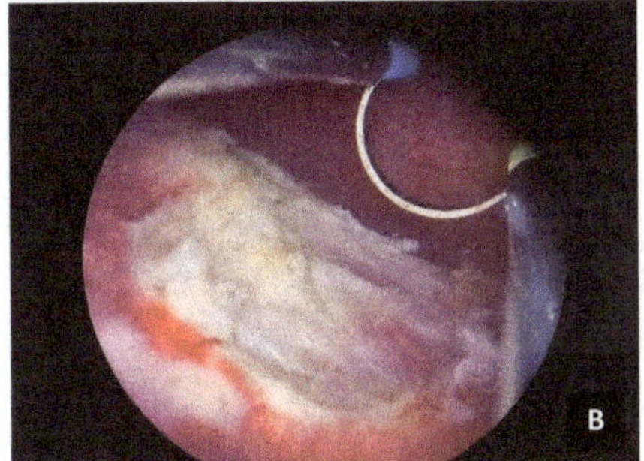

Q10.12

This is a 70-year-old male who had abdominal surgery for bladder cancer.

1. What is seen in the stoma bag?

2. What surgery was performed?

3. What are complications of this surgery?

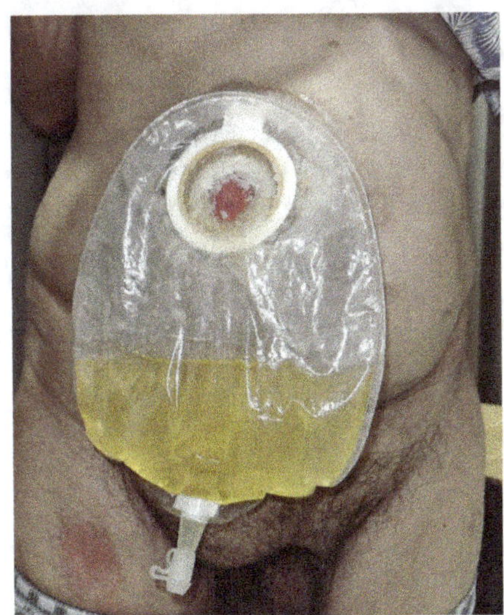

A10.11

1. There are frond-like papilliferous lesions with multiple vascularized projections. This is strongly suggestive of non-muscle invasive bladder carcinoma — Transitional cell carcinoma.

2. Haematuria, either gross or microscopic, is the most common initial symptom in patients with bladder cancer. Less common symptoms include painful micturition, increased urinary frequency and a pelvic mass.

3. A chronic indwelling catheter or foreign body, history of pelvic irradiation, chemotherapy, increasing age, male sex, smoking and toxic chemical exposure.

4. Transurethral resection of bladder tumour (TURBT). The resectoscope loop and tumour base are visible.

A10.12

1. Urine.

2. When a radical cystectomy is necessary, urinary diversion is required. An ileal conduit was created where the two ureters are anastomosed on to the ileal segment and the other end opened externally as a urostomy.

3. Prolonged conduit contact time with urine increases the risk of developing metabolic acidosis. Resection of a part of the terminal ileum can lead to patients developing vitamin B12 deficiency.

Q10.13

This is a 60-year-old male who had surgery for prostate cancer.

1. What special instrumentation is used in this surgery?

2. What are the advantages of using this instrumentation?

3. What are complications of this surgery?

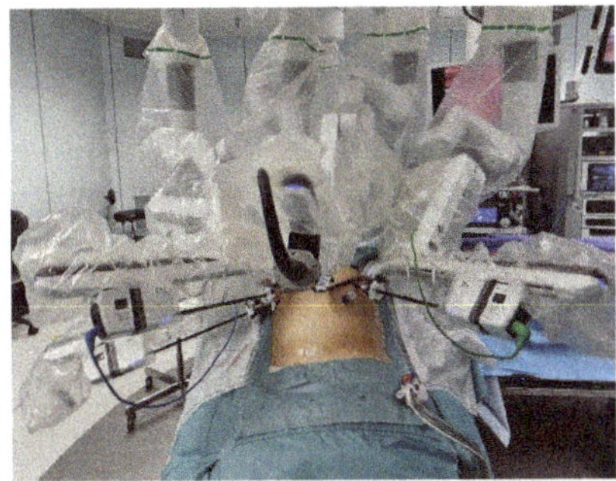

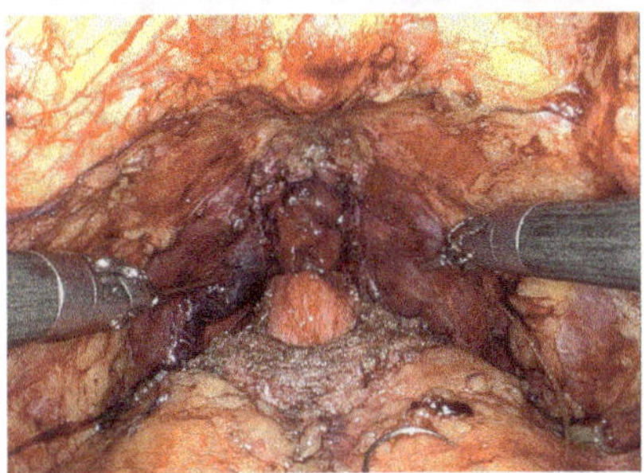

Q10.14

This is a 60-year-old male with an elevated serum prostate specific antigen (PSA).

1. What is PSA?

2. What surgery did the patient have based on the surgical specimen?

3. How common is this pathology?

4. What are the main prognostic indicators?

5. What score is used to prognosticate this pathology?

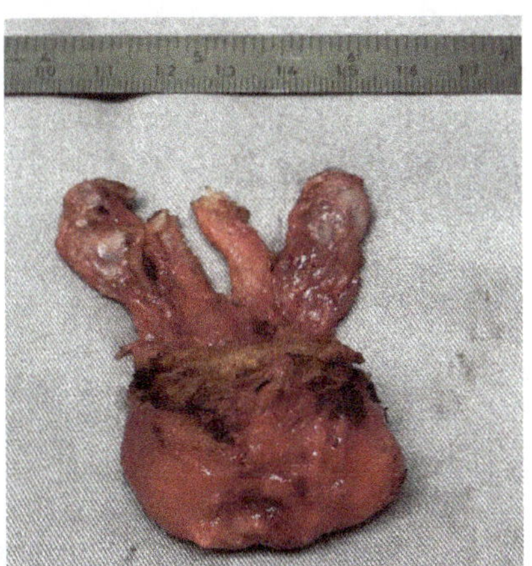

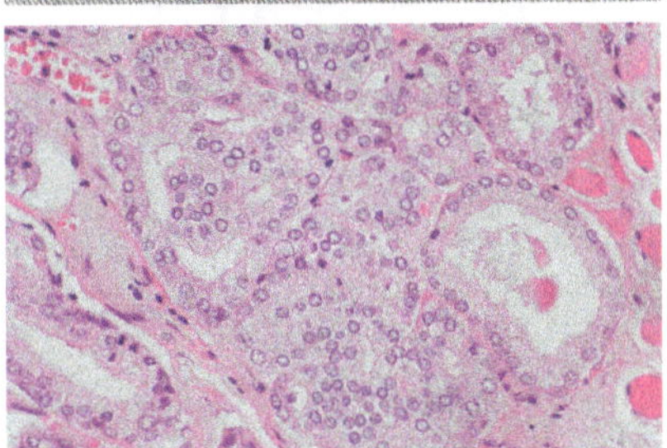

A10.13

1. Robotic-assisted prostatectomy.

2. The robotic surgical system has mechanical extensions arms with articulation and dexterity that replicate the movements of the surgeon's hands with remarkable precision. These arms are equipped with surgical instruments and can access tight spaces within the body, making them essential for intricate procedures.

3. Erectile dysfunction, urinary incontinence, urethral strictures and inguinal hernias.

A10.14

1. PSA is a glycoprotein produced by the prostate to liquify the ejaculate to assist with fertility. Increased levels of PSA are released into the blood as a result of tissue destruction from prostate cancer.

2. He had a radical prostatectomy.

3. Prostate cancer is one of the most common cancers in men.

4. PSA at presentation, tumour grade and stage.

5. The Gleason Score is the sum of two numbers. These two numbers represent the Gleason grade of the predominant pattern added to the grade of the next most common pattern. The Gleason grade is primarily based on the architecture or arrangement of the malignant cells within the tumour as well as other factors such as the degree of differentiation.

Q10.15

This is a 70-year-old male.

1. What is the pathology?
2. What procedure is being carried out?
3. What are potential side effects of this procedure?

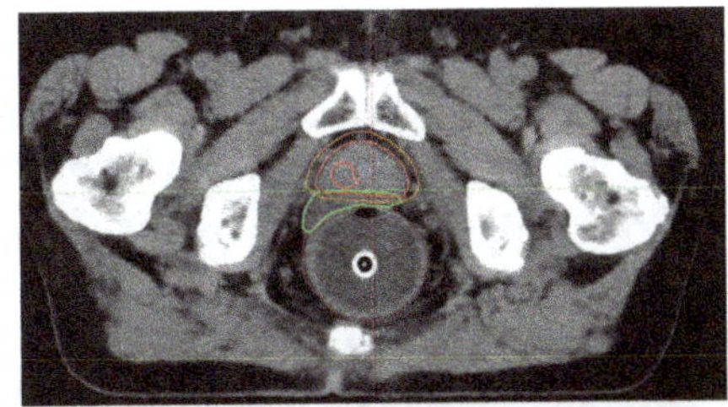

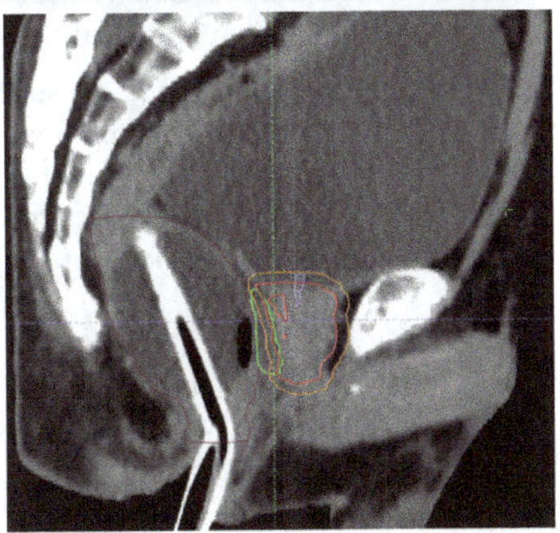

Q10.16

This is a 70-year-old male.

1. Describe the pathology seen on the penis?
2. What is the diagnosis?
3. What is the cell type?
4. What anatomical region should we examine?
5. What would the management for this patient be?

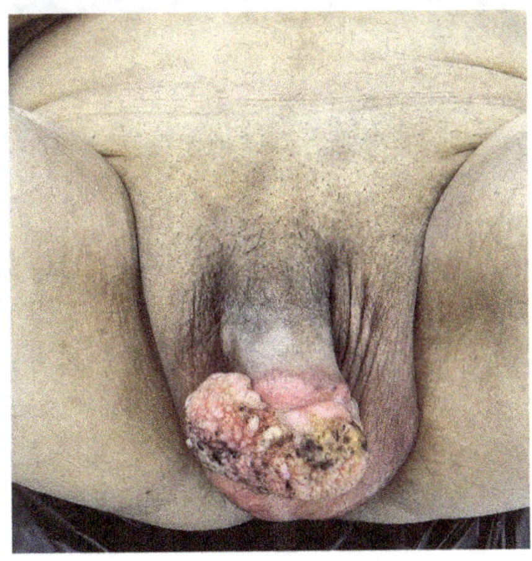

A10.15

1. The patient has localised prostate cancer.
   Acinar adenocarcinoma is the most likely histology.

2. The image shows CT simulation images for external beam radiotherapy planning.
   The entire prostate (contoured in red) and the target volume (orange contour) has been outlined. A rectal balloon filled with saline is present to help stabilise the prostate position.

3. Radiation cystitis is common, causing urinary frequency and urgency.
   Radiation proctitis is uncommon (5%) and may cause tenesmus or haematochezia. A hydrogel rectal spacer (outlined in green) displaces the rectum away from the prostate to reduce the risk of radiation proctitis. Erectile dysfunction is moderately common (50%).

A10.16

1. There is a large fungating ulcerative irregular lesion at the head of the penis. There is no active bleeding.

2. Penile cancer. It is an uncommon malignancy.

3. The most common is squamous cell carcinoma. Other uncommon ones include basal cell carcinomas, melanomas, sarcomas, and adeno-squamous carcinomas.

4. The bilateral inguinal lymph nodes are the lymphatic drainage basin for the penis.

5. A partial penectomy is recommended. Lymphatic clearance is needed if the lymph nodes are involved.

Q10.17

This is a 60-year-old male.

1. What is seen in the urethra at cystoscopy?

2. What is the likely clinical presentation?

3. What are possible aetiologies?

4. What other investigations can be done?

5. What surgery was performed for the patient?

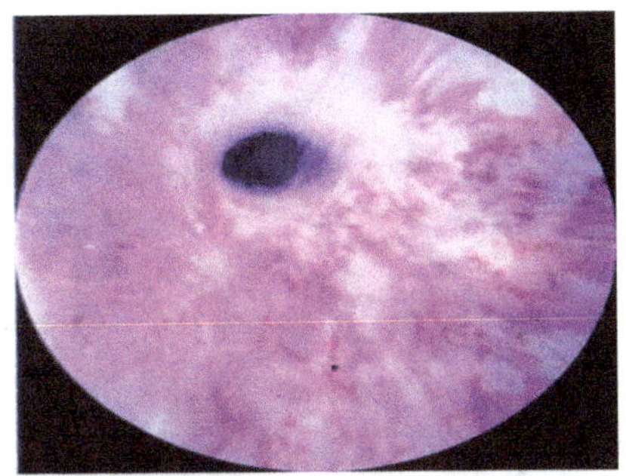

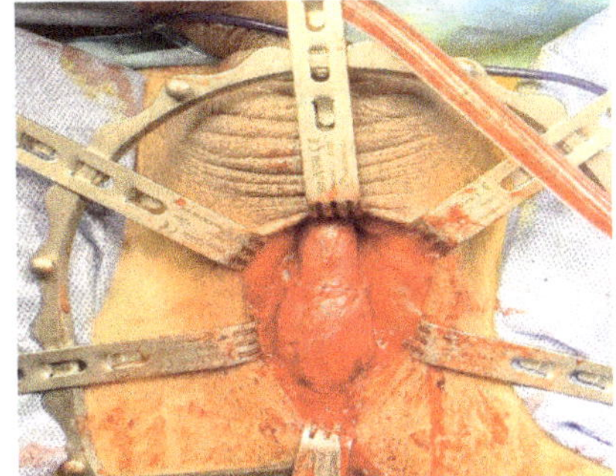

Q10.18

This is a 40-year-old male who was involved in a road traffic accident. He was unable to pass urine.

1. What procedure was performed on him?

2. What was the indication for the intervention?

3. What radiological investigation was performed and what does it show?

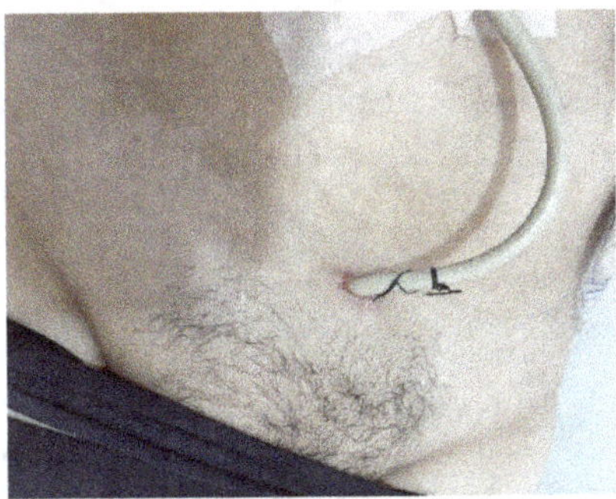

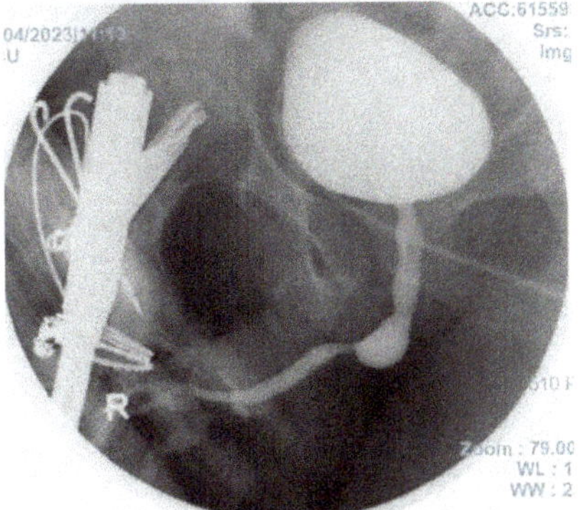

A10.17

1. The urethra lumen is narrowed, suggestive of a urethral stricture.

2. He may experience dysuria, a weak urinary stream, incomplete emptying, increased post-void residual urine volume, or a urinary tract infection.

3. Idiopathic.
   Iatrogenic: post transurethral resections, prolonged catheterization, cystoscopy.
   Inflammatory: post-infection.
   Post traumatic: compression of the bulbar urethra against the symphysis pubis (saddle injuries).

4. Uroflowmetry, post-void residual urine volume and retrograde urethrography.

5. The stricture was resected and primary anastomosis was performed.

A10.18

1. Suprapubic urinary catheterization.

2. Transurethral catheterization was not possible.

3. Retrograde urethrography shows a urethral stricture.

Q10.19

This is a 55-year-old male.

1. What is seen in the scrotum?

2. What is seen in the ultrasound?

3. What is the most likely diagnosis?

4. What can be detected on clinical examination?

5. What is the management?

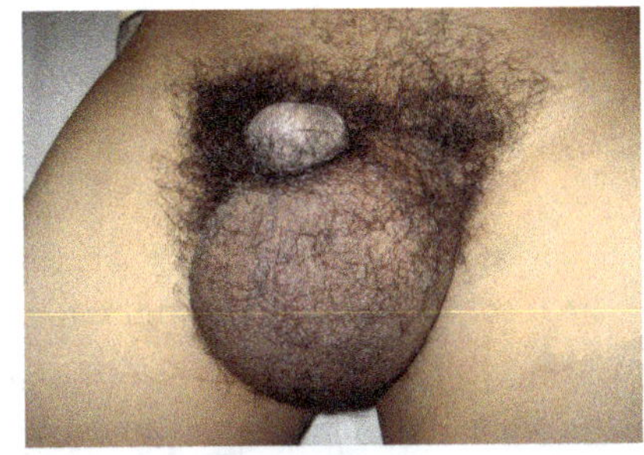

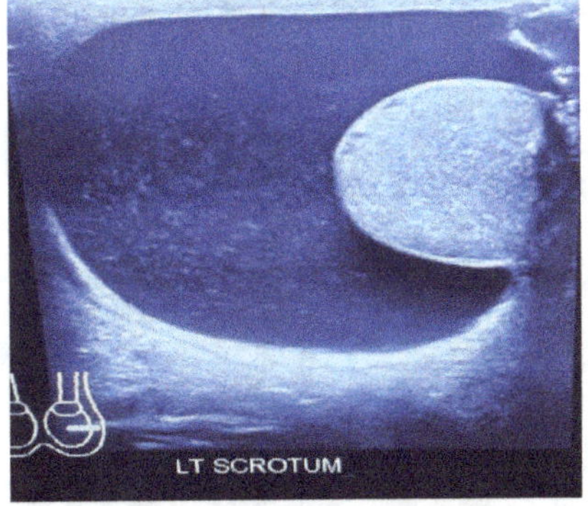

Q10.20

This is a 60-year-old diabetic who presented with fever and scrotal pain.

1. Describe the pathology.

2. What is the diagnosis?

3. What is the pathophysiology?

4. What is the management?

5. What is the prognosis?

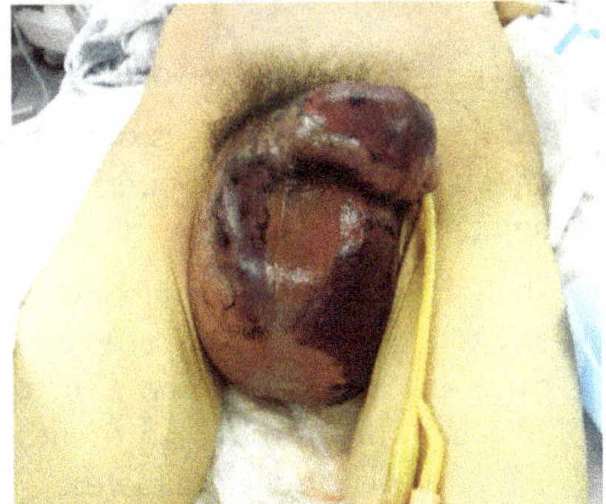

A10.19

1. The scrotum is larger on the left as compared to the right.

2. There is an echo-lucent area suggestive of large fluid filled lesion in the scrotum.

3. Left hydrocele. Hydroceles arise from an imbalance of secretion and reabsorption of fluid from the tunica vaginalis.

4. The scrotal swelling is painless and the testes impalpable. There will be positive transillumination and fluctuation.

5. Surgery is warranted when hydrocele becomes complicated or symptomatic. Plication or excision of tunica vaginalis and everting the sac behind the testes.

A10.20

1. The entire scrotum is swollen and inflamed. The skin has patches of necrosis.

2. Fournier's gangrene. It is a relatively rare form of necrotizing fasciitis that affects the deep and superficial tissues of the perineal, anal, scrotal, and genital regions.

3. The bacterial infection starts with an initial insult such as a perineal abscess or cellulitis. Endotoxins are released and this ultimately causes ischemic gangrene of the involved structures and rapid spread of the infection to adjacent and surrounding tissues. Most patients have other comorbidities like poorly controlled diabetes.

4. Fournier's gangrene is a surgical emergency.
   Medical intervention: broad spectrum antibiotics.
   Surgical intervention: aggressive and radical excision of all necrotic and gangrenous tissue.

5. The mortality rate is 40%. A significant contributor to this high mortality rate is the delay in diagnosis and treatment.

Q10.21

This is a 30-year-old male.

1. What is seen in picture A?
2. What is demonstrated in picture B?
3. What is the diagnosis?
4. What is the management?

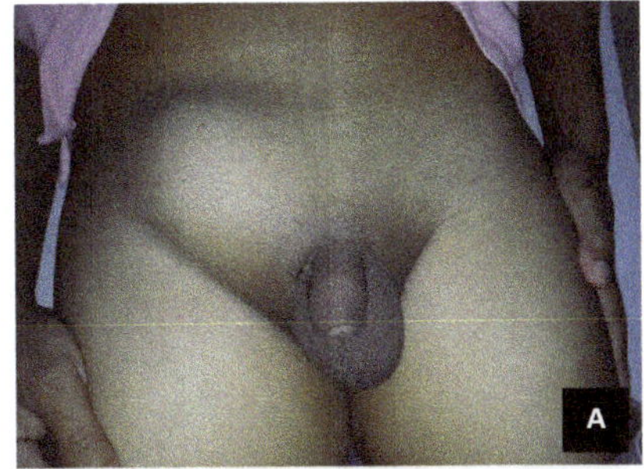

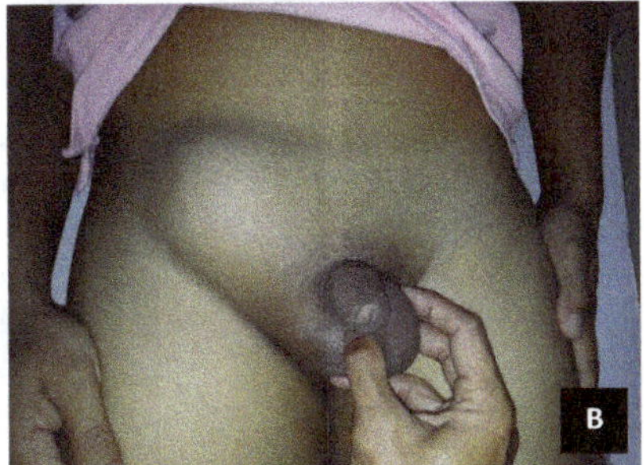

Q10.22

This is a 20-year-old male who had surgery on his left testis.

1. What is the most likely diagnosis?
2. Which age group of patients is affected?
3. What is the clinical presentation?
4. What is the histological cell type?
5. What serum tumour markers might be elevated?

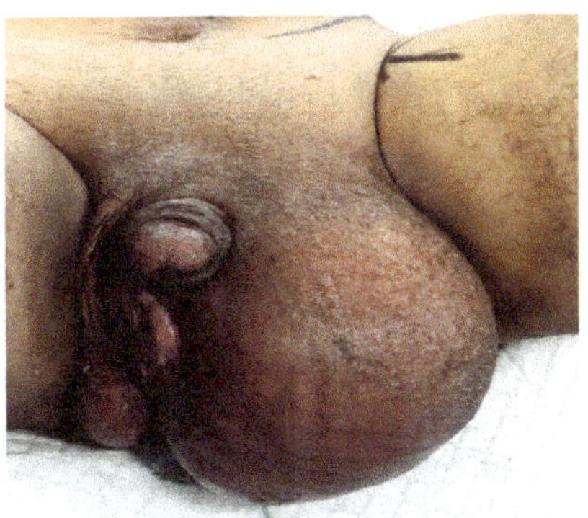

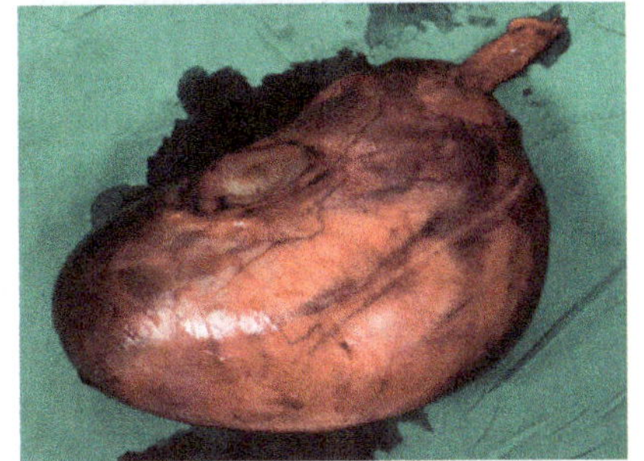

A10.21

1. There is a large mass in the right groin. There are no overlying skin changes.

2. The presence of a left testis and absence of the right testis in the scrotum.

3. An undescended right testis that has developed into a testicular germ cell tumour.

4. Radical right inguinal orchidectomy.

A10.22

1. Testicular tumour.

2. They are most common between the ages of 15 and 35 years.

3. A dull ache or heavy sensation in the lower abdomen could be the presenting symptom. A painless swelling in one testicle is the most common presenting sign.

4. Approximately 95% of testicular tumours are germ cell tumours. These are divided into two types: pure seminoma and non-seminomatous germ cell tumours.

5. Lactate dehydrogenase (LDH), alpha fetoprotein (AFP), and beta subunit of human chorionic gonadotropin (beta-hCG).

Q10.23

This is a 15-year-old boy who had emergency surgery on his left testis.

1. What does the intra-op picture show?
2. What is the likely clinical presentation?
3. What investigation can be useful in the diagnosis?
4. What pathology is often mistaken for this?
5. What surgery was performed?

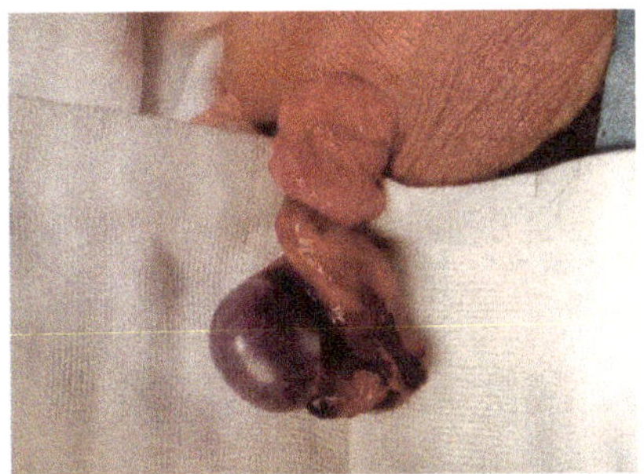

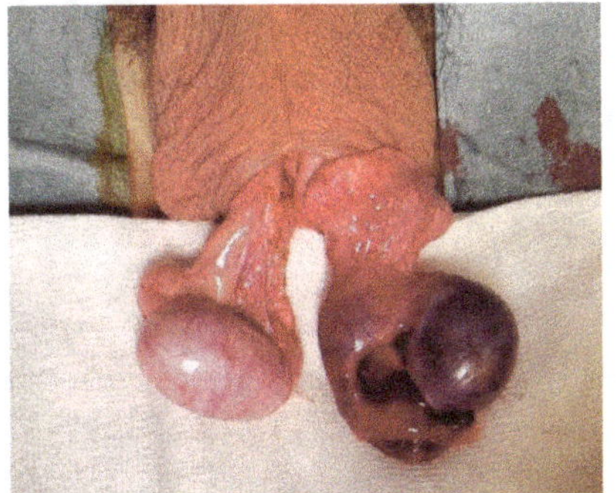

Q10.24

This is a 50-year-old female who had surgery.

1. What surgery did she have?
2. What are possible sources of donor kidneys?
3. What are complications of this surgery?
4. What complication did this patient have?

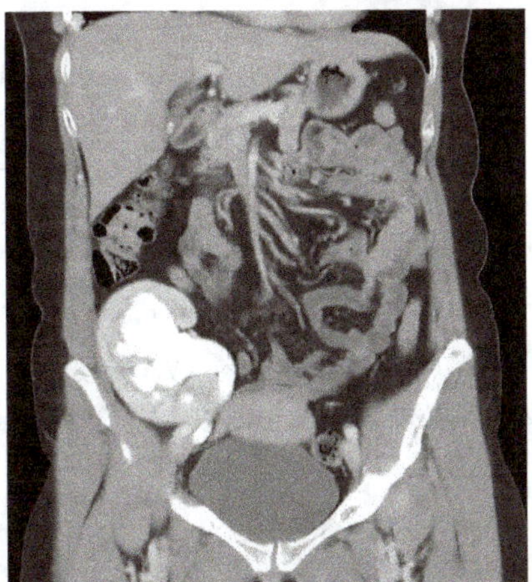

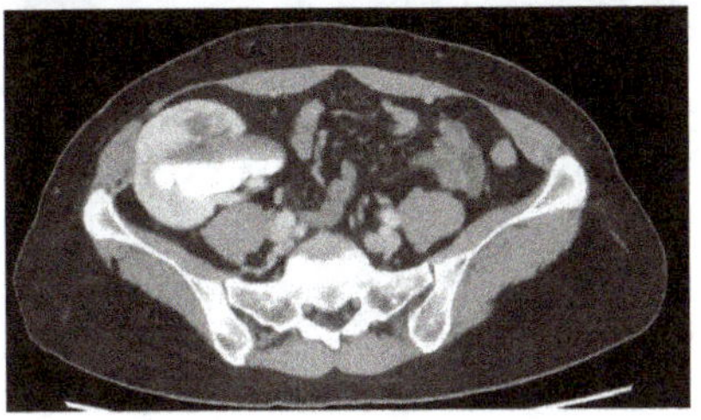

A10.23

1. The left testis is necrotic due to the torsion of the spermatic cord.

2. Sudden onset of severe testicular pain often after some physical activity. There may be some associated localised central abdominal pain (the testis retains its embryological nerve supply).

3. Ultrasound of the testis.

4. Acute epididymitis.

5. Emergency exploration and untwisting of the testis. Orchidectomy was performed as the testis was not viable.
   The contralateral testis is anchored to prevent torsion in future.

A10.24

1. Kidney transplantation.

2. There are two types of kidney donors: living or deceased.

3. Rejection: The body's immune system may recognize the transplanted kidney as foreign and attack it.
   Side effects of the immunosuppressive drugs.
   Surgical complications: bleeding, thrombosis of the renal vein, urine leak from the ureteroneocystostomy.

4. Hydronephrosis of the transplanted kidney.

11 Neurosurgery

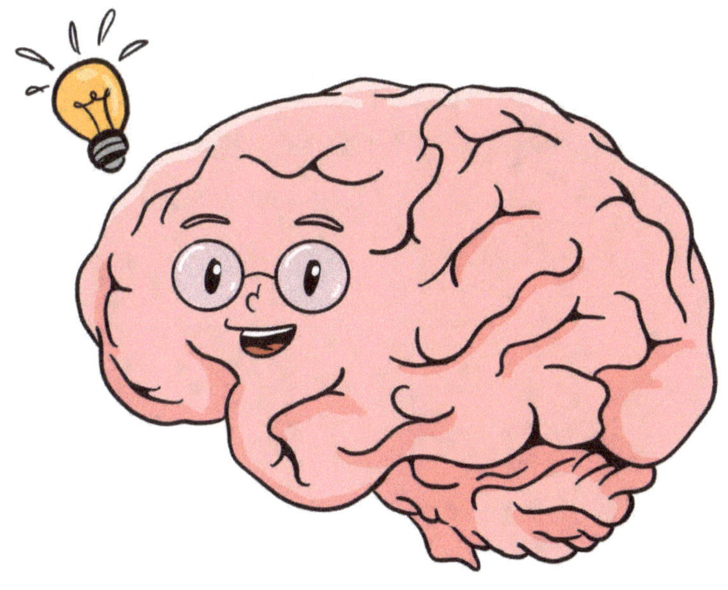

Q11.1

This is a 32-year-old female.

1. What is seen in the MRI scan?

2. What further test was performed for the patient and what does it show?

3. What other cranial nerves can be affected?

4. What hormonal disturbances can occur?

5. What is the management?

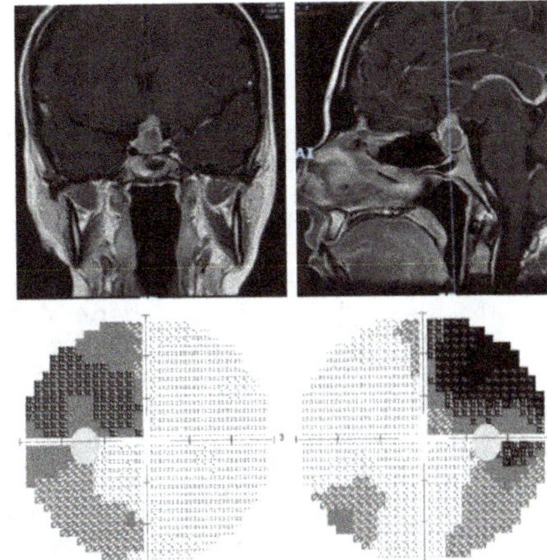

Q11.2

This is a 70-year-old male who presented with headache and left sided weakness.

1. What abnormality is seen on the CT scan?

2. What is the diagnosis?

3. What are other possible clinical presentations?

4. Why are patients at this age prone to this?

5. What is the management?

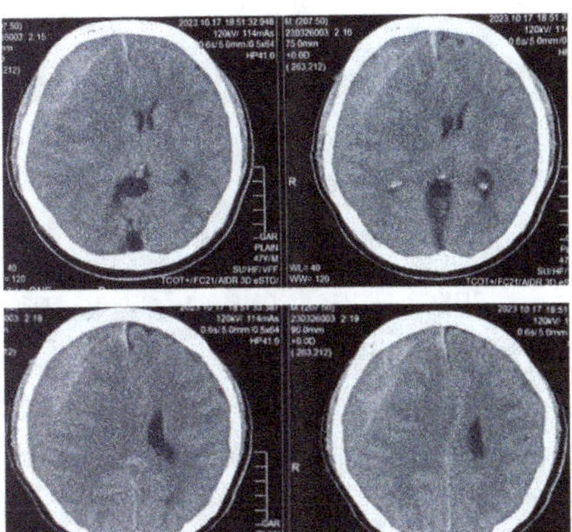

A11.1

1. There is a tumour arising from the pituitary gland.

2. A visual field test was performed and it shows bitemporal hemianopia. This results from mass effect on the optic chiasm due to tumour growth superiorly through the diaphragma sellae.

3. Cranial nerves within the cavernous sinus include the oculomotor nerve (III), trochlear (IV), trigeminal nerve (V1, V2), and the abducens nerve (VI). If a pituitary tumour invades the cavernous sinuses, it can result in ptosis, diplopia, facial numbness or loss of corneal sensation.

4. A pituitary mass can affect the levels of hormones produced by the gland itself. The patient may present with pan-hypopituitarism due to the mass effect on the normal pituitary gland within the sella.

5. Prolactinomas can be treated with bromocriptine. In most other cases, surgical resection via either the transsphenoidal or transcranial approach, is usually recommended.

A11.2

1. There is a hypodense lesion on the right side suggesting a subdural haematoma. It is causing midline shift with mass effect giving rise to effacement of the ventricles.

2. Chronic subdural haematoma.

3. Nausea and vomiting, dysarthria, visual change, dizziness, memory loss, personality changes.

4. With increasing age, there is cerebral atrophy. As the space between the skull and brain widens, the tiny bridging veins in the dura mater and arachnoid mater have greater propensity to tear.

5. Treatment of a subdural hematoma depends on its size and rate of progression.
   Small hematomas can be managed by careful monitoring as the blood clot is eventually resorbed naturally.
   Large or symptomatic hematomas require a craniotomy to remove the clot.

Q11.3

This is a 50-year-old male.

1. What is seen on the MRI?

2. What is the clinical presentation?

3. How are these tumours classified anatomically?

4. What was the management for this patient as seen in the surgical picture?

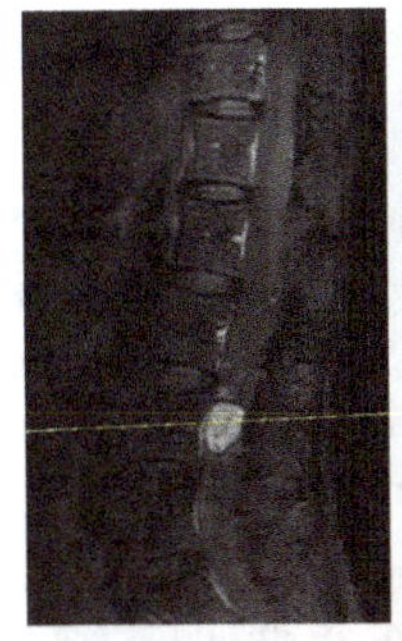
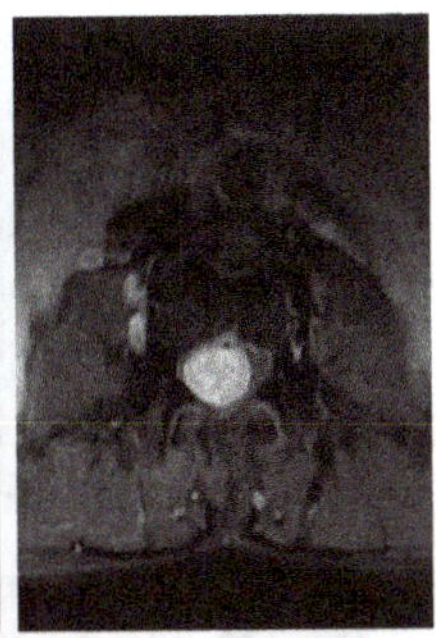
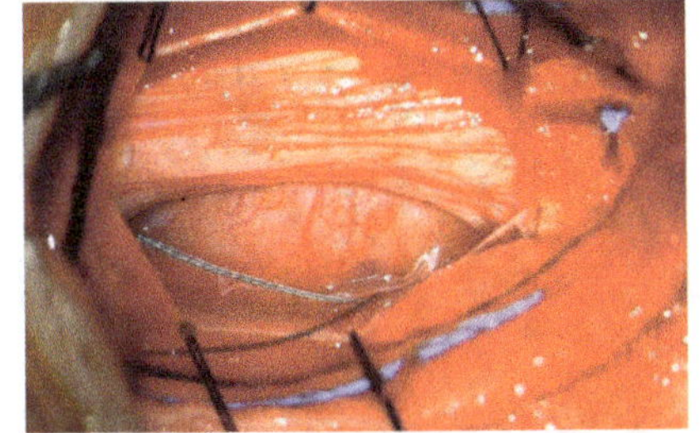

Q11.4

This is a 60-year-old male who suffered a head injury.

1. What is seen in the CT scan?

2. What is the diagnosis?

3. What is the clinical presentation?

4. What will happen if left untreated?

5. What surgical procedure was performed?

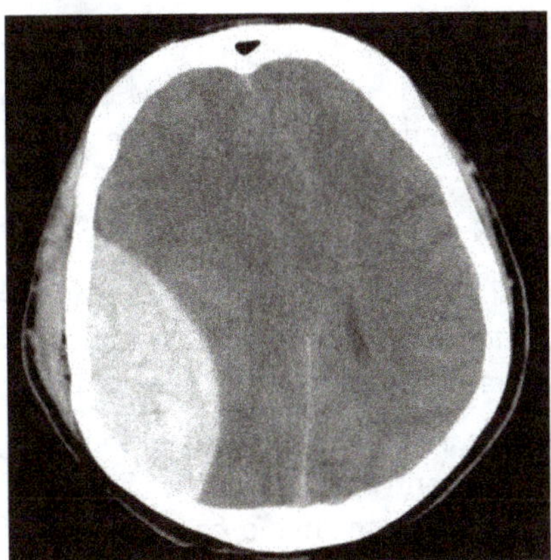
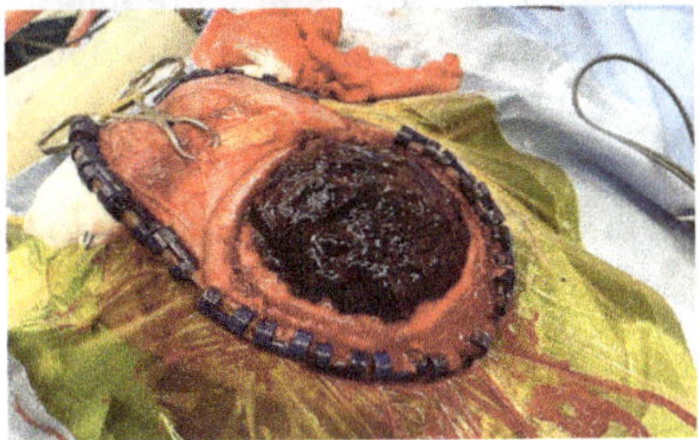

A11.3

1. There is a tumour at the L2-3 level of the spinal cord.

2. Small tumours are often asymptomatic. Larger ones can cause pain, which can be diffuse or radicular, and paraesthesia. This patient had weakness in the right lower limb.

3. Spinal tumours can be classified based on their locations — extradural, intradural-extramedullary, and intramedullary.

4. Surgical resection was performed. Conservative management can lead to further neurological deficits, some of which are irreversible. The primary objectives of surgical resection are to obtain tissue diagnosis, maximize safe tumour resection, and improve neurologic function.

A11.4

1. There is a biconvex mass on the right side of the brain. This is due to the limited ability of blood to expand within the fixed attachment of the dura to the cranial sutures.

2. Extradural haematoma (EDH).

3. The typical presentation is an initial loss of consciousness following trauma, followed by a complete transient recovery ("lucid interval"), culminating in rapid neurological deterioration.

4. An enlarging hematoma leads to elevation of intracranial pressure which will present with ipsilateral pupil dilation (secondary to uncal herniation and oculomotor nerve compression). The presence of elevated blood pressure, slowed heart rate, and irregular breathing is known as "Cushing's reflex." Immediate intracranial intervention is necessary.

5. Craniotomy and hematoma evacuation.

Q11.5

This is a 40-year-old male.

1. What neurosurgical procedure is performed here?

2. What are the indications for this type of surgery?

3. What is seen in the surgical field?

4. What type of anaesthesia is used?

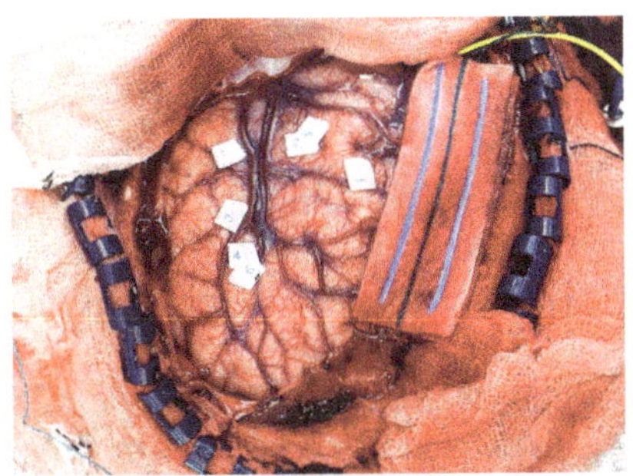

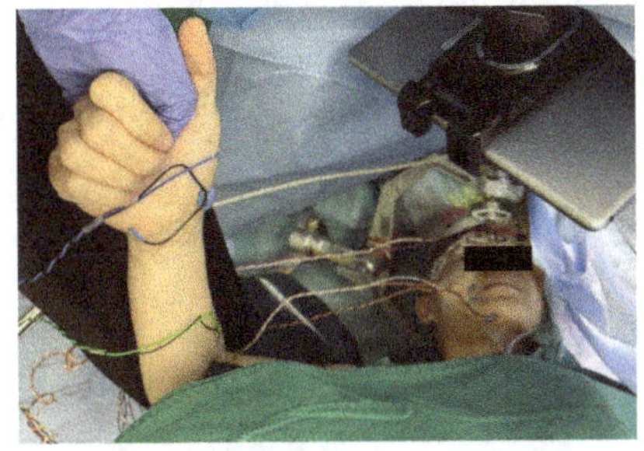

Q11.6

This is a 50-year-old female.

1. What is the diagnosis as seen in the CT scan?

2. What are risk factors?

3. What is the clinical presentation?

4. What surgery was performed?

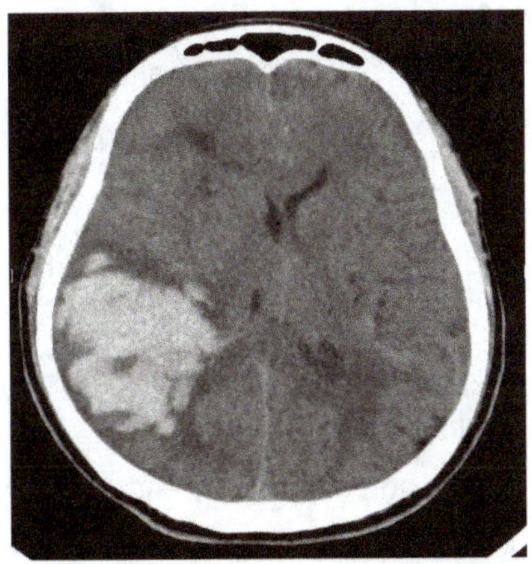

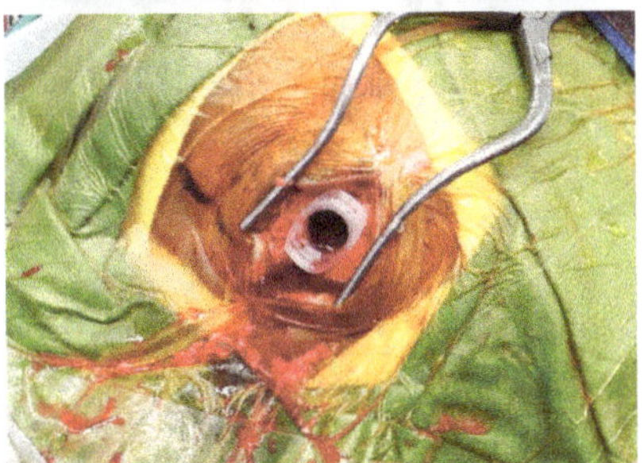

A11.5

1. Awake craniotomy. The patient is awake and holding the hand of a medical staff.

2. It is most commonly used to map and resect tumours involving vitally important areas like the motor and language cortex. The goal of awake craniotomy is to remove as much diseased tissue as possible without impairing critical function.
   It is also used for deep brain stimulation surgery classically for Parkinson's disease and other central movement disorders.

3. Intra-operative mapping of the brain.

4. Conscious sedation throughout the surgery.
   General anaesthesia with an intraoperative awakening for brain mapping.

A11.6

1. There is a large right parietal intracerebral haemorrhage (ICH).

2. Chronic hypertension, amyloid angiopathy, anticoagulation (medication), and vascular malformations.

3. The most common feature of ICH is the sudden onset of focal neurological deficits, the nature of which is determined by the location of the haemorrhage and subsequent oedema. This is often associated with a decrease in the patient's conscious level. Other common symptoms and signs include headache, nausea/vomiting, seizures, and a raised diastolic blood pressure.

4. Burr hole craniotomy and evacuation of the ICH.

Q11.7

This is a 60-year-old male.

1. What abnormality is seen in the CT scan?

2. What are the aetiologies?

3. What are possible clinical presentations?

4. What was the management for this problem as seen in the chest X-ray?

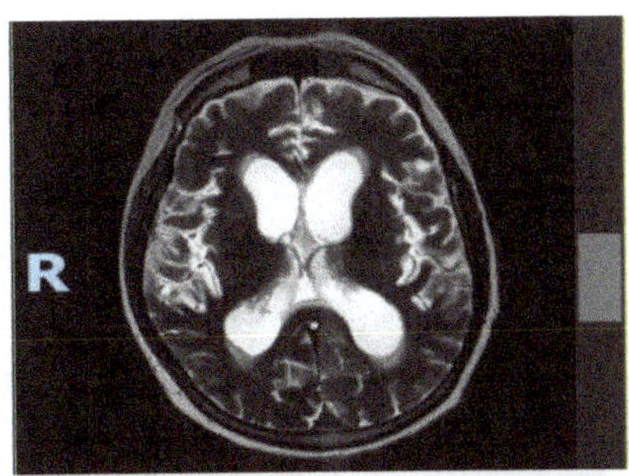

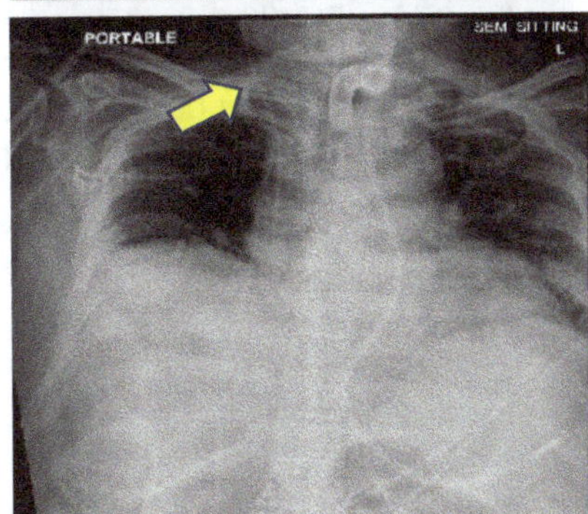

Q11.8

This is a 35-year-old male.

1. What is seen on the cerebral MRA?

2. What is the clinical presentation?

3. What does the surgical photo show?

4. What surgery is likely to be performed?

5. What is another treatment option for this pathology?

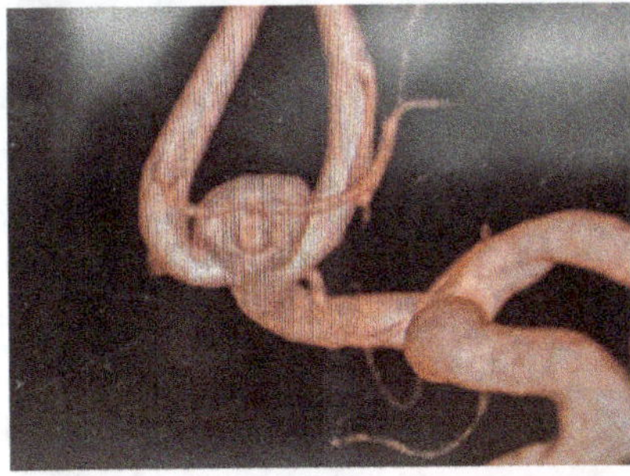

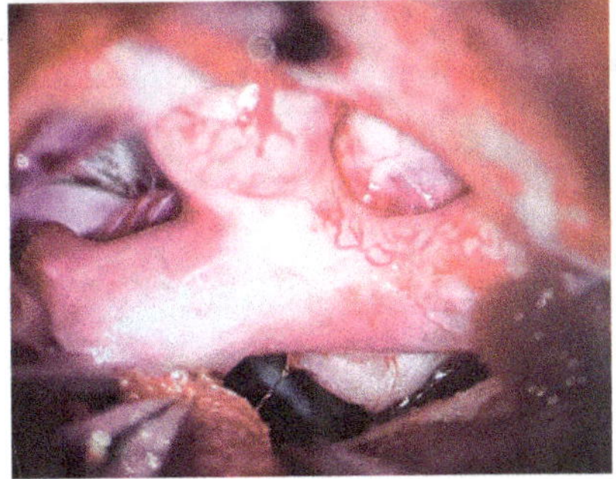

A11.7

1. Hydrocephalus. There is increased accumulation of cerebrospinal fluid (CSF) inside the cerebral ventricles, which are dilated.

2. This accumulation may be due to:
   - obstruction in the normal flow CSF.
   - problems with CSF absorption into the venous system by the arachnoid granulations.
   - excessive production of CSF.

3. Symptoms include headache, neck pain, nausea, vomiting, drowsiness, lethargy, irritability, seizures, confusion, disorientation, blurred vision, diplopia, urinary and bowel incontinence, gait instability, balance problems, lack of appetite, personality changes, and memory problems.

4. A ventriculoperitoneal (VP) shunt was placed on the right side of the patient (arrow). It drains CSF from the lateral ventricle to the peritoneal cavity.

A11.8

1. There is a saccular aneurysm.

2. Smaller ones can be asymptomatic. Larger ones can cause localized mass effect on adjacent structures. When ruptured, they present with a sudden onset of severe headache, classically described as a "thunderclap headache". The headache may be accompanied by a brief loss of consciousness, nausea, vomiting and signs of meningeal irritation.

3. The neck of the aneurysm.

4. Clipping of the aneurysm.

5. Endovascular coiling of the aneurysm.

Q11.9

This is a 60-year-old female with breast cancer.

1. What abnormality is seen on the MRI?

2. What is the diagnosis?

3. What is the clinical presentation?

4. What was the management as seen in the scans?

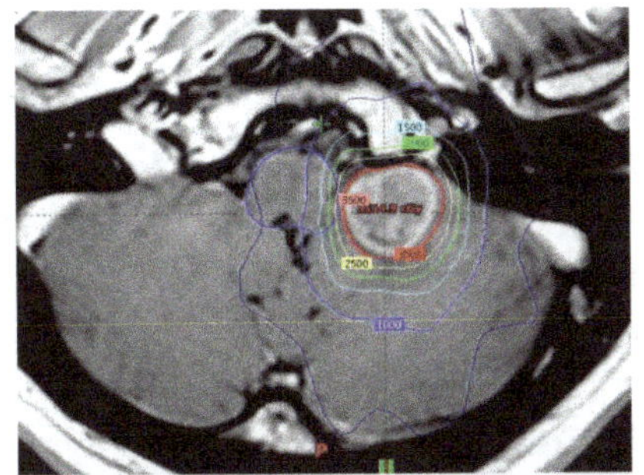

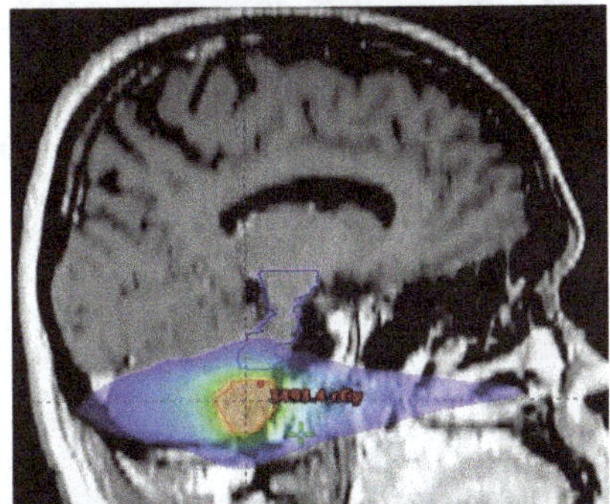

Q11.10

This is an 80-year-old male.

1. What has happened to the patient based on the CT scans?

2. What is the clinical presentation?

3. How is the neurological status assessed?

4. What are contributory risk factors?

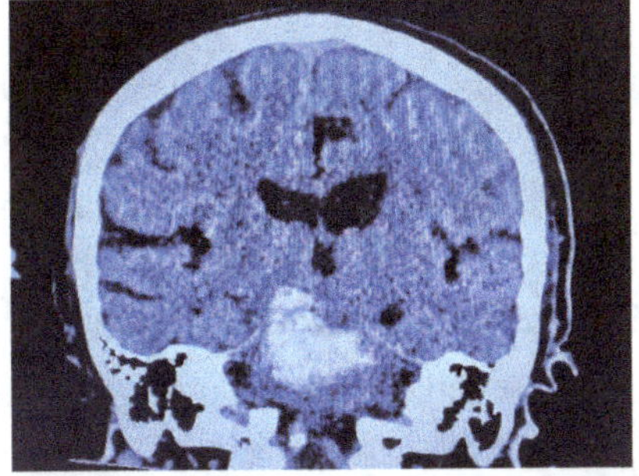

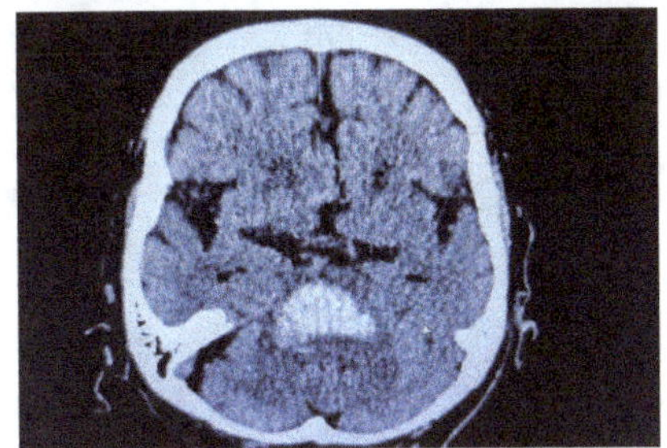

A11.9

1. There is a contrast enhancing lesion in the left cerebellum.

2. A solitary left cerebellar metastasis from breast cancer. In about one third of HER2+ patients, one third of 'triple negative' receptor patients with metastatic breast cancer will develop brain metastases.

3. Patients may be asymptomatic and detected on staging imaging. They may complain of headache, gait disturbance or dizziness.

4. Treatment options include systemic therapy, whole brain radiotherapy, radiosurgery, open surgery, or a combination of the above.
   This patient was treated with radiosurgery to the left cerebellar metastasis. This image shows a linear accelerator-based radiation plan delivering 30Gy in 5 fractions of radiation over 1 week to the left cerebellar metastasis.

A11.10

1. A haemorrhagic stroke has occurred at the brainstem. The brainstem is composed of the midbrain, the pons, and the medulla oblongata.

2. Acute loss of consciousness, altered mental status, altered respiratory drive, hypoxia and vomiting.

3. Glascow coma scale and pupillary reflexes.

4. Hypertension (90%), anticoagulant therapy and arteriovenous malformations.

Breast

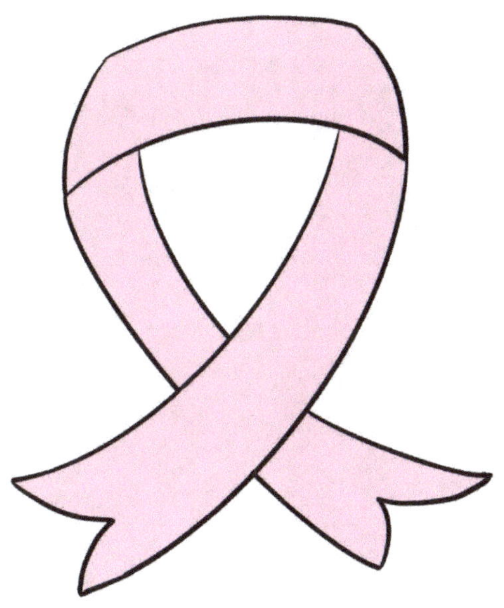

Q12.1

This is a 50-year-old female who presents with left nipple discharge.

1. What is the discharge?
2. What are causes of nipple discharge?
3. What other clinical signs should we examine for?
4. What is the management?

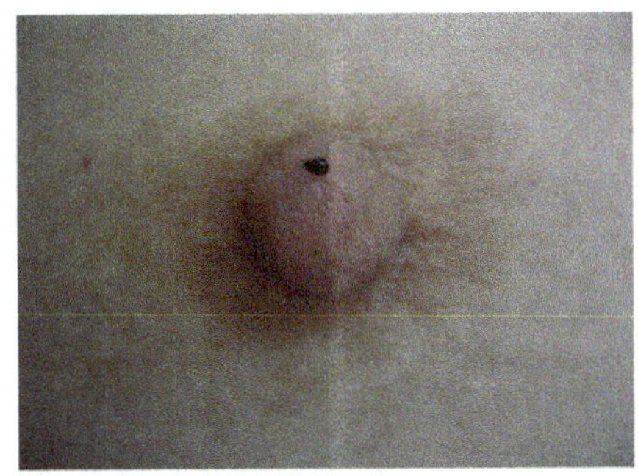

Q12.2

This is a 25-year-old female.

1. Describe the abnormality.
2. How common is it?
3. How can the pathology be classified?
4. What pathology needs to be ruled out?

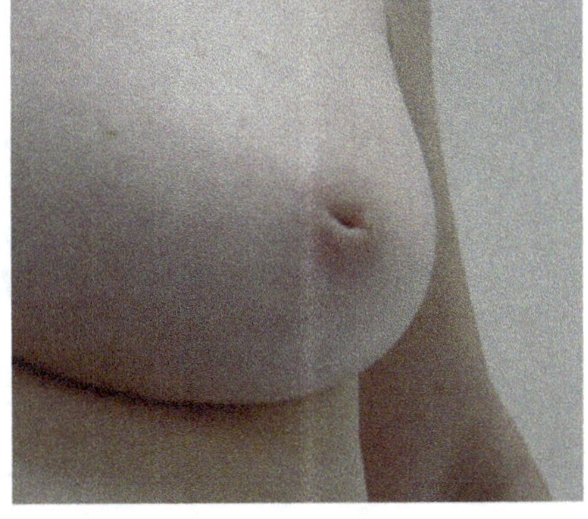

A12.1

1. Blood. Nipple discharge originates from the 15 to 20 milk ducts in a human breast.
   It can be clear, milky, yellow or brown.

2. Physiological — pregnancy, lactation, fibrocystic change, duct ectasia, intraductal papilloma.
   Pathological — infection, neoplasia, prolactinoma.

3. Any breast masses, asymmetry or skin changes.

4. Women over the age of 40 are at higher risk of having pathological discharge.
   She needs an ultrasound and mammogram to rule out neoplasia.

A12.2

1. The left nipple is inverted.

2. It affects 10-20% of females.

3. It is classified based on degree of fibrosis, ease of manipulation and extent of damage by the lactiferous ducts.
   Grade 1: can project with manipulation and still able to breastfeed.
   Grade 2: there is some fibrosis, hence breastfeeding may be difficult.
   Grade 3: fibrosis has caused soft tissue deficiency, lactiferous ducts are constricted and atrophied. Nipple cannot be everted.

4. Malignancy or other acquired causes.

Q12.3

This is a 54-year-old female who presented with a right breast lump.

1. What investigation was performed?

2. What "views" were they taken in?

3. What abnormality was detected?

4. What classification is used to report imaging?

5. What is the next investigation to confirm the diagnosis?

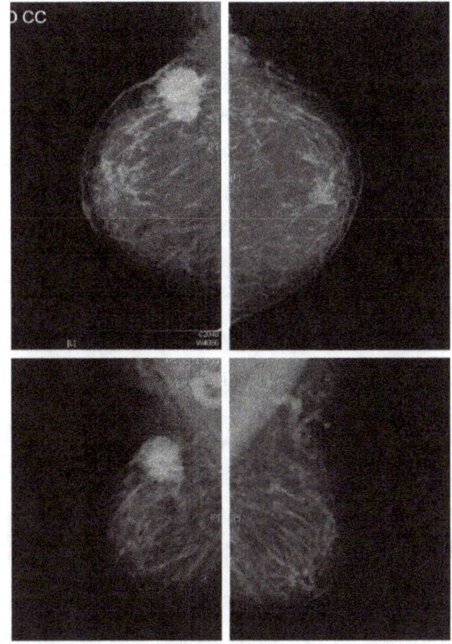

Q12.4

This is a 25-year-old female who presents with a left breast lump.

1. What is seen on the ultrasound?

2. What is the diagnosis?

3. What is the clinical presentation?

4. What is the management?

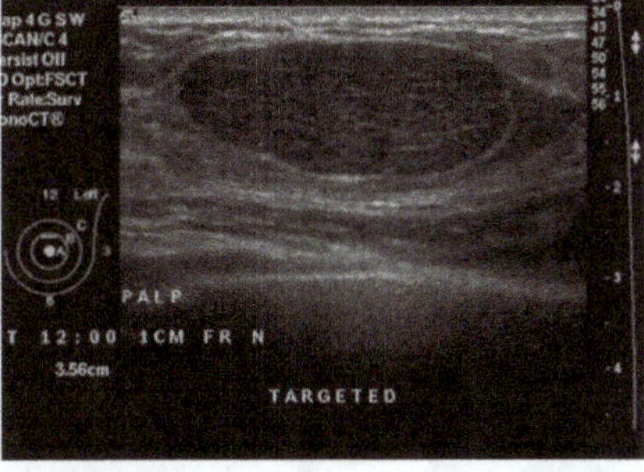

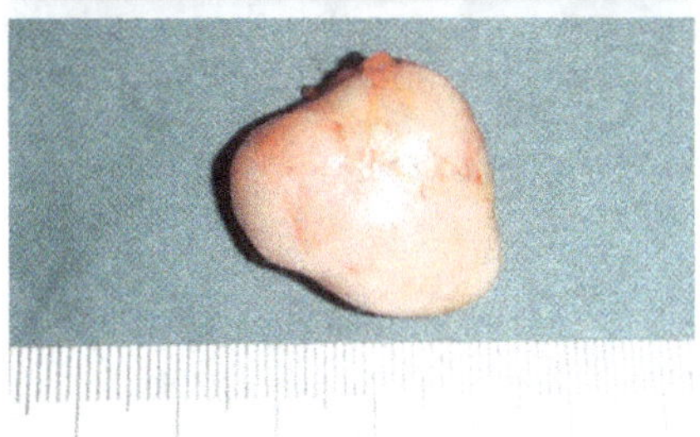

A12.3

1. Breast mammogram.

2. Craniocaudal (CC) and mediolateral oblique (MLO) views. Acquiring 2 views is imperative to adequately image the whole breast.

3. A large rounded radiodense lesion is seen in the upper outer quadrant of right breast, showing mildly spiculated borders.

4. All abnormalities in the mammograms are reported using the standard Breast Imaging–Reporting and Data System (BI-RADS) descriptors. They are classified into one of the standard BI-RADS categories 0-6.

5. Obtain histological confirmation with a core biopsy.

A12.4

1. There is a well circumscribed ovoid lesion measuring 3.5 cm with uniform hypoechogenicity.

2. Fibroadenoma. It is a benign solid lesion in the breast. It is commonly found in adolescents and less commonly in postmenopausal women.

3. They often present as a painless "marble-like" mobile mass in the breast, often referred to as a 'breast mouse'.

4. In most cases, fibroadenomas can be managed conservatively. They shrink and disappear over time. The lesions have no long-term risk of malignancy. Surgery is indicated if the fibroadenomas are large, increasing in size or when the lump could be malignant.

Q12.5

This is a 40-year-old female.

1. Describe the pathology.
2. What is the diagnosis?
3. What is the clinical presentation?
4. What is the management for this patient?

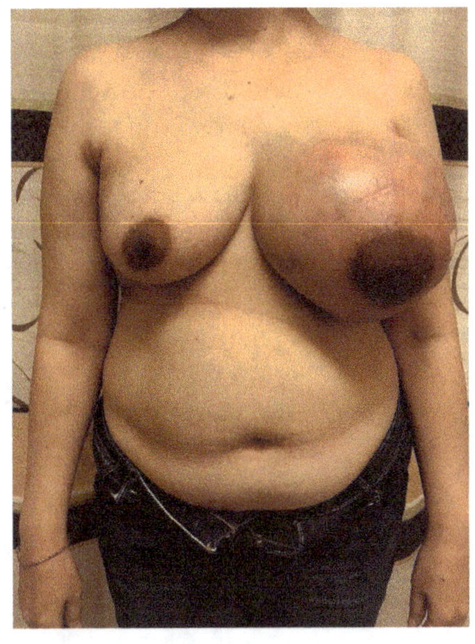

Q12.6

This is a 35-year-old female who presents with a fever for 4 days.

1. Describe the abnormality seen.
2. What is the diagnosis?
3. Which group of patients are prone to developing this?
4. What surgical procedure is being performed for this patient?

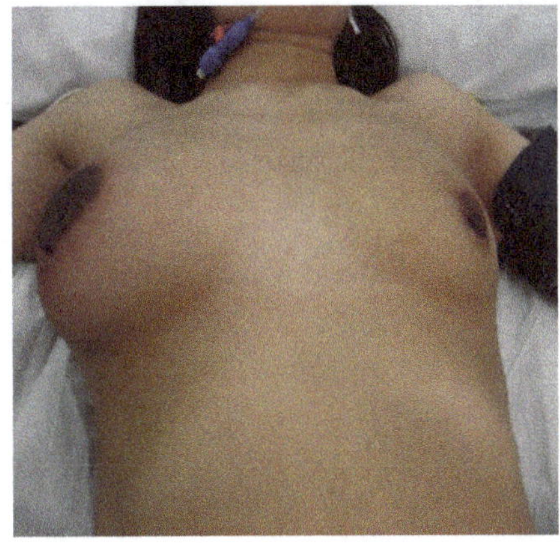

A12.5

1. There is a very large lesion in the left breast. There is erythema over the skin which remains intact. The right breast looks normal. (The erythema is due to the large mass stretching the overlying skin with distension of the superficial veins)
2. Phyllodes tumour. It is an infrequently encountered fibroepithelial neoplasm.
3. They present as a painless enlarging firm mass.
4. Ultrasound or mammogram will not be helpful as this lesion it is too large. MRI can be used to evaluate the depth of invasion and the contralateral breast.
   Core biopsy can confirm the histology.
   The patient would require a mastectomy with soft tissue reconstruction.

A12.6

1. The right breast is larger compared to the left. The overlying skin is erythematous.
2. Right breast abscess.
3. Lactating women.
4. Incision and drainage of the abscess.

Q12.7

This is a 50-year-old female.

1. What abnormality is seen in the mammogram?

2. How would this mammogram finding be classified under the standard reporting system (BI-RADS)?

3. What is the possible pathology?

4. What is the likely clinical presentation?

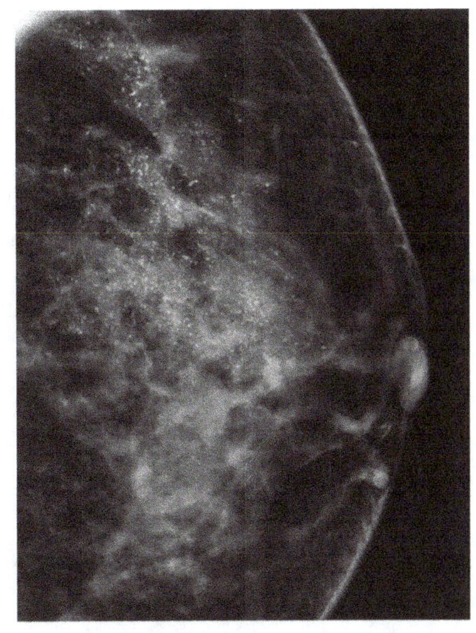

Q12.8

This is a 40-year-old female with right triple negative breast cancer.

1. What is triple negative breast cancer?

2. What abnormality is seen in the MRI?

3. What are the advantages in using MRI for imaging breast lesions?

4. What further information can an MRI provide in breast cancer patients?

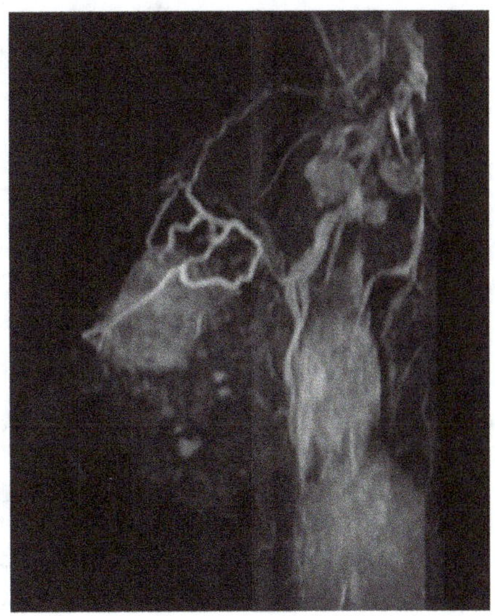

A12.7

1. There are multiple specks of microcalcification. The calcium deposits are considered as robust markers of breast cancer.

2. These macrocalcifications exhibit suspicious morphological characteristics for malignancy and are classified as BI-RADS 4.

3. Ductal carcinoma in situ or invasive ductal carcinoma.

4. Most patients are asymptomatic and the pathology is often detected on screening mammogram.

A12.8

1. Triple negative breast cancer (TNBC) is diagnosed based on immunohistochemistry staining. It is oestrogen receptor (ER), progesterone receptor (PR) and human epidermal growth factor receptor 2 (HER2) negative.
   TNBC is characterized by its aggressive nature and lack of targeted therapies.

2. There is a highly suspicious lesion in the upper part of the breast. There are multiple smaller enhancing masses inferiorly that are suggestive of satellite lesions.

3. MRIs have a higher sensitivity rate in the detection of breast cancer compared to mammograms and ultrasonography.

4. Preoperative assessment of cancer extent (multifocal and multicentric).
   Screening of contralateral breast for cancer.
   Accurate tumour size assessment for staging.
   Monitoring tumour response to neoadjuvant therapy.

Q12.9

This is a 70-year-old female.

1. Describe the pathology seen?

2. What is the most likely diagnosis?

3. What diagnostic tool is used as seen in the pictures to confirm the diagnosis?

4. What information can we obtain from it?

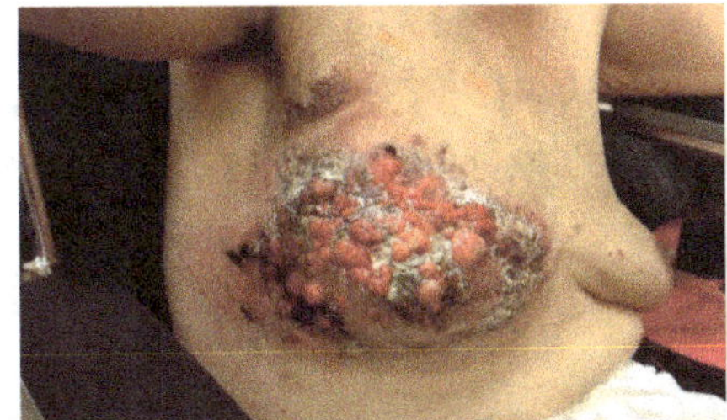

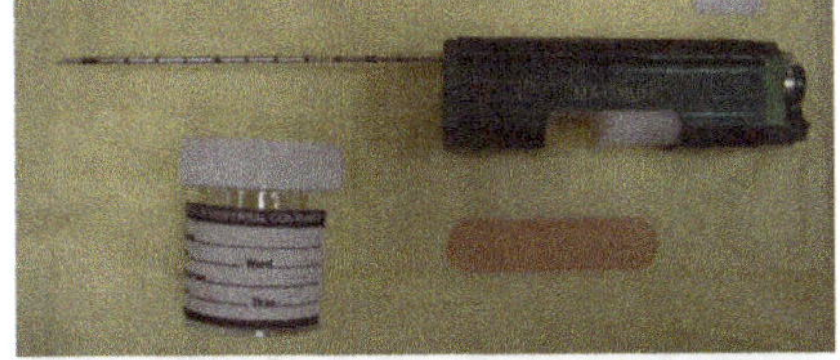

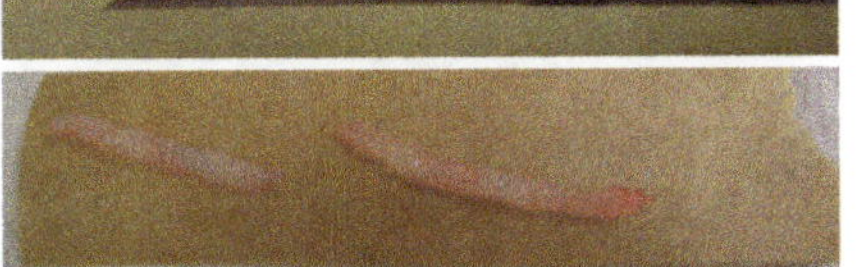

Q12.10

This is a 40-year-old female who presented with a right breast lump.

1. What is seen on the breast ultrasound?

2. How would this ultrasound finding be classified under the standard reporting system (BI-RADS)?

3. What is seen in the PET-CT scan?

4. Why was a PET-CT scan performed for this patient?

5. What the next step in management for the patient?

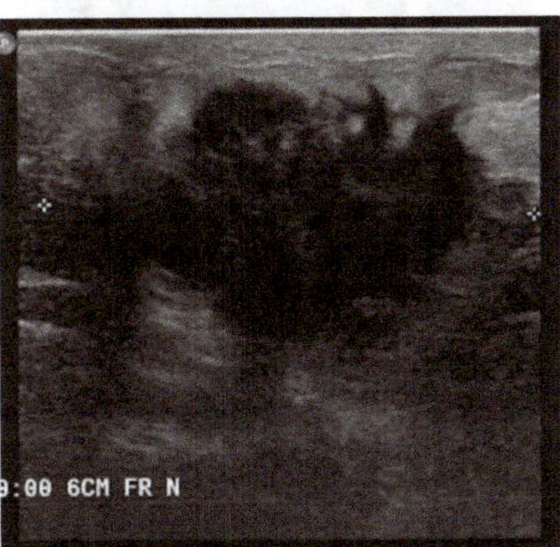

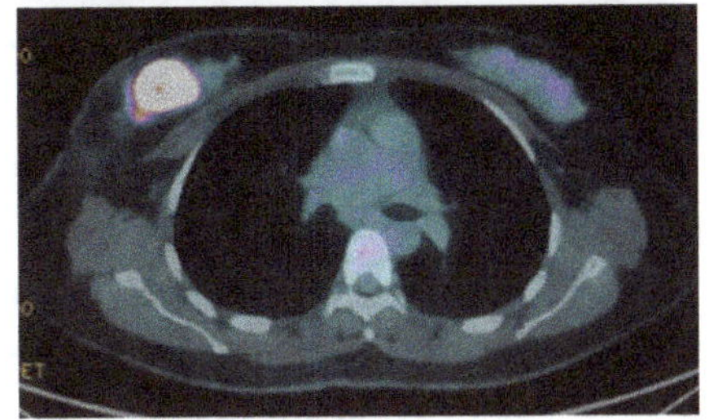

A12.9

1. There is a necrotic ulcerative mass in the right breast with multiple erythematous nodules on the skin surface.

2. Locally advanced breast carcinoma.

3. Core biopsy needle.

4. Core biopsy is better than fine-needle biopsy as it provides adequate tissue for histology and specialized staining for hormonal receptors (ER, PR and HER2).

A12.10

1. There is a hypoechoic lesion with irregular borders which exhibits posterior shadowing.

2. This is a Category 5 BI-RADS lesion.

3. There is a FDG-avid right breast lesion.

4. Metastatic workup.

5. Obtain histological diagnosis.

Q12.11

This is a 60-year-old female.

1. What procedure has been performed in picture A?

2. How is it accurately inserted?

3. When and why is it used?

4. What is seen in picture B?

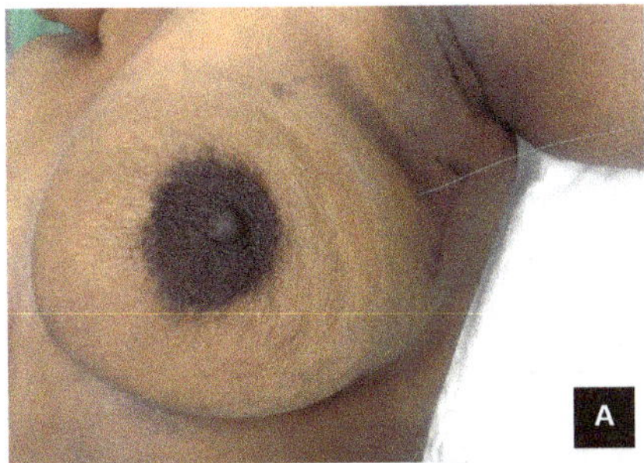

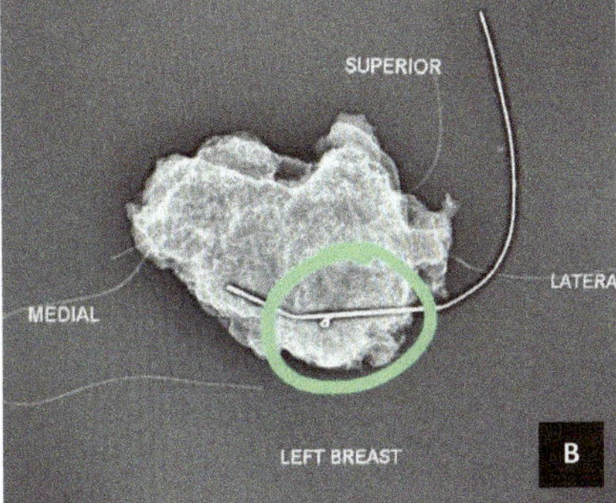

Q12.12

This is a 70-year-old female.

1. Describe the abnormality seen.

2. What is the diagnosis?

3. What are possible clinical symptoms?

4. What are differential diagnoses?

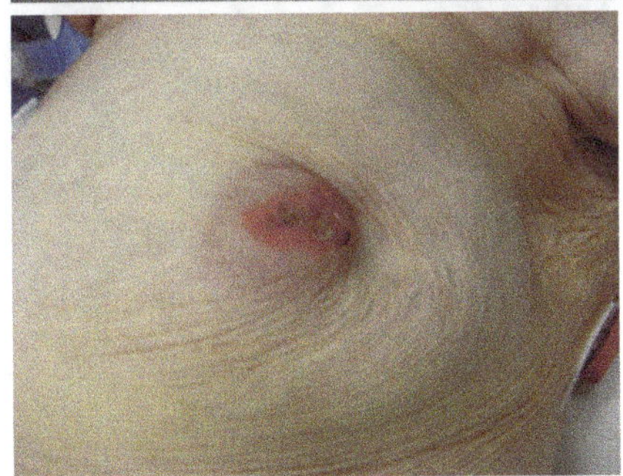

A12.11

1. Hookwire localisation of a lesion in the left breast.

2. It is inserted under radiological guidance — either mammogram, ultrasound or MRI.

3. It is used to locate non-palpable suspicious lesions for excision.

4. After excision, an x-ray is performed on the specimen to confirm the presence of the localized lesion (clip or calcifications).

A12.12

1. There is an ulcerative erythematous patch around the left nipple with irregular borders.

2. Paget's disease of the breast. It is a manifestation of underlying breast cancer in postmenopausal women.

3. Patients may experience itching and eczema-like symptoms.

4. Inflammatory skin conditions — atopic or contact dermatitis or other forms of eczema.
Skin cancers — squamous cell or basal cell carcinoma.
Benign nipple pathology.

Q12.13

This is a 60-year-old female undergoing surgery for a right breast cancer.

1. What is being injected to the areola?

2. What surgical procedure is carried out?

3. What is the advantage of this surgery versus conventional axillary lymph node clearance surgery?

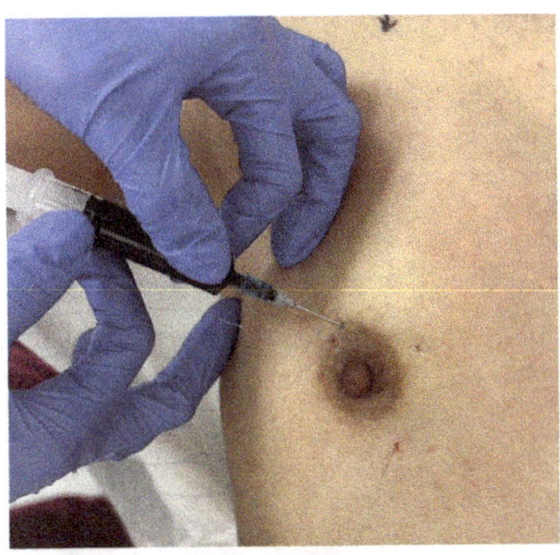

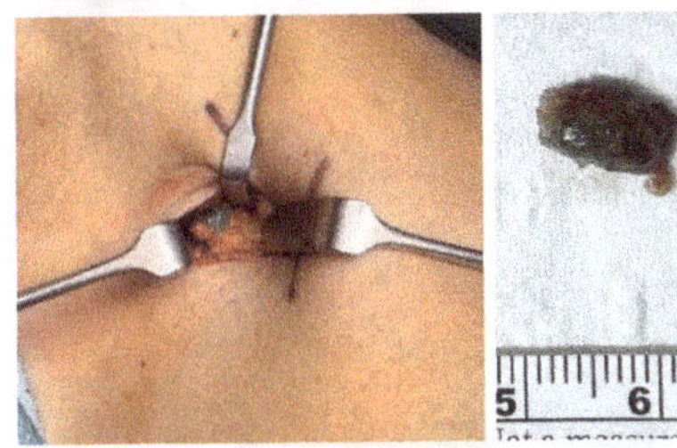

Q12.14

This lady had a right mastectomy and axillary clearance.

1. What problem has she developed post-surgery?

2. How often does this occur post axillary clearance?

3. What are risk factors to developing this condition after surgery?

4. How is the condition treated?

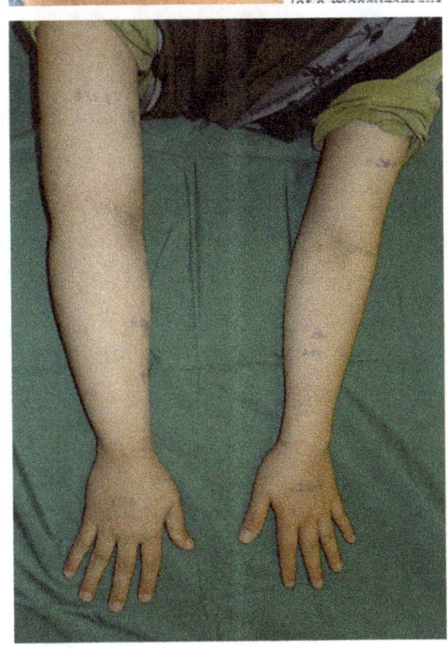

A12.13

1. Blue dye. It is injected either near the tumour or under the areola. This is done just before surgery because the blue dye is a small molecule that moves quickly in the lymphatic system.

2. Sentinel lymph node biopsy of the axillary lymph node basin.
   The node removed is dyed blue.

3. It allows assessment of cancer spread to axillary lymph nodes without the need for formal axillary node dissection, which is associated with higher morbidity.

A12.14

1. Secondary lymphedema due to damage/dysfunction of the normally functioning axillary lymphatic system.

2. It occurs in 15–20% of patients after axillary lymph node clearance.

3. Patients who had previous inflammation/infection in the chest, breast or arm and higher body mass index (BMI).

4. Conservative: Manual lymphatic drainage (massage) and compression garments.
   Surgery: microsurgical lympho-venous or lympho-lymphatic anastomosis.

Q12.15

This is a 54-year-old female who presents with a right breast lump that is increasing in size for the last 6 months.

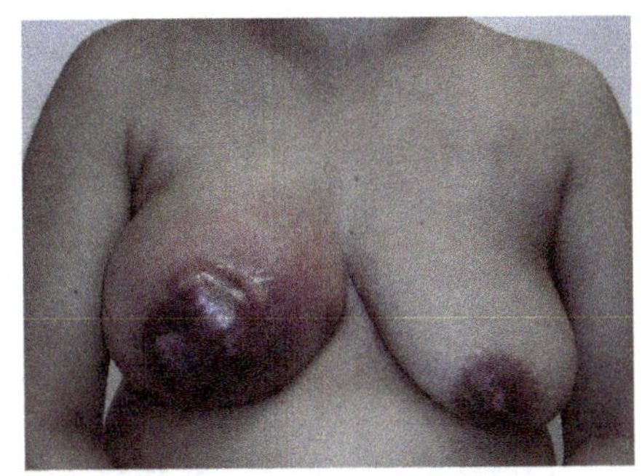

1. Describe the pathology seen.
2. What is the likely diagnosis?
3. What is a differential diagnosis?
4. What is the pathogenesis?
5. What is the management?

Q12.16

This is a 60-year-old female.

1. Describe the pathology seen.
2. What is the diagnosis?
3. What symptoms would she be experiencing?
4. What investigation was performed on her?
5. What is the management?

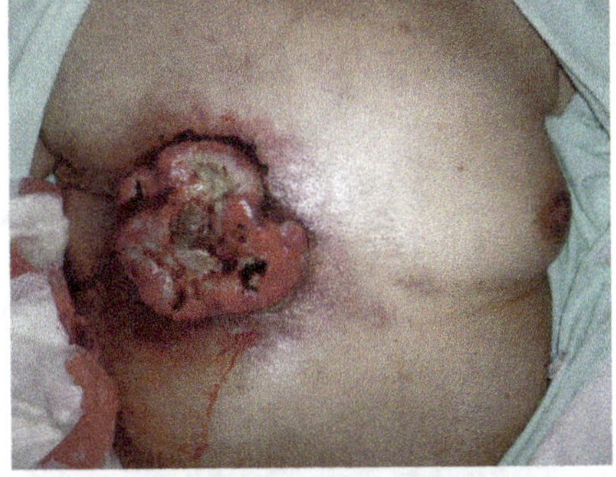

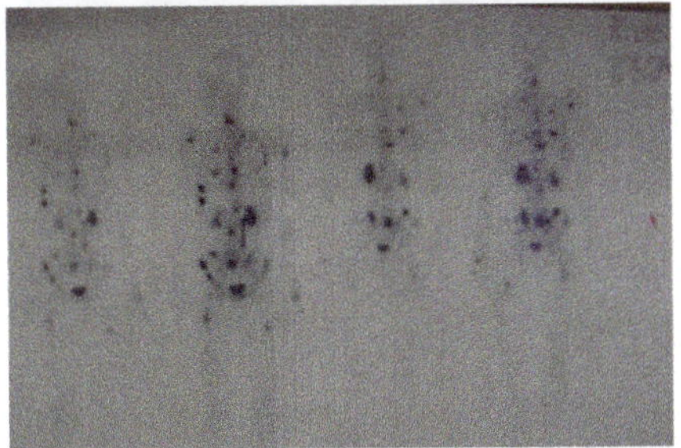

A12.15

1. The right breast is larger than the left breast. The peri-areolar area appears red/purple and the surrounding skin is reddish-pink.

2. Inflammatory Breast Cancer (IBC).

3. Because of its aggressive behaviour and unusual appearance, IBC can be easily misdiagnosed for a bacterial infection (mastitis or breast abscess) and hence treated inappropriately.

4. The increased size of the breast is the result of oedema caused by tumour blockage of the lymphatic channels. The oedema is associated with exaggerated hair follicle pits, causing a characteristic peau d'orange (orange peel) appearance of the skin.

5. Systemic chemotherapy.

A12.16

1. There is a large fungating mass arising from the right breast that is actively bleeding.

2. Breast cancer.

3. The fungating tumour can cause pain, malodour, and itchiness.

4. Bone scan to identify presence of metastases.

5. This patient is not a surgical candidate, as there is extensive involvement of the dermis and chest wall.
   She can be treated with a multimodality approach via systemic chemotherapy or hormonal therapy and radiation for locoregional control.

Q12.17

This 60-year-old female had surgery done on her right breast, followed by adjuvant treatment.

1. What surgery was previously done?

2. What adjuvant treatment was given?

3. What are the visible signs of the adjuvant treatment?

4. What are the indications for this adjuvant treatment?

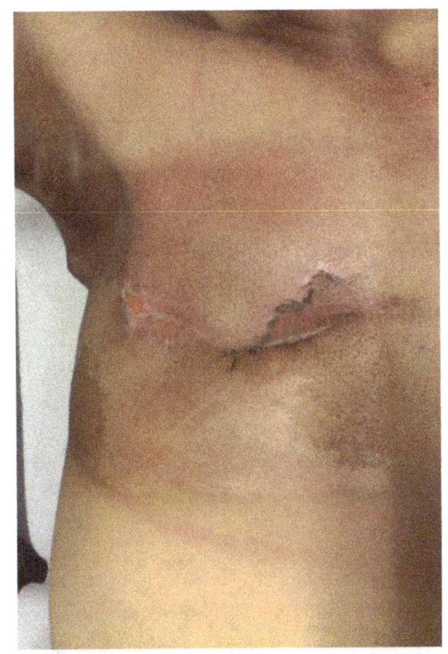

Q12.18

These are two different patients who are preparing for treatment for breast cancer.

1. What previous surgery did patient A undergo?

2. What procedure is being performed for these patients?

3. What are the advantages over external beam radiotherapy?

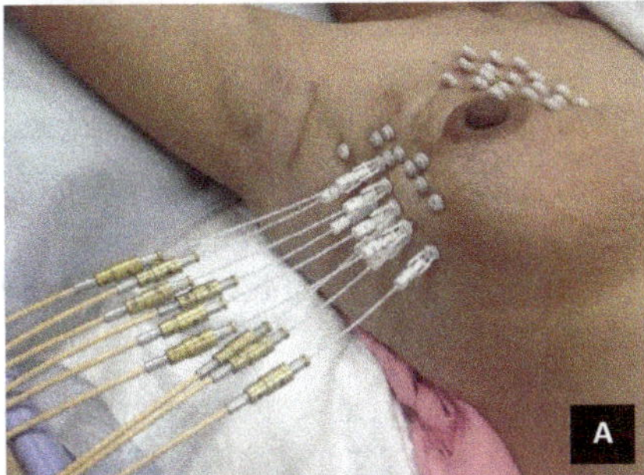

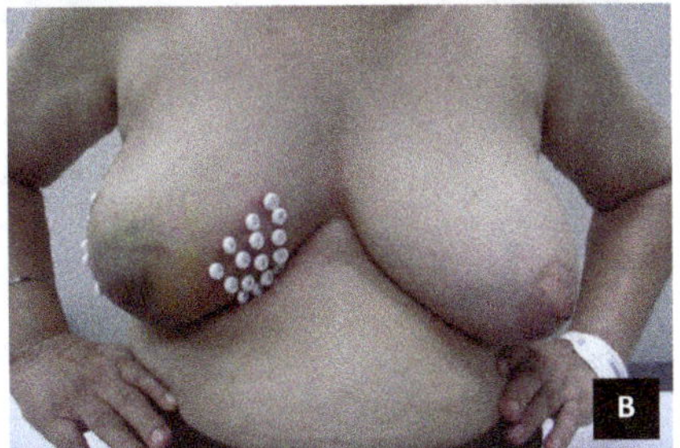

A12.17

1. Right mastectomy and clearance of axillary lymph nodes.

2. Adjuvant post-mastectomy right chest wall radiotherapy.

3. Patient has acute radiation dermatitis.
    There is erythema and pigmentation with demarcation corresponding to the radiation field borders. There is also patchy desquamation.

4. Tumour >5cm (T3).
    Positive surgical margins.
    Regional node metastases.

A12.18

1. Patient A had a lumpectomy or wide excision for low-risk breast cancer. There is a scar in the axilla suggesting a prior sentinel lymph node biopsy.

2. The patients are receiving adjuvant accelerated partial breast irradiation using interstitial brachytherapy.
    Picture A shows the brachytherapy applicators attached to the guide tubes.
    Picture B shows the external plugs of guide tubes in-situ between fractions.

3. Radiation doses are reduced to the heart, lungs, and skin.
    Overall treatment time is shorter (about 5 days).

Q12.19

This is a 40-year-old female who had breast reconstruction surgery.

1. What surgery was performed?
2. What are considerations prior to breast reconstruction?
3. What are other options for breast reconstruction?
4. What further surgery may be performed for this patient?

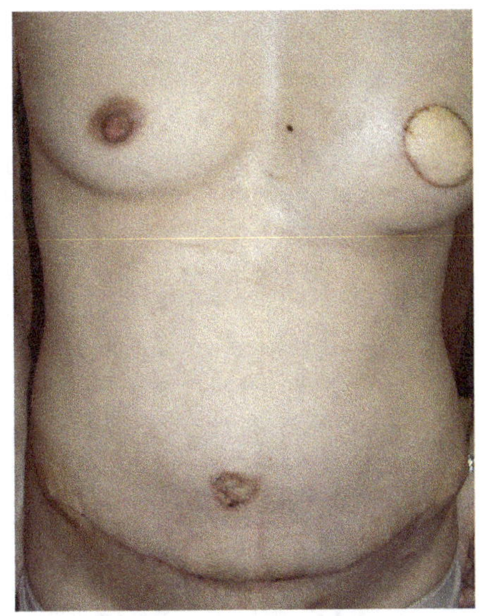

Q12.20

This is a 35-year-old male with a right chest lump.

1. What is the diagnosis?
2. What are the causes?
3. What pathology needs to be excluded?
4. Why was surgical resection performed?

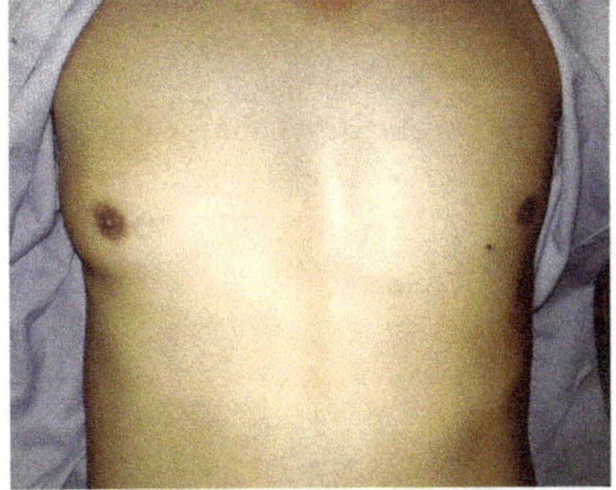

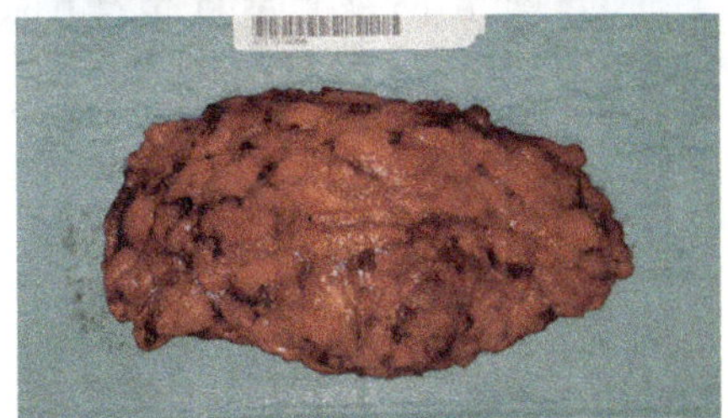

A12.19

1. Transverse rectus abdominus muscle (TRAM) or deep inferior epigastric perforator (DIEP) flap.

2. Amount of tissue resected: skin or pectoralis muscle.
   Symmetry: volume of contralateral breast.
   Donor site availability.
   Patient's preference.
   Adjuvant treatment.

3. Tissue expanders and implants.
   Autologous: Latissimus Dorsi flap.

4. Creation of the nipple areolar complex.

A12.20

1. Right gynaecomastia.
   It is the abnormal non-cancerous enlargement of breasts in males due to the growth of breast tissue as a result of hormonal imbalance between oestrogens and androgens.

2. Oestrogen excess.
   Androgen deficiency or resistance.
   Medications (eg cimetidine, calcium channel blockers).

3. Breast cancer.

4. Men with gynecomastia may have psychosocial issues due to concerns about its appearance and the possibility of having breast cancer. Surgical resection would address both issues.

13 Paediatric Surgery

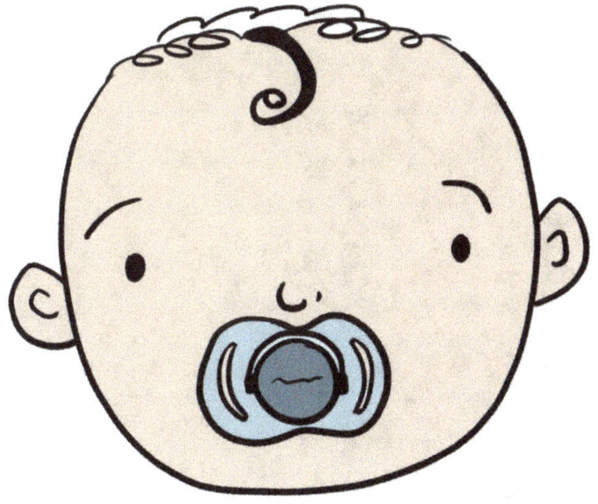

Q13.1

This is a 5-year-old boy.

1. Describe the abnormality seen in his groin?

2. What is the diagnosis?

3. What is the pathophysiology?

4. What surgery was performed?

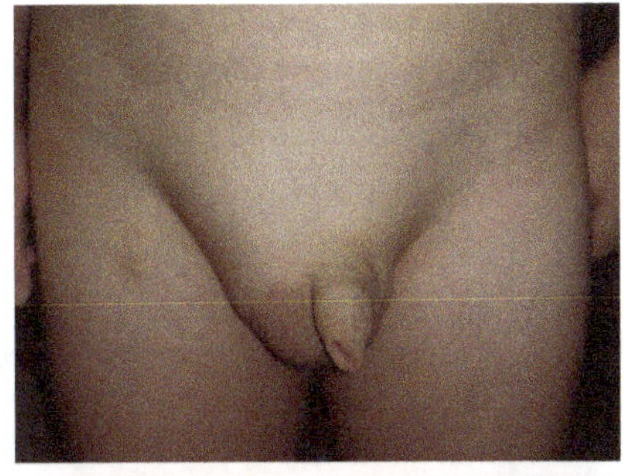

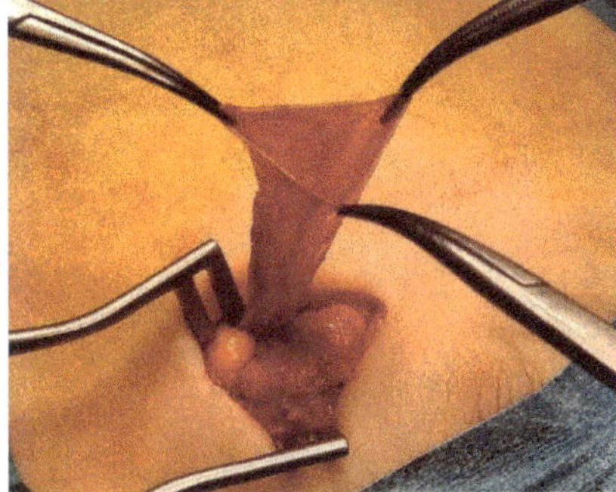

Q13.2

This is a 9-year-old boy.

1. Describe the lesion seen?

2. What is the diagnosis?

3. How common is it?

4. What is the classification based on depth?

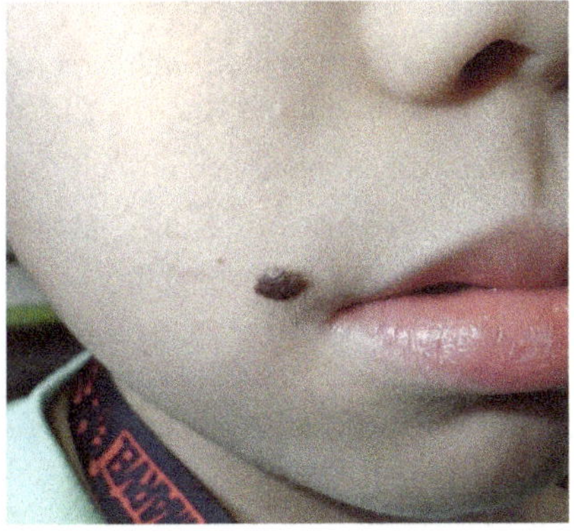

A13.1

1. There is a right inguinal scrotal swelling.

2. Right inguinal hernia.

3. Most paediatric inguinal hernias are indirect due to a patent processus vaginalis (outpouching of the peritoneum).

4. Open right inguinal hernia with herniotomy. The sac is demonstrated in the surgical picture and ligated at the internal ring.

A13.2

1. There is a pigmented, well-circumscribed ovoid lesion seen lateral to the left commissure of the lips. The surface is smooth and the colour uniform.

2. Melanocytic nevus, commonly known as a mole.

3. It occurs in 1% of babies. Majority of moles appear during the first two decades of a person's life.

4. Junctional: along the junction of the epidermis and dermis.
Compound: involving both epidermis and dermis.
Intradermal: within the dermis (A classic mole or birthmark. It typically appears as an elevated, dome-shaped bump on the surface of the skin).

Q13.3

This is a 15-year-old male.

1. Describe the pathology seen.
2. What is seen in the intra-op photos?
3. What is the diagnosis?
4. What is its aetiology?
5. What is the management?

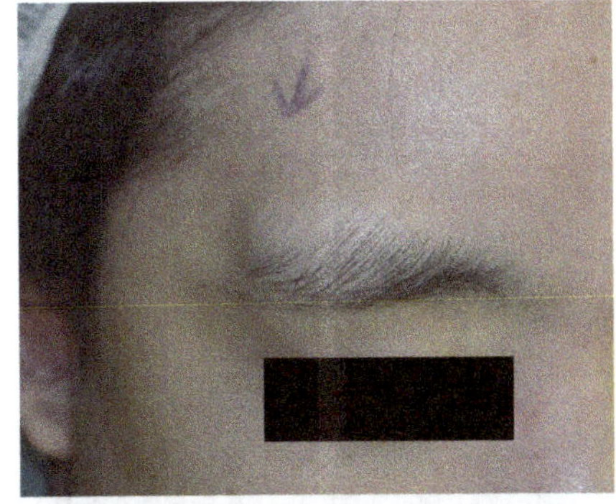

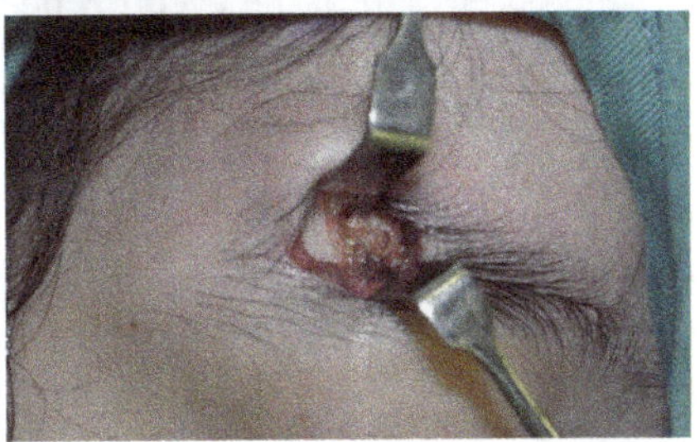

Q13.4

This is a 6-year-old boy.

1. Describe the lesion seen on the face.
2. What is the diagnosis?
3. What is the malignant potential of this lesion?
4. What is the management?

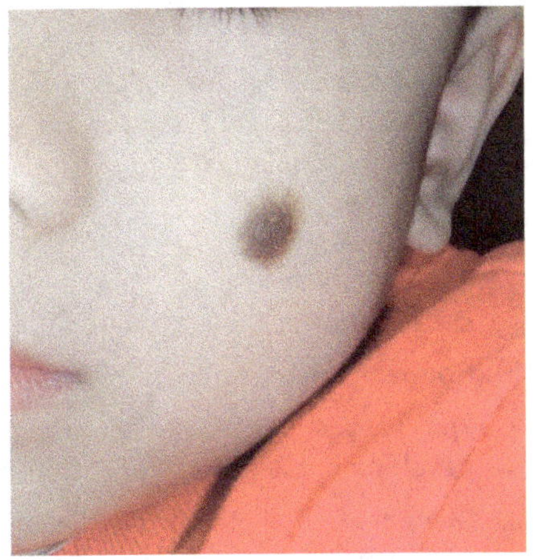

A13.3

1. There is a well-circumscribed lesion over right eyebrow. There are no overlying skin changes.

2. The lesion involves the orbital bone.

3. Dermoid cyst.

4. A dermoid cyst is a benign cutaneous developmental anomaly that arises from the entrapment of ectodermal elements along the lines of embryonic closure.
   They are commonly seen in the frontal, occipital, and supraorbital areas, with the outer third of the eyebrow being the most frequently affected region.

5. Dermoid cysts usually tend to grow slowly. They have the potential to cause bony deformities, extending intracranially. Early resection is recommended.

A13.4

1. Size: 2 x 2 cm.
   Location: left aspect of face.
   Borders: irregular.
   Surface: with hair.
   Shape: round.
   Colour: brown.
   Distribution: single (vs multiple).

2. Congenital hairy naevus.

3. The naevus expands with growth of the child. The risk of melanoma development is proportional to the size of the congenital nevus.

4. Management depends on the lesion's size, location, and propensity for malignant transformation. Aesthetic considerations are important. Procedures used in surgical treatment include serial excision and reconstruction with skin grafting, tissue expansion, local rotation flaps, and free tissue transfer.

Q13.5

This is a newborn baby.

1. What is the abnormality seen in the x-ray?

2. What is the diagnosis?

3. How common is it?

4. What other abnormalities is this pathology associated with?

5. What is the likely clinical presentation of this patient?

6. What is the management?

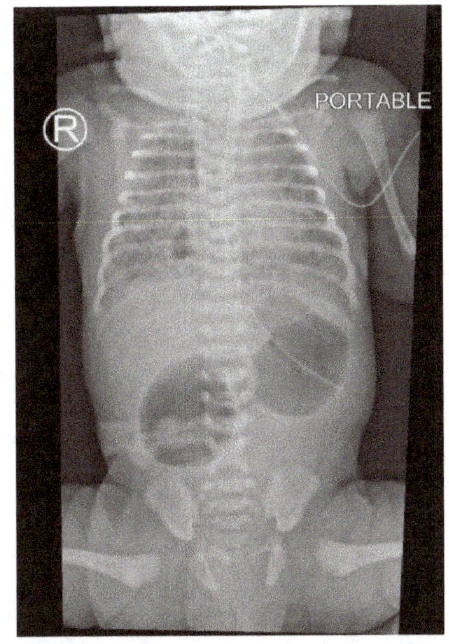

Q13.6

This is a newborn baby. There was an attempted insertion of a nasogastric tube (NGT).

1. Where is the location/position of the NGT as seen on chest x-ray?

2. What is the diagnosis?

3. What is its aetiology?

4. How are they diagnosed?

5. What is the management?

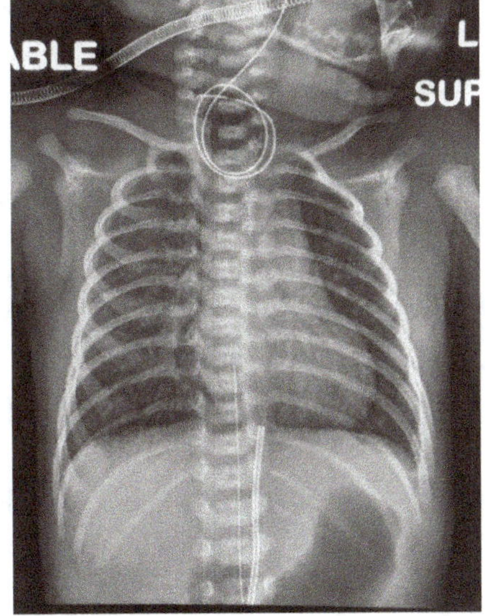

A13.5

1. A double bubble sign. The first bubble is a radiolucent (air-filled) stomach in the normal position to the left of the midline, and the second bubble to the right of the midline represents a post-pyloric dilated duodenum.

2. Duodenal atresia.

3. Duodenal atresia occurs in 1 in 5000 live births.

4. It is associated with trisomy 21(Down's syndrome), cardiac malformations and other small bowel atresias.

5. Duodenal atresia is often suspected antenatally on ultrasound. It presents early in life as vomiting, usually occurring within the first 24 to 38 hours of life after the first feed. Clinical examination will reveal epigastric fullness due to dilation of the stomach and proximal duodenum.

6. Duodenoduodenostomy.

A13.6

1. The tube has coiled up in the upper oesophagus.

2. Oesophageal atresia. There is air in the stomach suggestive of a distal trachea-oesophageal fistula.

3. Oesophageal atresia with or without an associated trachea-oesophageal fistula is the failure of separation or incomplete development of the foregut.

4. 1/3 of cases are diagnosed prenatally with polyhydramnios seen on sonography. The other cases are symptomatic soon after birth, presenting with increased oral secretions which leads to choking, respiratory distress, or cyanotic episodes during feeding.

5. Evaluation for other abnormalities.
   No oral feeding and frequent oral suctioning.
   Surgical anastomosis of the two ends of the oesophagus and ligation of the fistula.

Q13.7

This 9-year-old boy presented with right sided abdominal pain and had emergency surgery performed on him.

1. What is the diagnosis as seen in the surgical photos?

2. What is the classical clinical presentation?

3. What determines the position of pain/tenderness in a patient with this diagnosis?

4. What surgery was performed?

5. What complications can occur if the pathology is not promptly treated?

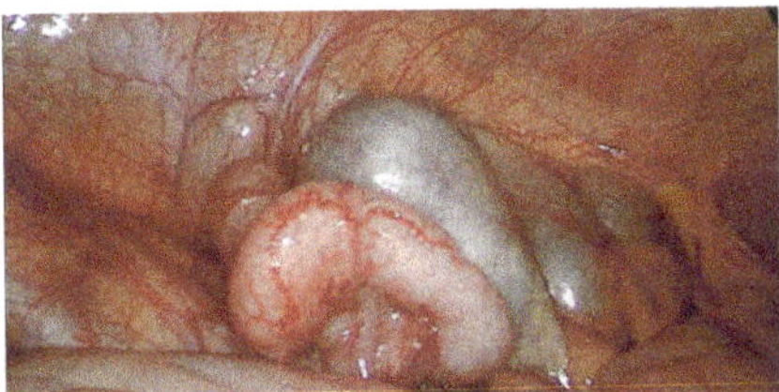
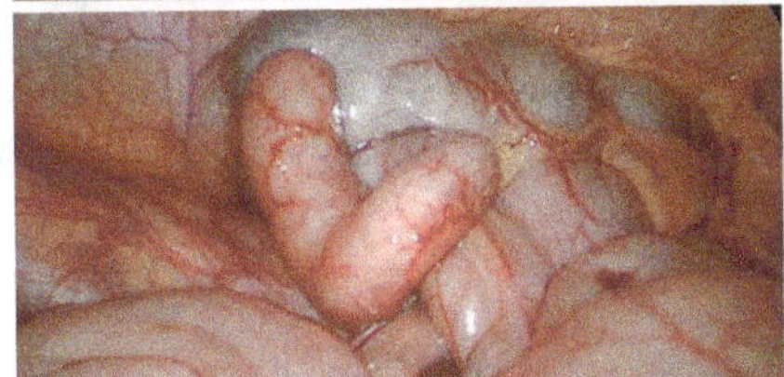
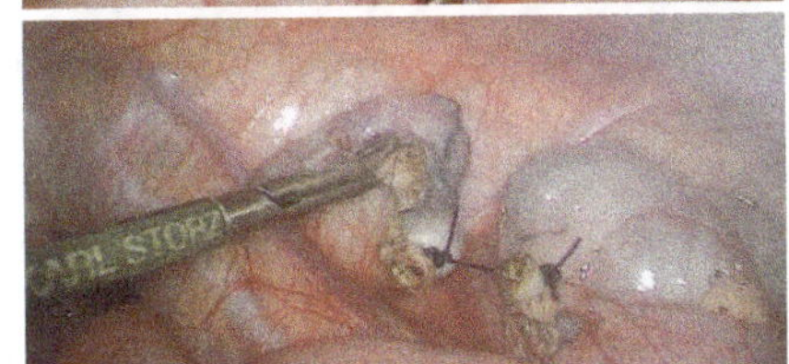

Q13.8

This is a neonate.

1. What is seen on the AXR?

2. What are possible clinical presentations?

3. What is the management?

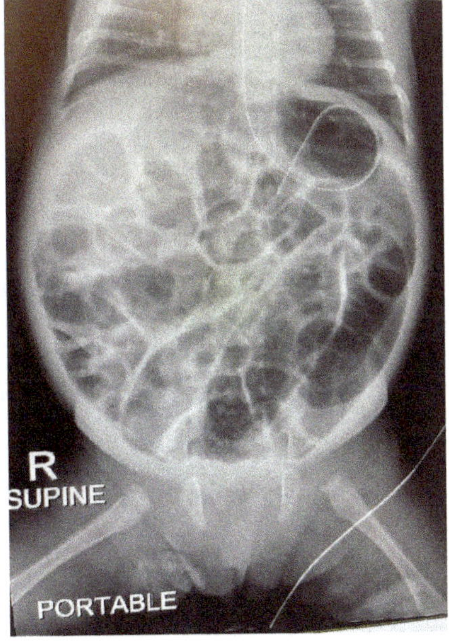

A13.7

1. Acute appendicitis.

2. In the early stages, the visceral afferent nerve fibres at T8 through T10 are stimulated, leading to vague centralized abdominal pain. As the appendix becomes more inflamed and irritates the adjacent parietal peritoneum, the pain becomes more localized to the right lower quadrant.

3. The position of the inflamed appendix determines the presentation.
    *   Intraperitoneal: classic McBurney's point tenderness.
    *   Retrocaecal: the tenderness may be "dampened" by the overlying caecum.
    *   Adjacent to psoas muscle: pain on hip flexion and walking.

4. Laparoscopic appendectomy.

5. Perforation of the appendix leading to abscess formation or frank peritonitis.

A13.8

1. There is gas-filled dilated small and large bowel suggestive of intestinal obstruction. A fine-bore naso-gastric tube has been inserted.

2. Maternal polyhydramnios.
    Feeding intolerance.
    Bilious emesis.
    Abdominal distention.
    Delayed passage of meconium.

3. If the obstruction does not resolve with conservative management, surgical exploration is necessary to preserve intestinal viability.

Q13.9

These are two newborn babies.

1. What is the diagnosis?
2. How common is this?
3. What is VACTERL association?
4. What is the management?

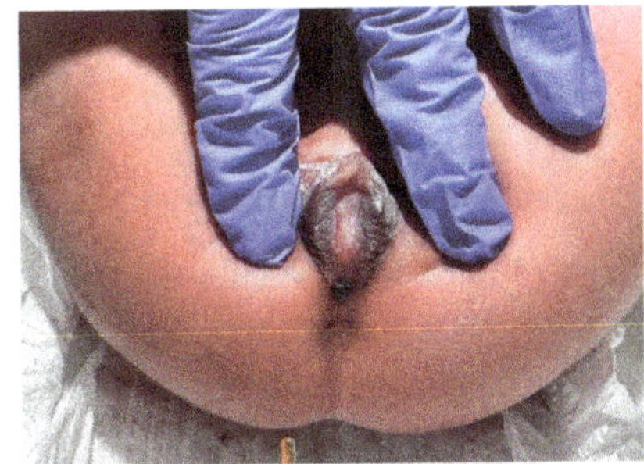

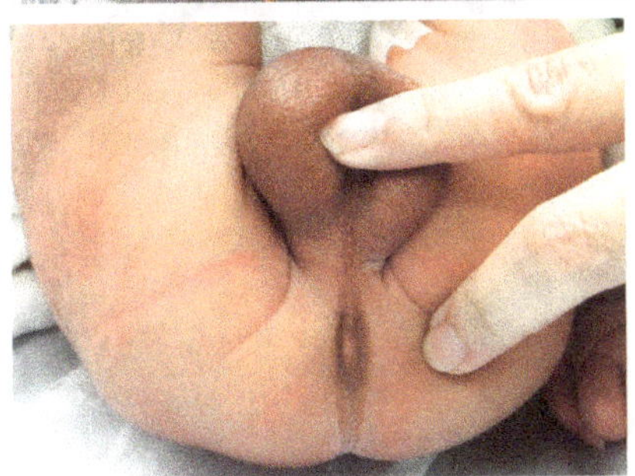

Q13.10

This is a 2-year-old child.

1. Describe the findings in the CT scan?
2. What is the diagnosis?
3. What is the clinical presentation?
4. What is the management?

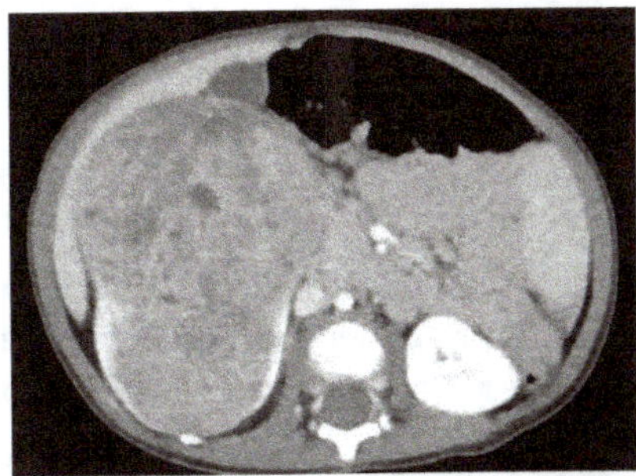

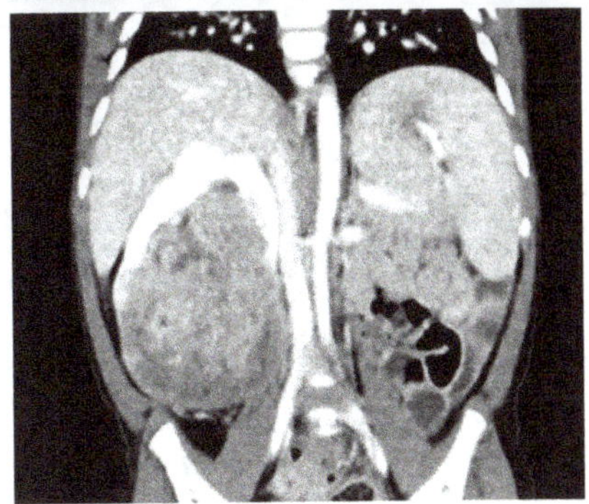

A13.9

1. Anorectal malformations. The babies have an imperforate anus.
   In the female baby, there is a fistula between the rectum and the vulval vestibule of the female genitalia (rectovestibular fistula).

2. About 1 in every 5,000 babies are born with anorectal malformations.

3. These patients have other associated Vertebral, Anal, Cardiac, Tracheal, Esophageal, Renal and Limb abnormalities.

4. Initial management is intestinal decompression.
   In males, colostomy is usually required in the neonatal period.
   The babies will need reconstructive surgery to reposition the rectum in the correct location and create an anal opening.

A13.10

1. There is a large mass seen in the right abdominal cavity. It appears to arise from the right kidney.

2. Wilms tumour or nephroblastoma.

3. They present as an asymptomatic abdominal mass in the majority of children. Other presentations include abdominal pain, gross haematuria, urinary tract infections and hypertension.

4. Nephrectomy with either neoadjuvant or adjuvant chemotherapy.

Q13.11

This is a 2-year-old boy with urine coming out of the visible orifice.

1. What is the diagnosis?
2. How is this pathology commonly classified?
3. What other abnormal conditions is it associated with?
4. What is the management?

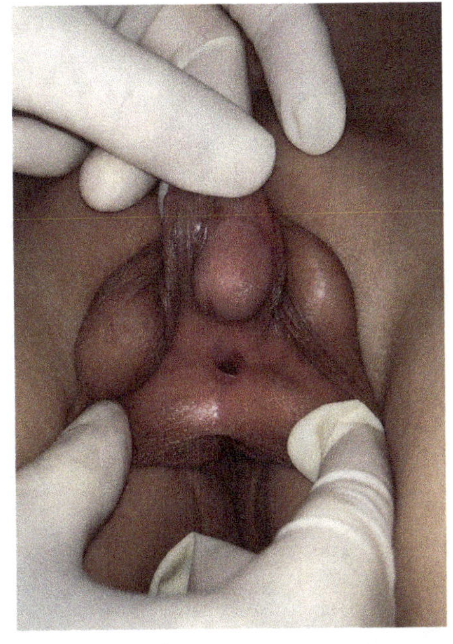

Q13.12

This is a one-month-old baby.

1. What is the diagnosis?
2. What problems will the baby have?
3. How common is it?
4. What is the management?

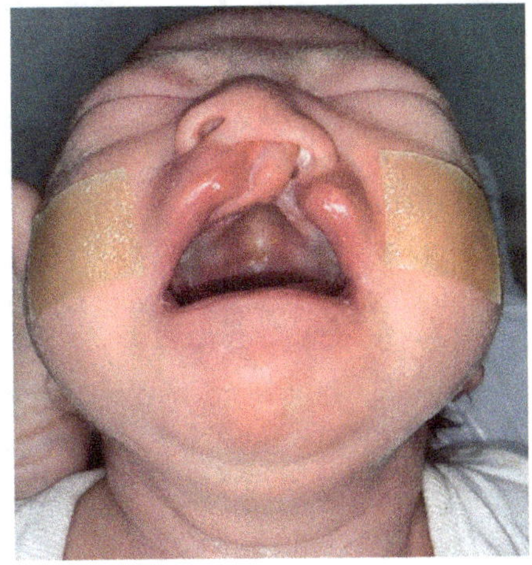

A13.11

1. Hypospadias. It is a congenital malformation of the male penis associated with an abnormal curvature (chordee).

2. They are classified by the abnormal location of the urethral meatus. This case has peno-scrotal hypospadias.

3. Hypospadias in most patients present as an isolated malformation.
   10% are associated with cryptorchidism and inguinal hernias.

4. Surgical correction is the mainstay of treatment.
   The aim is to straighten the penis and reposition the meatus to give an adequate functional and cosmetic result.

A13.12

1. Cleft lip and palate.

2. The newborn's ability to feed is affected. This includes increased nasal reflux, inability to form an adequate latch, and increased work of feeding leading to fatigue.
   There are negative cometic implications.

3. 1 in 700 live births. Asians being twice as affected as Whites. Males affected more than females (2 to 1).

4. Definitive management is achieved through surgical intervention. Repair is often staged, with the lip managed first, followed by the palate. The prognosis is good as feeding difficulties are resolved with the closure of the cleft.

Q13.13

This 2-year-old female is diagnosed with a 12 × 11 × 10 cm choledochal cyst (CC).

1. What does the AXR show?
2. What is seen on the ultrasound?
3. How common is it?
4. How is the pathology classified?
5. What is the likely clinical presentation of CCs?
6. What is the management?

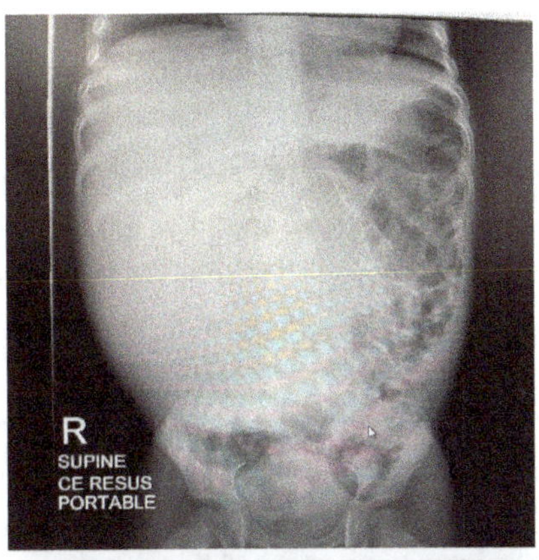

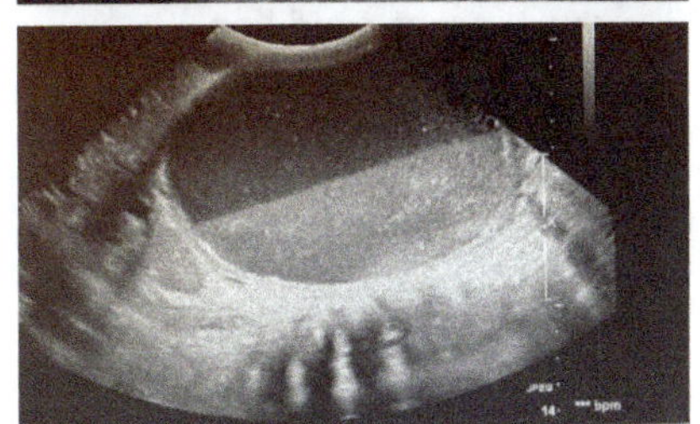

Q13.14

This is a 2-year-old boy with chronic constipation.

1. What is seen on radiology?
2. What is the likely diagnosis?
3. What is the pathogenesis?
4. What is the clinical presentation?
5. What was performed for this patient?

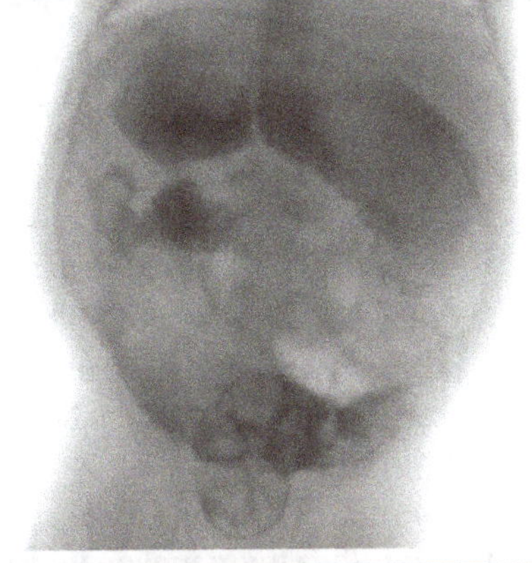

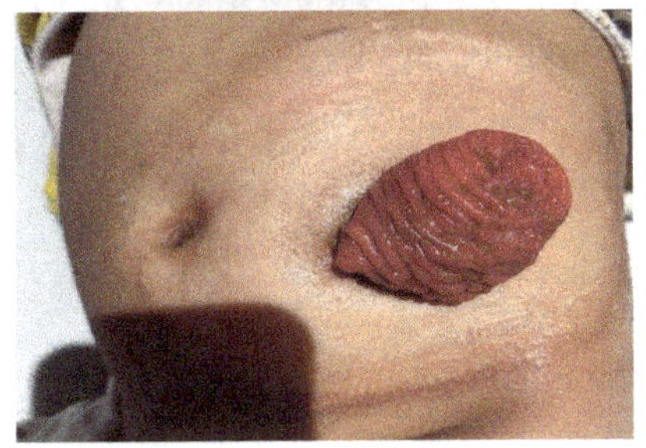

A13.13

1. There is a radio-opacity in the right side of the abdomen suggestive of a large abdominal mass.

2. There is a cystic lesion with a fluid level seen.

3. It occurs 1 in 1000 live births It is 10 times as common in the Asians as compared to the Western population.

4. Todani classification: 5 types based on the anatomical position of the cyst with respect to the biliary tree.

5. They are initially asymptomatic when small in size. They can present with a triad of abdominal pain, palpable abdominal mass, and jaundice.

6. All CCs should be resected with restoration of bile flow as it is considered a premalignant condition.

A13.14

1. The contrast enema demonstrates a dilated transverse colon. The sigmoid colon and rectum are collapsed.

2. Hirschsprung's disease (HD).

3. It is a congenital disorder characterized by the absence of ganglion cells at the Meissner's plexus (submucosa) and Auerbach's plexus (muscularis) most commonly affecting the distal large intestine.

4. A newborn with HD might present with failure to pass meconium in the first 48 hours of life. This patient had a mild case of HD and presented at 2-years-old with chronic intestinal obstruction.

5. A colostomy was performed to relieve the obstruction. A definitive pull-through (healthy ganglionated colon) procedure should be arranged 4–6 months later.

Q13.15

This is a 3-year-old boy. His serum alphafetoprotein is elevated.

1. What is seen in the CT scan?
2. What is the diagnosis?
3. What is the clinical presentation?
4. What is the aetiology?
5. What is the management?

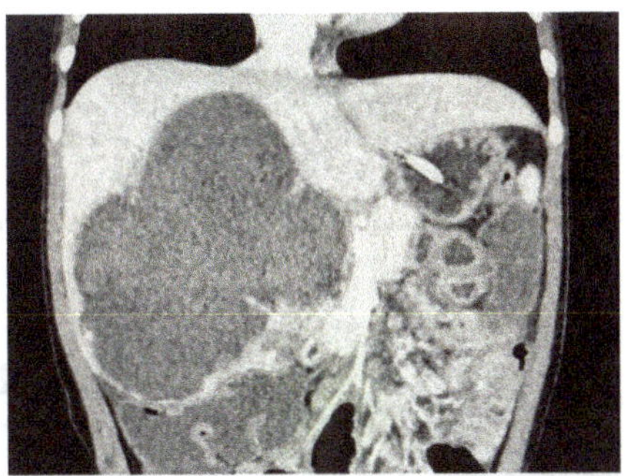

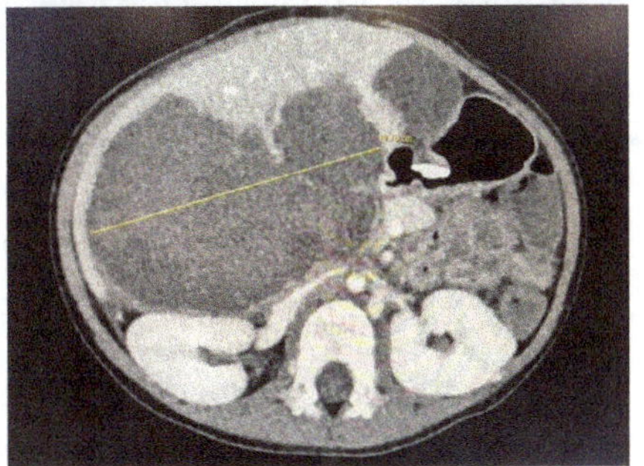

Q13.16

This is a 10-year-old boy.

1. What is the abnormality seen?
2. What anatomical structure is absent?
3. What is the diagnosis?
4. What is the management?

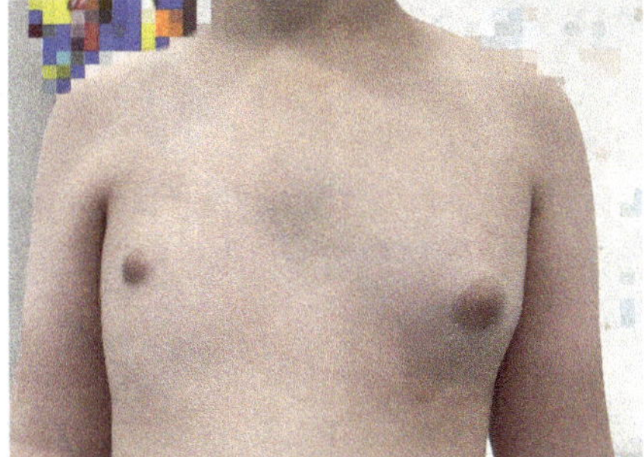

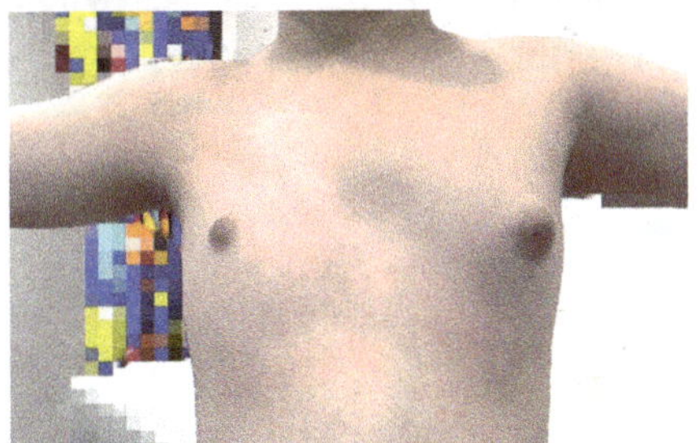

A13.15

1. There is a large homogenous lobulated lesion in the right lobe of the liver.

2. Hepatoblastoma.

3. It usually presents with as a single, mildly painful, rapidly enlarging abdominal mass. Less commonly, anaemia or tumour rupture.

4. Most tumours are sporadic, but 1/3 of cases may be associated with Beckwith-Weidemann, familial adenomatous polyposis (FAP), Edward syndrome (trisomy 18), nephroblastoma, and Down syndrome.

5. Surgical resection with neo-adjuvant or adjuvant chemotherapy.

A13.16

1. There is asymmetry of the chest wall musculature. The left chest is larger than the right.

2. There is absence or hypoplasia of the right pectoralis major muscle and/or pectoralis minor muscle. Defects are often unilateral.

3. Poland syndrome.

4. Most cases are managed conservatively.
   Surgical intervention can be indicated for reasons including paradoxical movement of the chest wall, hypoplasia or aplasia of the female breast, and aesthetic asymmetry.

14 Plastics

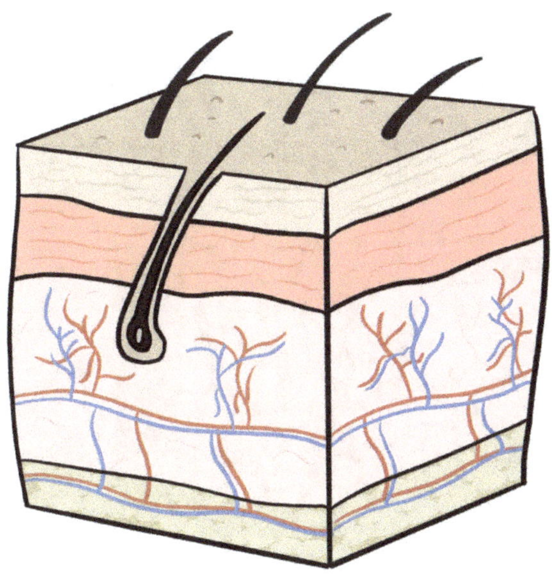

Q14.1

This is a 45-year-old male.

1. What is seen on his forehead?
2. What scan was performed and what does it show?
3. What is the diagnosis?
4. What is the natural history of this pathology?
5. What is the management?

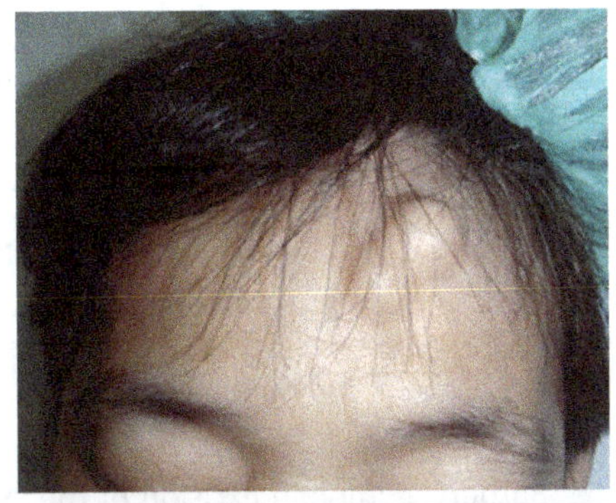

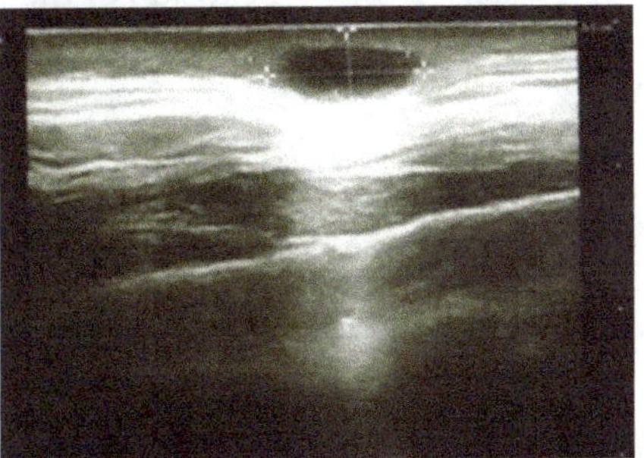

Q14.2

This is a 44-year-old male.

1. What is seen on his forehead?
2. What does the ultrasound show?
3. What is the diagnosis?
4. What is the management?

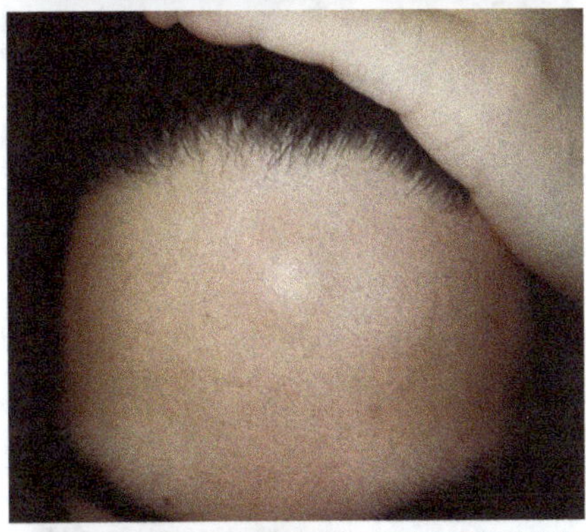

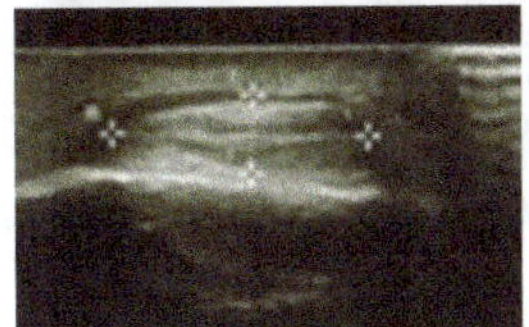

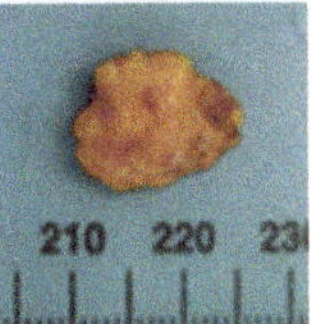

A14.1

1. There is a multilobulated lesion on the left side of his forehead. There are no overlying skin changes.

2. An ultrasound scan demonstrates a well-circumscribed hypodense lesion within the skin layer.

3. Epidermal/skin cyst.

4. It is a benign lesion. It can increase, decrease or remain the same in size. If left alone, it may get infected.

5. Conservative: watchful waiting.
    Surgery: complete excision of the cyst to prevent recurrence.

A14.2

1. There is a well-circumscribed lesion at the centre of his forehead. There are no overlying skin changes.

2. There is a hyperechoic elliptical mass with linear echogenic lines deep to the skin

3. Lipoma.

4. Lipomas are benign tumours that do not resolve spontaneously.
    This patient had the lesion surgically removed for cosmetic reasons and for histological confirmation.

Q14.3

This is a 50-year-old male.

1. What is seen on his forehead?
2. What is seen on the ultrasound?
3. What are the likely findings on clinical examination?
4. What is the diagnosis and its natural history?

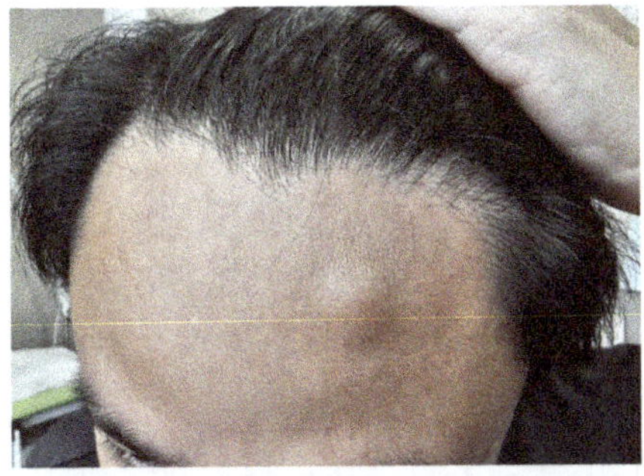

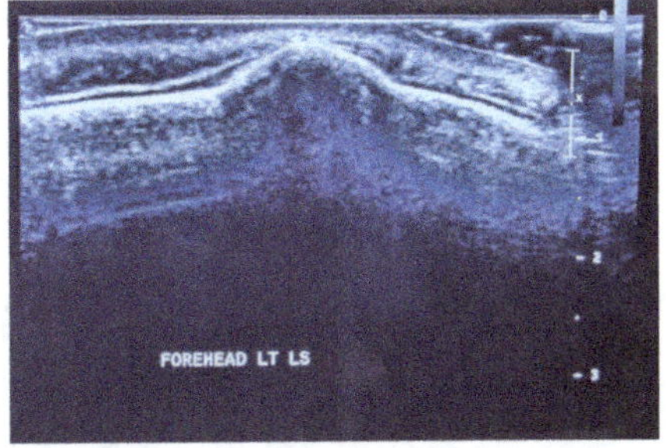

Q14.4

This is a 50-year-old male.

1. What is seen on his abdominal wall?
2. What is the diagnosis?
3. What is the clinical presentation?
4. What is the management?
5. What is seen in the surgical specimen?

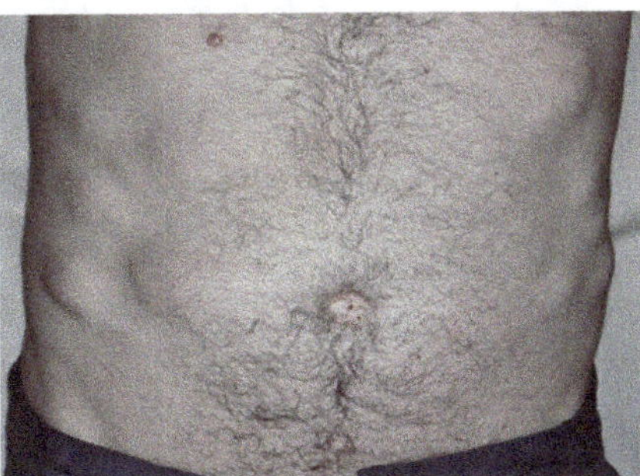

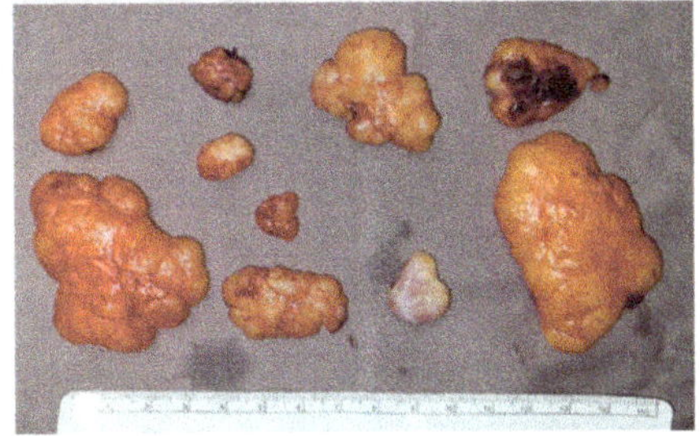

A14.3

1. There is a well-circumscribed lesion on the left side of his forehead. There are no overlying skin changes.

2. There is a smooth protrusion from the bone.

3. There will be a non-tender, hard, immobile subcutaneous mass.

4. It is an osteoid osteoma, which is a benign bone tumour that has no potential to become malignant. It may slowly enlarge over time.

A14.4

1. There are multiple subcutaneous lumps in the abdominal wall. There are no overlying skin changes.

2. Multiple lipomas. If there is a family history, it can be classified as familial multiple lipomatosis.

3. They are often asymptomatic. Occasionally patients may experience discomfort or pain if the lipomas compress a sensory nerve.

4. They can be often left alone as they are benign. Surgical excision is recommended if the lipomas become symptomatic.

5. Surgical excision of the multiple lipomas.

Q14.5

This is a 70-year-old male with a lesion on his left forearm.

1. What is the diagnosis?
2. What is its aetiology?
3. What is the clinical presentation?
4. What is being performed for this patient?

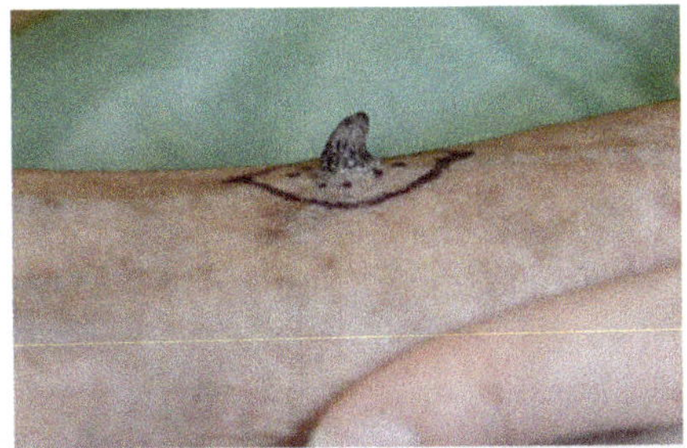

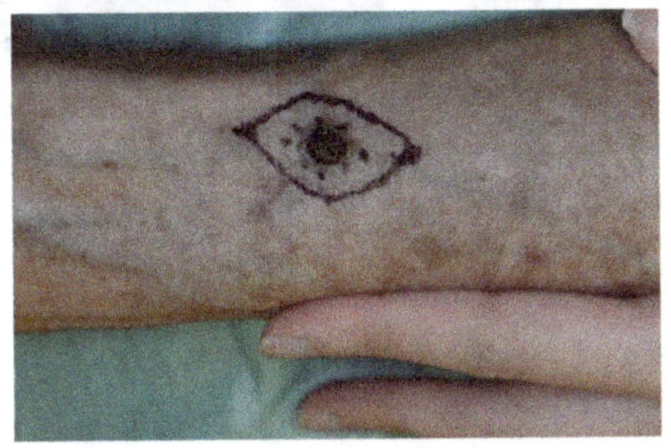

Q14.6

This is a 60-year-old male.

1. Describe the lesion.
2. What is the diagnosis?
3. Where is this pathology often located in the body?
4. What is the prognosis if left alone?
5. What is the management?

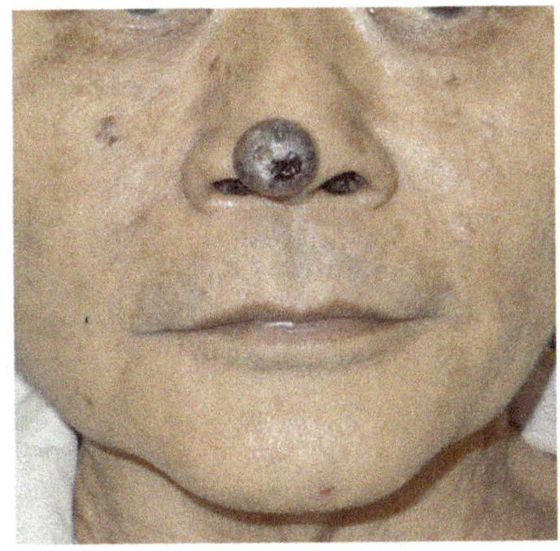

A14.5

1. A cutaneous horn (cornu cutaneum). It is an uncommon, hyperkeratotic epithelial lesion.

2. The aetiology varies as it is a secondary manifestation of a benign (seborrheic or lichenoid keratoses), premalignant (actinic keratoses), or malignant lesion (squamous cell carcinoma).

3. Patients are usually asymptomatic.
   Appearance: straight or curved, hard, yellow-brown projection from the skin.
   Location: most seen over the sun-exposed areas like the face, eyelids, and forearms.
   Size: Typically, the horn is taller than twice the width at the base.

4. Surgical excision with adequate radial margins (markings are drawn out).

A14.6

1. There is a dome-shaped skin lesion with a centralized keratinous plug over his nose.

2. Keratoacanthoma (KA). The lesions begin as a small, round, pink or skin-coloured papule that undergoes rapid growth into a dome-shaped nodule with a central keratin plug.

3. Most lesions occur on sun-exposed areas like the face, head, neck, and dorsum of extremities.

4. While KA is benign, treatment is recommended due to their association with squamous cell carcinoma (SCC). KA shares similar histopathological features with SCC.

5. Surgical excision with 4mm margins.
   Mohs micrographic surgery can be considered for lesions in cosmetically sensitive areas that require tissue sparing.

Q14.7

This is a 50-year-old male.

1. Describe the lesion seen.
2. What is the diagnosis?
3. What is the pathogenesis?
4. What is the management?
5. What are potential complications if left alone?

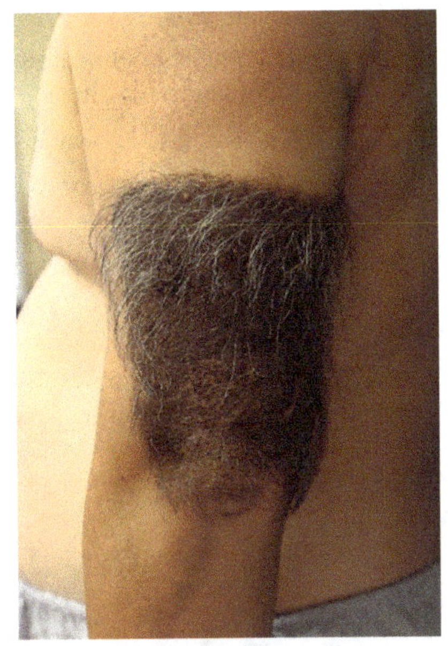

Q14.8

This is a 30-year-old female.

1. What is seen in picture A?
2. What is seen on her back in picture B?
3. What is the diagnosis?
4. Describe the genetics of this disorder.
5. What is the management?
6. What other pathologies are these patients at risk of developing?

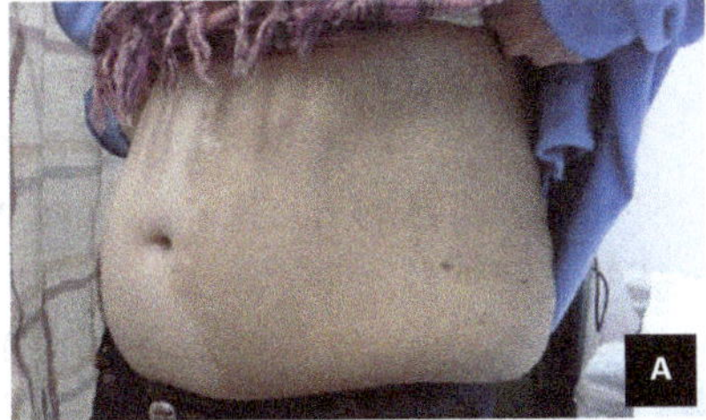

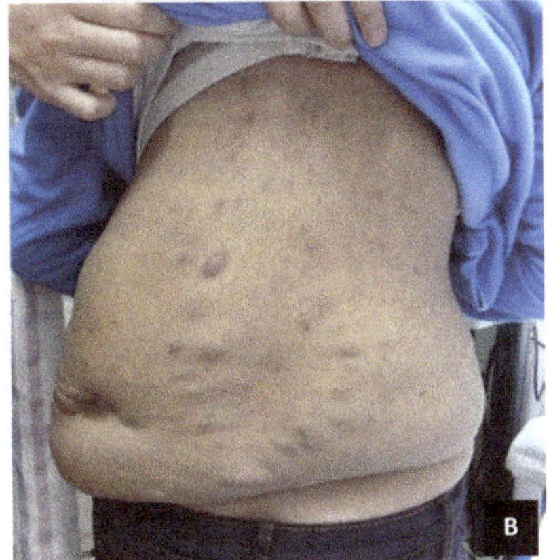

A14.7

1. There is a large hairy pigmented lesion over the posterior lateral aspect of his arm extending to the elbow.

2. Giant hairy nevus, also known as a congenital melanocytic nevus.

3. It is caused by abnormal growth of melanocytes. This is often accompanied by the presence of excessive hair growth.

4. Regular skin surveillance with skin biopsy of suspicious parts of the lesion. Surgical excision is the main treatment option. The resultant defect will need to be covered.

5. Risk of malignant change. The risk of developing a melanoma with a large congenital melanocytic nevus is around 10–15%.

A14.8

1. There is a large area of light brown pigmentation on the skin ("café au lait") over the left aspect of her abdominal wall.

2. There is a large plexiform neurofibroma that extends over her entire lower back and left flank.

3. Neurofibromatosis type 1 (NF1), also known as von Recklinghausen's disease.

4. NF1 is caused by a loss of function mutation on the neurofibromin 1 (NF1) gene, that is located on band 17q11.2 which codes for neurofibromin. It has an autosomal dominant pattern of inheritance.

5. Plexiform neurofibromas have 10% risk of developing into malignant peripheral nerve sheath tumours. This should be suspected if there is pain, new neurologic deficits, change of the neurofibroma from soft to hard, or a rapid increase in size.

6. Optic glioma, rhabdomyosarcomas, myeloid leukaemia and phaeochromocytomas.

Q14.9

These are 2 different patients with the same pathology.

1. Describe the lesion on the right lower abdominal wall.
2. Describe the lesion on the lip.
3. What are the diagnoses?
4. What is the clinical presentation?
5. What is the management?

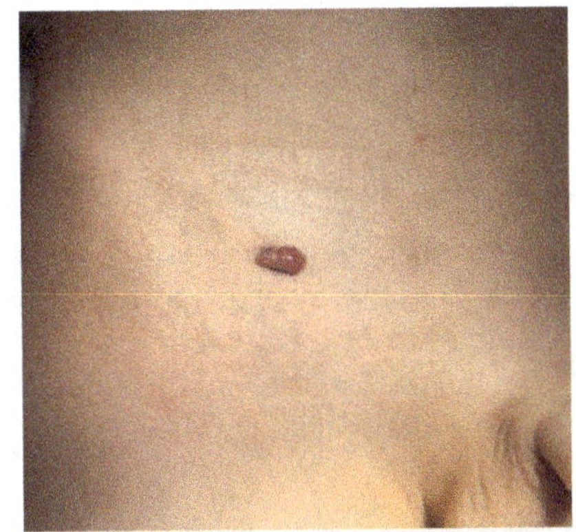

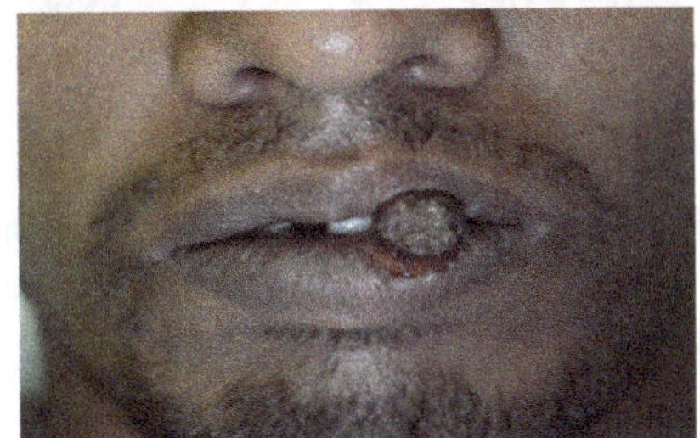

Q14.10

This 7-year-old boy had an uneventful open right inguinal hernia surgery.

1. What has happened to the surgical wound?
2. Which group of patients are prone to it?
3. What is the pathophysiology?
4. What is the management?

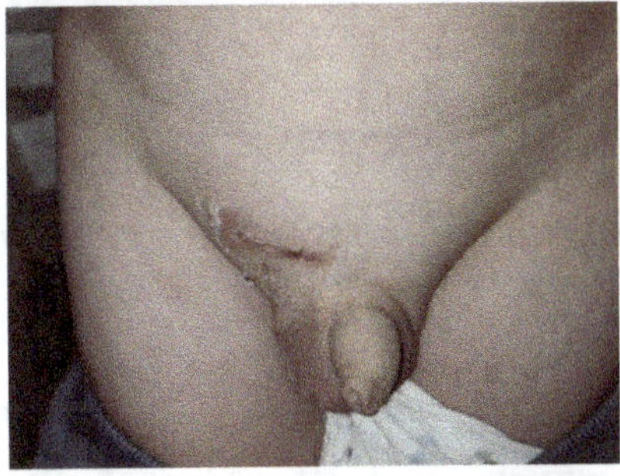

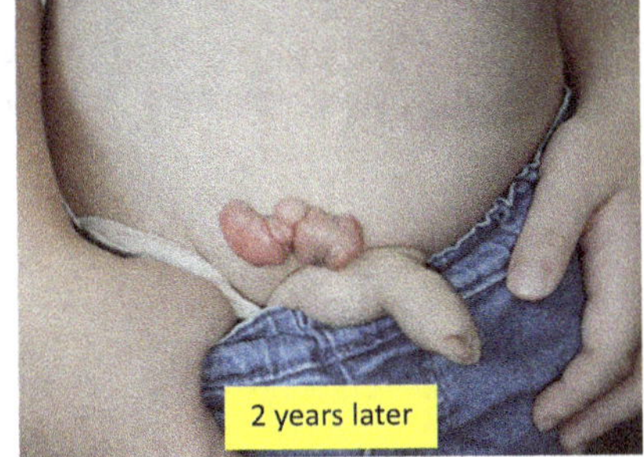

A14.9

1. There is a smooth small red nodule arising from the skin of the right abdominal wall.

2. There is an irregular pea-sized nodule arising from the lip.

3. Pyogenic granuloma, also known as lobular capillary haemangioma.
   It is a common acquired benign vascular tumour that arises from the skin and mucous membranes.
   In the past, it was thought to be an exaggerated granulomatous reaction to an infectious or pyogenic insult, which led to terms such as 'pyogenic granuloma'.

4. It starts as a small red papule that undergoes exophytic growth phase eventually stabilizing in size. The colour may vary from red to reddish-brown or purple.
   The surface is often friable and bleeds with minor trauma.

5. Small lesions can be managed with non-operative modalities such as pulsed dye laser, CO_2 laser ablation, or electrocautery.
   Large lesions should be excised and sent for histology.

A14.10

1. Keloid formation. They present as firm, rubbery nodules.

2. Higher incidence is seen in darker skinned individuals.

3. Keloids are a result of aberrant wound healing. Standard wound healing consists of three phases: (1) inflammatory, (2) fibroblastic, and (3) maturation. In keloids, the fibroblastic phase continues unchecked, persists longer and has a lower rate of apoptosis. This results in collagen overproduction.

4. Keloids remain a difficult to treat as recurrence is high.
   Options include:
   Intralesional steroids are considered first line therapy.
   Surgical excision with adjuvant radiotherapy.

Q14.11

This is a 65-year-old female.

1. Describe the pathology seen.
2. What is the diagnosis?
3. What is the main risk factor?
4. How was the lesion managed?

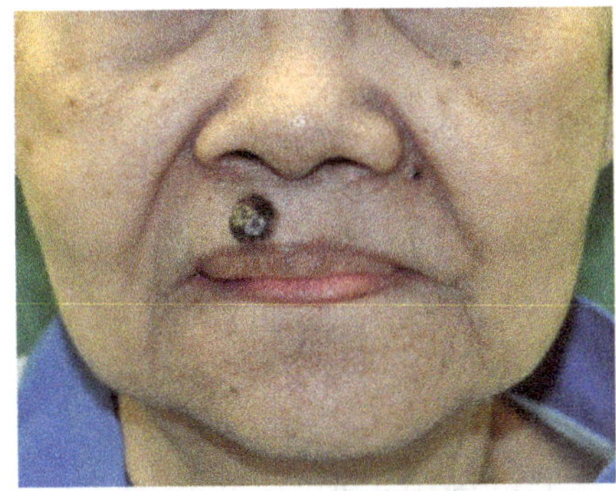

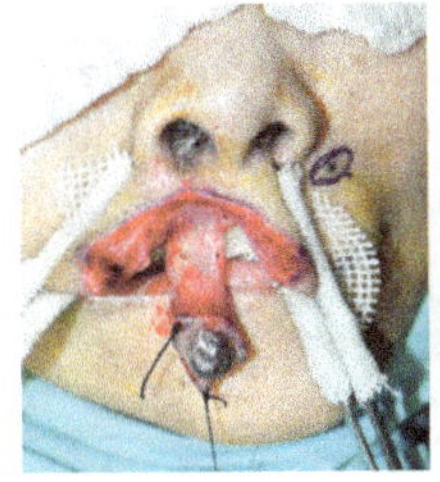
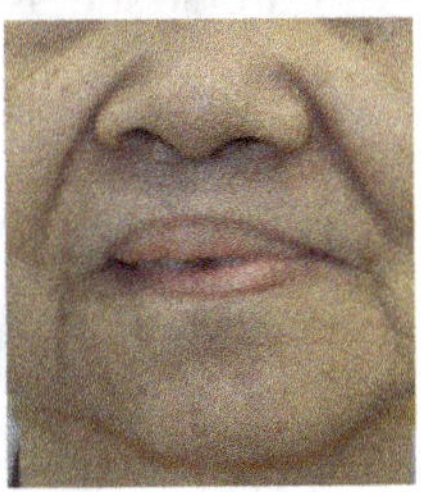

Q14.12

This is a 60-year-old man.

1. Describe what you see.
2. What are his likely symptoms?
3. What is the diagnosis?
4. How can the diagnosis be confirmed?
5. How is the pathology managed?

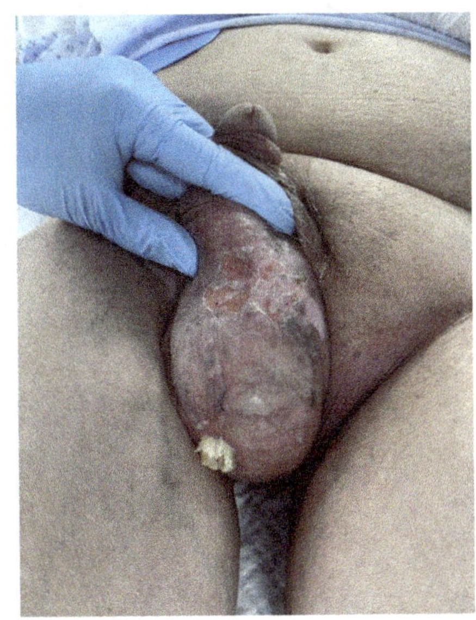

A14.11

1. Site: right upper lip.
   Size: 2 x 2 cm.
   Shape: circular.
   Borders: regular.
   Colour/surface: smooth and black.
   The tumour may enlarge and ulcerate, giving the borders a rolled or rodent ulcer appearance.

2. Basal cell carcinoma (nodular).

3. Chronic sun exposure.

4. Treatment depends on the patient's age and gender as well as the site, size, and type of lesion. Surgical excision was performed with adequate margins and aesthetic/functional skin cover.

A14.12

1. The scrotal skin has red, crusty and scaly patches with irregular borders. There is a yellowish dry exophytic lesion at the inferior aspect.

2. He may experience a burning sensation, itch or pain (akin to eczema).

3. Extramammary Paget's disease (EMPD). It is a rare slow-growing intraepithelial malignant neoplasm that occurs around the perineum, a region rich in apocrine skin glands.

4. A skin biopsy will show abnormal large cells with distinctive characteristics called Paget cells.

5. Wide local excision or Mohs micrographic surgery is standard of care.

Q14.13

This is a 70-year-old male with a lesion on his scalp.

1. Describe the lesion.
2. What is the likely diagnosis?
3. What is the main risk factor?
4. What surgery was planned as seen in picture A?
5. How was the defect closed as seen in picture B?

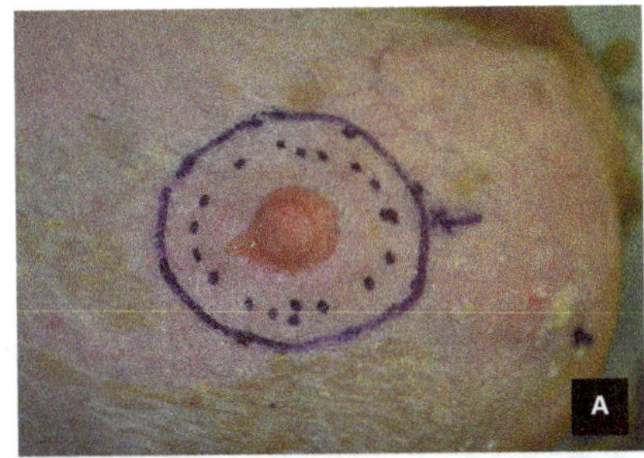

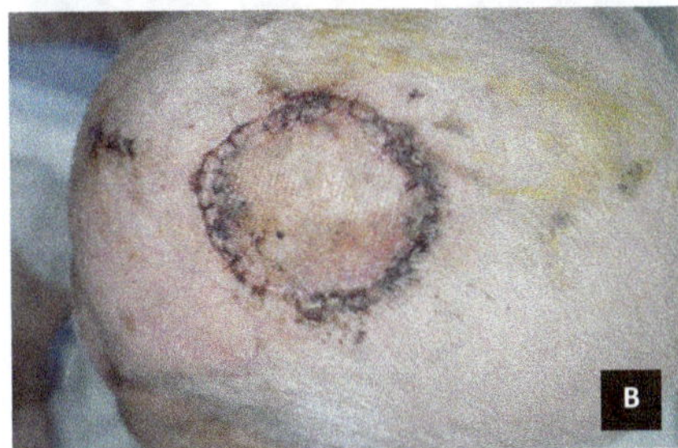

Q14.14

This is a 94-year-old male.

1. Describe the pathology seen.
2. What is the most likely diagnosis?
3. What is a pre-malignant form of this lesion?
4. How was this lesion managed?

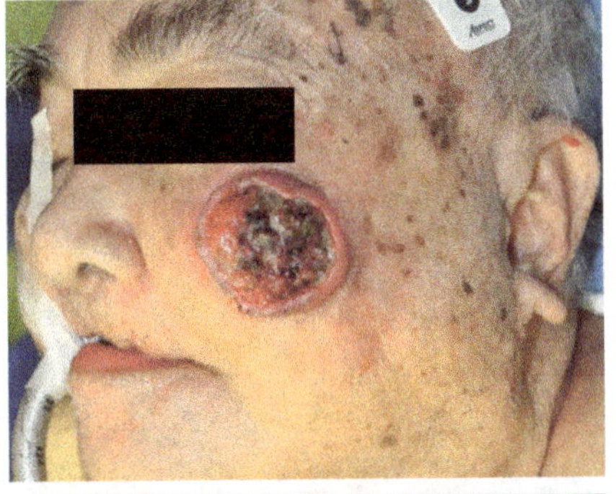

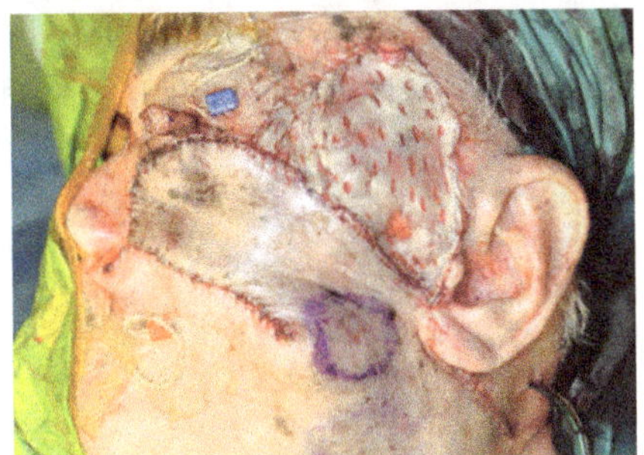

A14.13

1. There is a red raised circular lesion over his scalp. There is no active bleeding.
2. Squamous cell carcinoma.
3. Ultraviolet radiation exposure.
4. Wide local excision with adequate margins.
5. It was closed with a full thickness skin graft.

A14.14

1. Site: left cheek.
    Size: 5 x 5 cm.
    Shape: circular.
    Borders: regular with rolled edges.
    Colour/surface: non-uniform — slough, necrosis with erythema.
2. Squamous cell carcinoma (SCC).
3. Bowen's disease — Carcinoma in situ. SCC can also develop from pre-existing lesions such as actinic keratosis, chronic wounds (Marjolin ulcer), Human Papillomavirus infection and discoid cutaneous lupus erythematosus.
4. After surgical excision with clear margins, there was a remaining 8 cm skin and soft tissue defect with exposed zygoma bone. The defect was closed with a fasciocutaneous rotation flap. The flap donor site was then covered with split skin graft.

Q14.15

This is a 70-year-old male who presents with a lesion over the scalp that is increasing in size.

1. Describe the lesion seen on his scalp.
2. What is the diagnosis?
3. What is the management?
4. What treatment did he receive as seen in the picture?

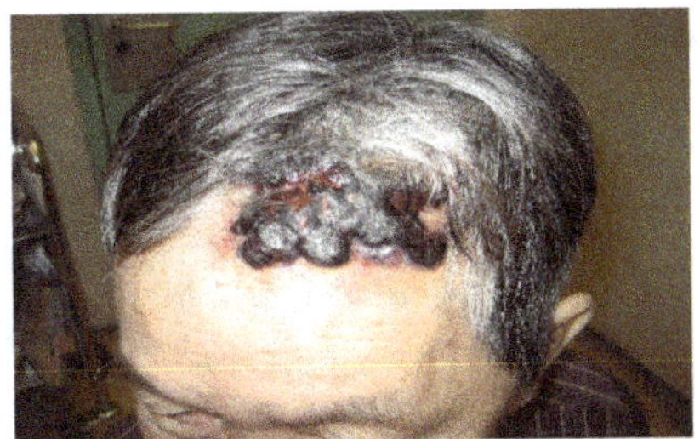

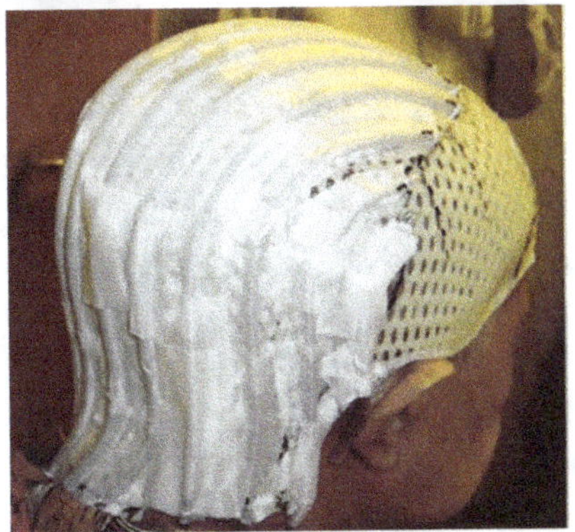

Q14.16

This is a 70-year-old male.

1. Describe the clinical findings.
2. What is the likely diagnosis?
3. How can we confirm the diagnosis?
4. What is the management?

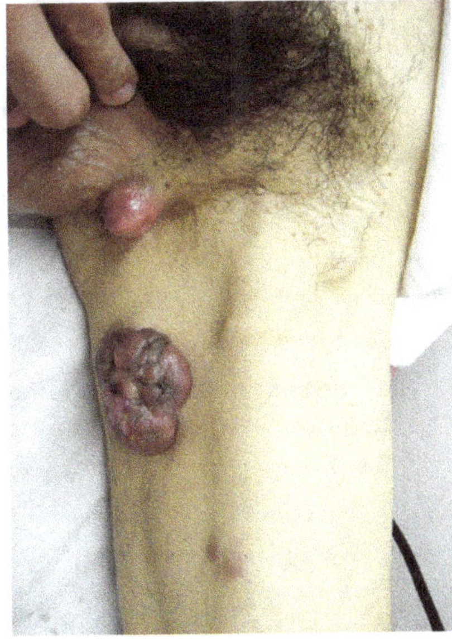

A14.15

1. There is a large multilobulated, pigmented lesion over his forehead with bleeding at the edges.

2. Angiosarcoma. It is a rare and highly aggressive malignant tumour, originating from lymphatic or vascular endothelial cells.

3. Radical surgery with clear margins remains the cornerstone of all treatments for angiosarcoma.
   Adjuvant radiotherapy following surgery is offered to control the risk of local recurrence.
   Cytotoxic chemotherapy is reserved for metastatic angiosarcoma.

4. The patient is prepared with guide tubes on thermoplastic shells over the scalp for surface brachytherapy.

A14.16

1. There are multiple red nodular lesions of different sizes over the left lower limb. They are not actively bleeding.

2. Cutaneous lymphomas.
   It is an uncommon cancer of lymphocytes that primarily involves the skin. They are classified based on B-lymphocyte (B-cell) or T-lymphocyte (T-cell) lineage.
   This patient had a cutaneous B-cell lymphoma (CBCL).

3. Obtain histology of the lesion, either with incision or excision biopsy.

4. Management is based on the histology, immunohistological staining and staging of the disease. It can be treated with radiotherapy and systemic therapy.

Q14.17

This is a 50-year-old female.

1. Describe the lesion on her abdominal wall.

2. What is the likely diagnosis?

3. What mnemonic is used to describe the clinical signs of this pathology?

4. What surgery was performed for her?

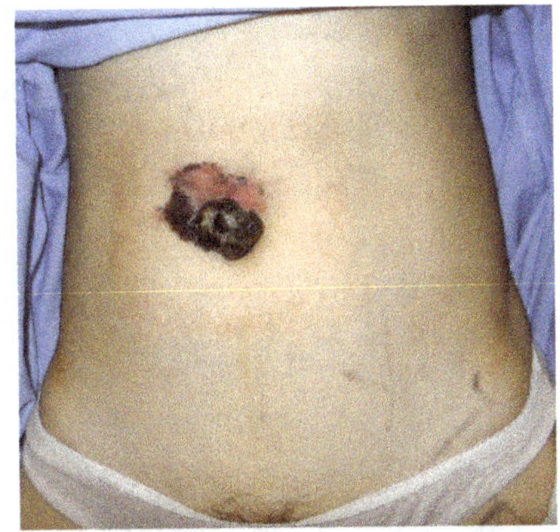

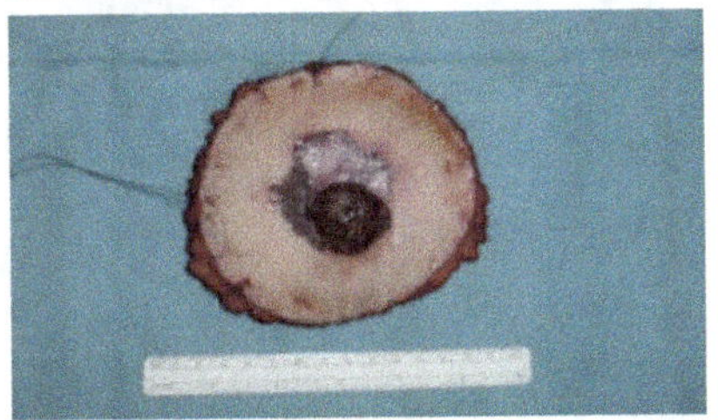

Q14.18

This is the same patient in question Q14.17.

1. How was the extensive wound closed?

2. Where was the donor site?

3. How are tissue flaps classified?

4. What are complications from this reconstructive surgery?

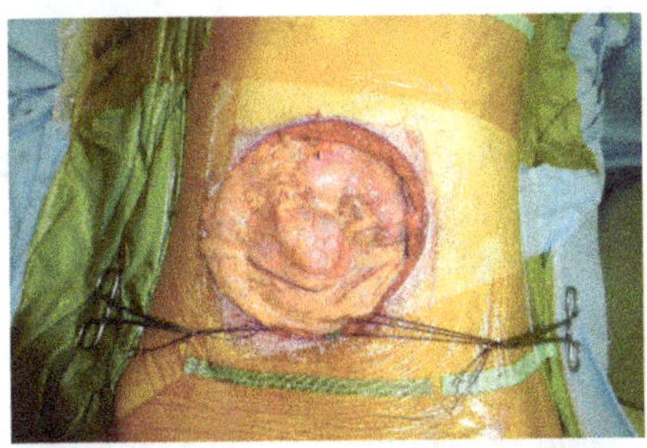

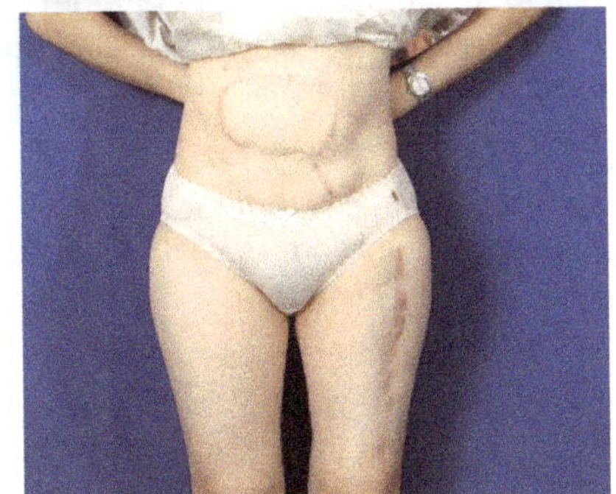

A14.17

1. There is a multilobulated pigmented lesion in the middle of her abdominal wall that involves the umbilicus. Superior to it is an erythematous patch.

2. Malignant melanoma.

3. **A**symmetry
   Border
   Colour
   Diameter
   Evolving: changes in size, shape, or colour

4. Wide local excision with clear radial and deep margins. The excised surgical specimen in the picture is 15cm in diameter.

A14.18

1. Primary closure was not possible due to the large defect. Closure with secondary intention was also not possible due to exposed abdominal viscera.
   This wound was closed with a flap.

2. A distant tissue flap was raised from the left thigh.

3. Flaps are classified based on:
   Blood supply — axial vs random.
   Tissue type — muscle, fascial or composite (multiple).
   Distance of the harvest site from the tissue defect — distant, regional or local.

4. Donor site — bleeding, infection and functional impairment.
   Flap — compromise of the flap's blood supply leading to necrosis.

Q14.19

This is a 60-year-old male.

1. Describe what you see on his foot.
2. What is the diagnosis?
3. What are the next steps in managing the patient?
4. What surgery was performed for this patient?

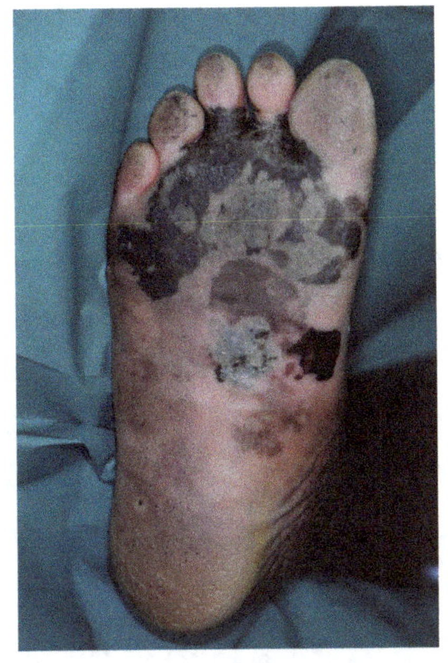

Q14.20

This is a 50-year-old male.

1. What is seen on the left flank in picture A?
2. What surgery was planned for him as marked out?
3. What is the lymphatic drainage of the lesion?
4. What surgery was performed as seen in picture B?

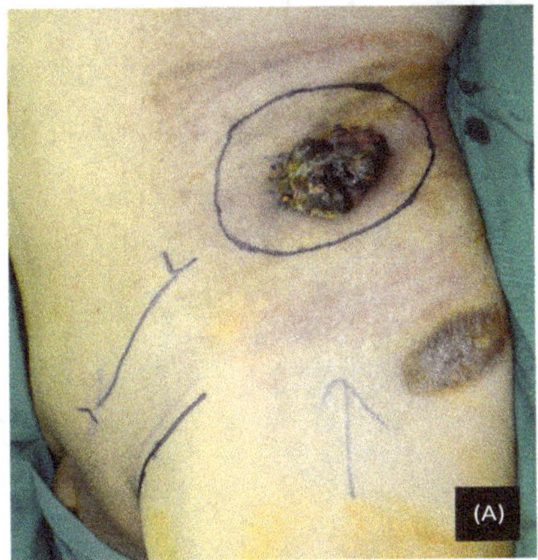

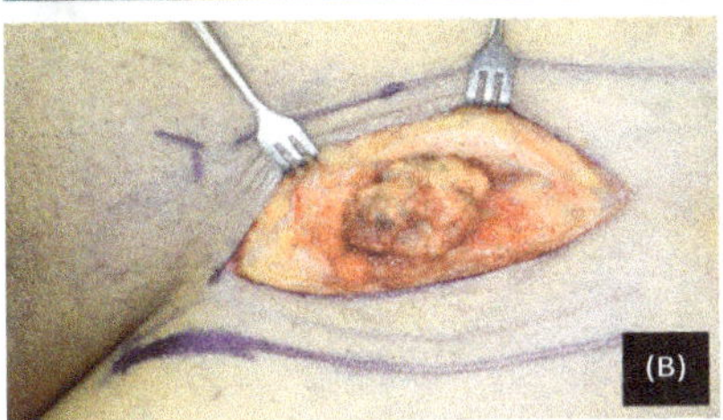

A14.19

1. There are large areas of black-grey skin discolouration involving the distal aspect of the plantar regions of his foot. The borders are irregular. There is no skin ulceration or bleeding.

2. Acral lentiginous melanoma.

3. Confirm the diagnosis with a biopsy and exclude distal metastases.

4. Excision of the lesion with clear surgical margins was not possible. A below-knee amputation was performed.

A14.20

1. There is a well-circumscribed nodular pigmented lesion at the left flank.

2. Wide local excision with adequate margins.

3. Left inguinal lymph nodes.

4. Sentinel lymph node biopsy of the inguinal lymph nodes.

Q14.21

This is a 35-year-old male.

1. What is seen in picture A?
2. What is the diagnosis?
3. What is the management?
4. How was this patient treated as seen in picture B?

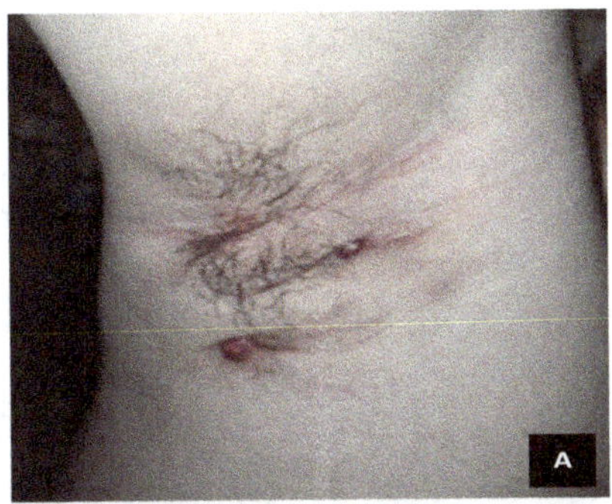

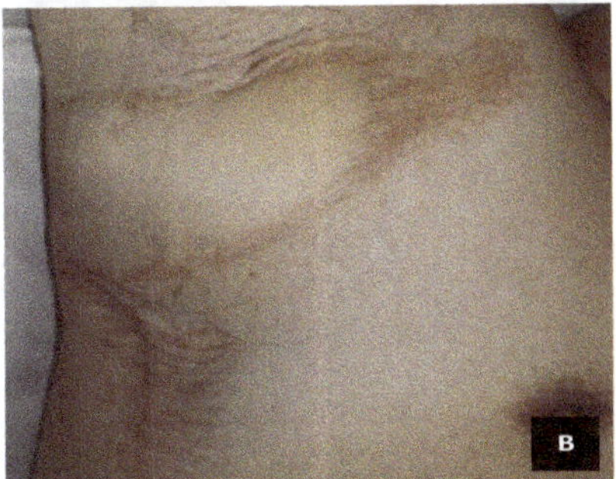

Q14.22

This is a 40-year-old male with repeated infections at the right axilla.

1. What type of skin cover was used post-excision?
2. What are the advantages of this type of skin cover?
3. What are the disadvantages of its use?

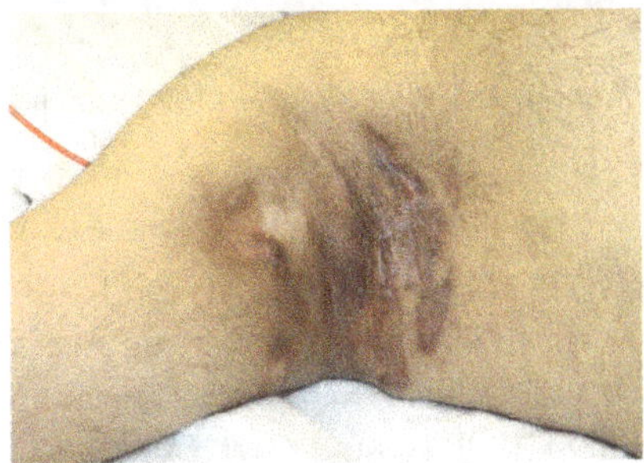

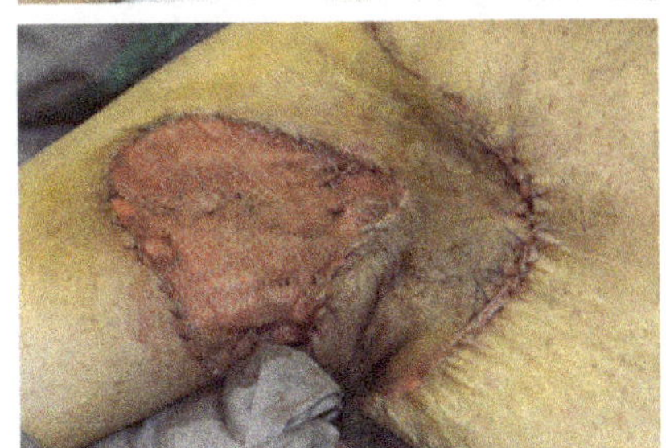

A14.21

1. There are multiple sinuses in the right axilla.

2. Hidradenitis suppurativa. It is a chronic inflammatory skin condition of hair follicles characterized by repeated infections (deep-seated sinuses and abscesses).

3. Topical and systemic antibiotics can be used to treat acute infections. Small abscesses may need surgical drainage.

4. The affected area was excised, and the defect covered with a flap.

A14.22

1. Split-thickness skin graft (STSG). It can be identified by the "mesh" appearance.

2. A smaller donor graft can be used to cover a larger recipient bed. The donor skin can be meshed to increase its surface area to cover larger wounds.

3. STSG are more fragile and need a healthy well-vascularised soft tissue recipient bed. They can contract and become hypo or hyperpigmented over time. STSG donor sites must re-epithelialize and often cause significant discomfort, and require ongoing wound care until healing is complete.

Q14.23

This is a 63-year-old male who became tetraplegic after a road traffic accident.

1. What is the diagnosis?
2. What is the pathogenesis?
3. What is the management?
4. What was performed for this patient?

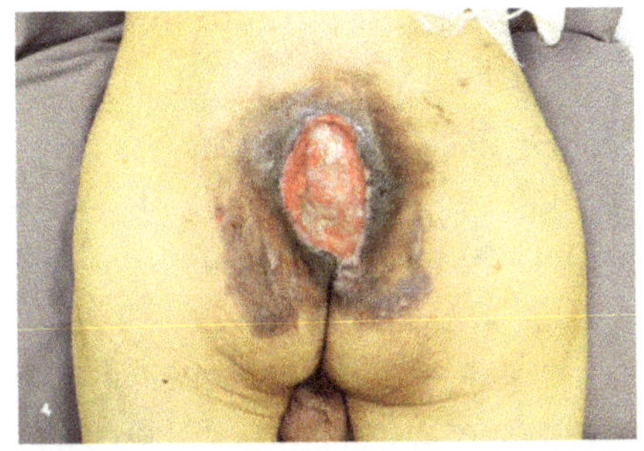

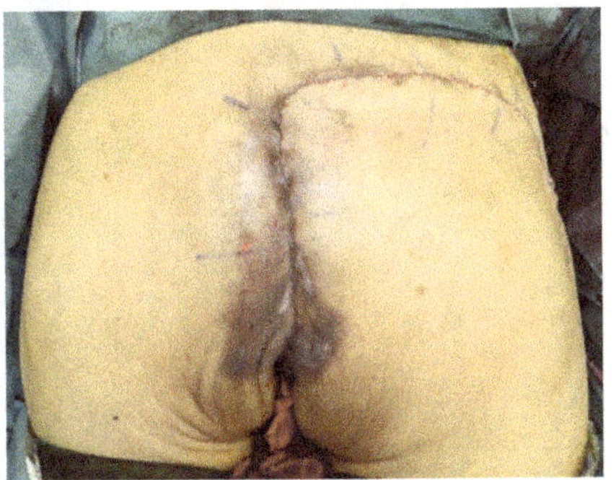

Q14.24

These are 2 separate patients with similar burn injuries.

1. What is seen in picture A?
2. What are the causes of burns?
3. How do we assess the extent of burns?
4. What surgical procedure was performed in picture B?

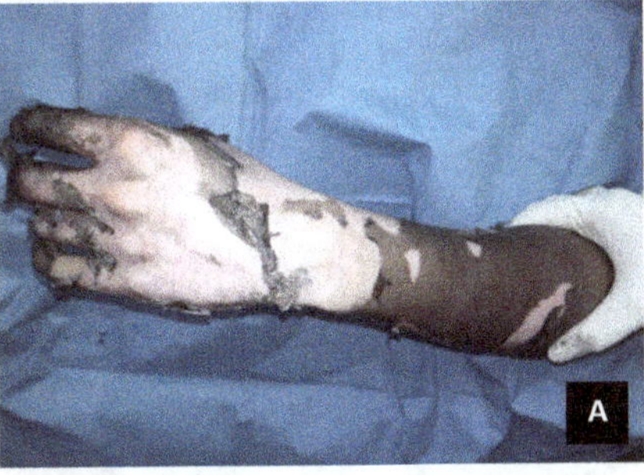

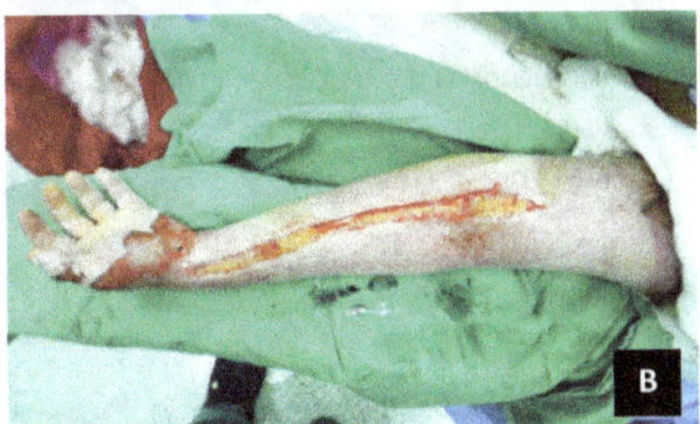

A14.23

1. There is a large pressure ulcer at the sacrum.

2. Pressure is exerted on the skin, soft tissue and muscle against the bone by the weight of the recumbent patient. This pressure is greater than the arterial capillary pressure, impairing blood flow for an extended time.

3. Superficial ulcers can be managed conservatively with wound care. Deep ulcers will need surgical intervention.

4. Local rotational myocutanous flap.

A14.24

1. The left upper limb had suffered full-thickness burns. This skin is charred and white. It should feel firm and leathery to palpation with no blanching.

2. Up to 80% are thermal. The remaining are electrical and chemical burns.

3. The extent of the burns is usually calculated by the percentage of total body surface area (% TBSA) involved and the estimated depth of the burns (superficial, partial thickness, or full thickness).

4. Escharotomy.
   The presence of circumferential full-thickness burns compresses the underlying structures, an effect that is exacerbated by the development of oedema resulting from fluid resuscitation. The resulting increase in tissue pressure can cause compartment syndrome.

www.ingramcontent.com/pod-product-compliance
Lightning Source LLC
Chambersburg PA
CBHW070503160726
48003CB00004B/1401

9 789881 980756